W9-AXP-942

WIDMANN'S CLINICAL INTERPRETATION OF LABORATORY TESTS

Edition 10

BY RONALD A. SACHER, MB, BCH, DTM&H, FRCP(C)

WIDMANN'S CLINICAL INTERPRETATION OF LABORATORY TESTS

Edition 10

RONALD A. SACHER, MB, BCH, DTM&H, FRCP(C)
Professor of Medicine and Pathology
Director, Transfusion Medicine
Associate Director, Department of Laboratory Medicine
Georgetown University Medical Center
Washington, D.C.

AND:

RICHARD A. MCPHERSON, MD
Director, Immunology Reference Laboratory
Scripps Clinic and Research Foundation
LaJolla, California
and
Clinical Professor of Pathology
University of California, San Diego

WITH:

JOSEPH M. CAMPOS, PHD
Associate Professor of Pediatrics and Child Health
George Washington University Medical Center
Director, Microbiology Laboratory
Children's Hospital National Medical Center
Washington, D.C.

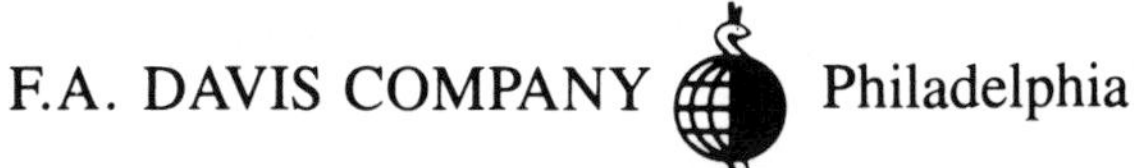

Copyright © 1991 by F. A. Davis Company

Copyright © 1949, 1952, 1954, 1958, 1964, 1969, 1973, 1979, and 1983 by F. A. Davis Company. All rights reserved. This book is protected by copyright. No part of it may be reproduced, stored in a retrieval system, or transmitted in any form or by any means, electronic, mechanical, photocopying, recording, or otherwise, without written permission from the publisher.

Printed in the United States of America

Last digit indicates print number: 10 9 8 7 6 5 4 3 2

Library of Congress Cataloging-in-Publication Data

Sacher, Ronald A.

Widmann's clinical interpretation of laboratory tests. — 10th ed. / Ronald A. Sacher, Richard A. McPherson.

p. cm.

Rev. ed. of: Clinical interpretation of laboratory tests / Frances K. Widmann. Ed. 9. c1983.

Includes bibliographical references.

ISBN 0-8036-7694-8

1. Diagnosis, Laboratory. I. McPherson, Richard A. II. Widmann, Frances K., 1935- Clinical interpretation of laboratory tests. III. Title. IV. Title: Clinical interpretation of laboratory tests.

[DNLM: 1. Diagnosis, Laboratory. QY 4 W641c]

RB37.S225 1990

616.07'5—dc20

DNLM/DLC

for Library of Congress 89-71420

CIP

Authorization to photocopy items for internal or personal use, or the internal or personal use of specific clients, is granted by F. A. Davis Company for users registered with the Copyright Clearance Center (CCC) Transactional Reporting Service, provided that the fee of $.10 per copy is paid directly to CCC, 27 Congress St., Salem, MA 01970. For those organizations that have been granted a photocopy license by CCC, a separate system of payment has been arranged. The fee code for users of the Transactional Reporting Service is: 8036-7694/91 0 + $.10.

DEDICATION

To Heather, Greg, and Sassy. Thanks for the love and many hours of support as well as cups of tea that have sustained me through the writing of this book. This book is dedicated to you.

PREFACE

Since the ninth edition of this book, major advances have taken place in both the understanding and the diagnosis of disease processes. These explosions in knowledge have occurred in all the realms of laboratory medicine. Consequently, this edition is intended to update the reader on these areas while keeping the comprehensive theme of past editions. To accomplish this goal, many sections have been totally rewritten, and pictorial presentations have been expanded. In these revisions, we have drawn extensively on our own experiences in the Department of Laboratory Medicine at Georgetown University Medical Center and in the teaching of medical students, residents, and fellows in medicine, hematology, and clinical pathology. In this book as in our daily teaching and practice, we recognize the theory of disease and biochemical abnormalities, while maintaining a practical approach to the use of laboratory testing in clinical medicine.

Among the new sections of this tenth edition, Chapter 1 discusses the features of sensitivity and specificity, reference ranges, predictive values, applications of panel profiles, and other basic test characteristics. The section on hematology has undergone extensive reorganization. There is comprehensive presentation of hematologic methods (Chapter 2) and detailed correlation with the diseases of erythrocytes (Chapter 3) and of leukocytes and lymphoproliferative disorders (Chapter 4). Similar in-depth development is afforded to the theory of hemostasis and coagulation testing (Chapter 5) and the clinical diagnosis and monitoring of bleeding disorders (Chapter 6).

The topics of humoral and cellular immunity, immunologic disorders, and autoimmune diseases are reviewed in Chapter 7. Chapter 8 continues with a presentation of immunohematology with emphasis on the testing for antibodies against blood group antigens and HLA types as practiced in transfusion therapy (blood banking).

The section on chemistry has been expanded to include all the commonly measured serum constituents plus the diagnostic significance of lipid fractionation and individual proteins (Chapter 9). In addition, there is comprehensive coverage of acid-base and electrolyte disturbances (Chapter 10), measurement of serum enzymes (Chapter 11), and extensive description of diagnostic tests important in liver diseases (Chapter 12).

Rapid advances in techniques of molecular biology have substantially transformed microbiologic diagnosis and the assessment and diagnosis of viral diseases. Consequently the section on microbiology (Chapters 13 to 15) has been totally reorganized and brought up-to-date with current diagnostic principles. This field continues to evolve at a feverish pace with new discoveries emerging almost daily that add to the diagnostic armamentarium of microbiology. The diagnosis of the human immunodeficiency virus and discoveries of other retroviruses as yet unrecognized may in the near future change our approach to infectious disease screening still more and particularly so in transfusion medicine. Molecular analysis of specific viral nucleic acid and protein sequences has enabled rapid diagnostic tests to be developed for use in both body fluids and in tissues. These technologies are also discussed in the microbiology section. Yet despite the complexity of these new innovations, the text is written in a narrative style conducive to easy reading.

Refinements in protein analysis and advances in immunoassays also have enhanced our ability to diagnose and monitor endocrine diseases. Chapter 16 delineates the test procedures practical for diagnosis of endocrine disorders, and Chapter 17 reviews applications of testing to the endocrinology of reproduction and perinatal diagnosis.

Chapter 18, which covers therapeutic drug monitoring and toxicology, is completely new to this edition. These fields have taken on more importance than ever before as automated methods for therapeutic drug analysis have been almost universally adopted. Toxicologic analysis also has assumed major significance both in diagnosis of emergency room patients and in the medicolegal sphere. In addition, exposure to enivronmental and industrial toxins is a major concern today.

The laboratory plays a crucial role in the biochemical, microscopic, and microbiologic analysis of body fluids other than blood. Chapter 19 provides a comprehensive and coordinated approach to the laboratory assessment of urine, cerebrospinal fluid, feces, sputum, gastric and duodenal fluids, peritoneal and pleural fluids (including diagnosis of exudates versus transudates), pericardial fluid, and joint fluid.

As our society becomes more involved in preventive medicine and as the population grows older due to longer life expectancy, there is a need for clinical appreciation of both the nutritional elements of good health and screening tests for the prevention and early detection of disease. These aspects are discussed in Appendix A (Nutrition) and in the specific chemistry sections on health profile screening and risk assessment. Cancer testing and monitoring of cancer therapy have been greatly aided in the last few years by the introduction of new analyses for tumor markers in blood or tissues including tumor antigens, ectopic hormones and enzymes, oncogenes, and rearrangement of key genetic elements. Appendix B summarizes the tumor markers most commonly used today.

Another major change from previous editions is the inclusion of a color plate section that highlights some of the morphologic features of hematologic disease and also microbiologic testing. This revision of the tenth edition also includes new interpretations and new applications of information from the past editions. The reader will find more figures, charts, lists, and tabular comparisons that present the details in simplest format. In addition, a glossary of normal values based on the reference intervals published from the *New England Journal of Medicine* is provided. It has proven to be a very useful reference source, and the publishers of the *Journal* have graciously granted permission to use this material. Furthermore, because reference ranges are substantially different in newborns and children, reference ranges for the pediatric age group also are provided in the Appendix.

Clearly this book cannot be a comprehensive textbook of medicine, but it is intended to present a practical approach to the understanding of pathophysiology and the application of laboratory testing in clinical diagnosis. It is meant to be a "hybrid" between the shorter handbooks that merely list disorders with associated abnormal test results and the more comprehensive texts that serve as essential reference sources. This challenge of revising a very successful past edition with updating of newer tests and providing information that was previously omitted has greatly enhanced our presentation of the material. We believe that this book will continue to be a useful addition to the personal libraries of busy clinicians, medical students, laboratory workers, and paramedical personnel who wish to have an understanding of the tests and methodologies used in clinical laboratory medicine.

Ronald A. Sacher, MB, BCh, DTM&H, FRCP(C)
Richard A. McPherson, MD

CONSULTANTS

VICTOR BUENDIA, MT, (ASCP), SBB (ASCP)
Assistant Chief Medical Techniogist
Columbia Hospital
Milwaukee, Wisconsin

MIKE DOWZICKY, MT (ASCP)
SmithKline Beckman Laboratories
Norristown, Pennsylvania

FRANCES TALASKA FISCHBACH, RN, BSN, MSN
Associate Clinical Professor
University of Wisconsin-Milwaukee
School of Nursing
Department of Health Restoration
Milwaukee, Wisconsin

ROBERT J. JACOBSON, MD
Professor, Medicine & Pathology
Division of Hematology
Georgetown University Hospital
Washington, D.C.

STANLEY PODLASEK, MD
Department of Laboratory Medicine
Georgetown University Hospital
Washington, D.C.

GEORGE PURCELL, PHD
Manager, Special Chemistry
SmithKline Beckman Laboratories
Norristown, Pennsylvania

CONTENTS

SECTION FIVE: CLINICAL MICROBIOLOGY

SECTION SIX: ENDOCRINE SYSTEM

SECTION SEVEN: MISCELLANEOUS

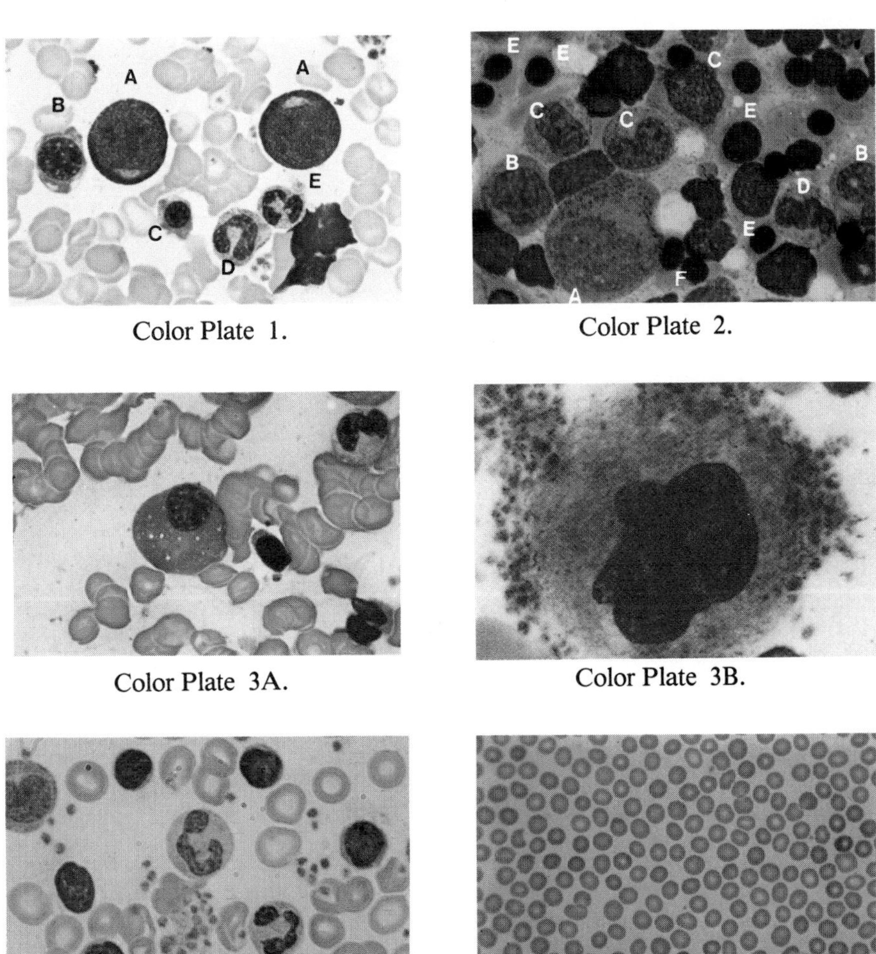

Color Plate 1. Color Plate 2.

Color Plate 3A. Color Plate 3B.

Color Plate 4. Color Plate 5.

Color Plate 1. Developing red blood cells showing: *A)* basophilic erythroblasts; *B)* polychromatophilic erythroblasts; *C)* orthochromatic erythroblasts; *D, E)* polymorphonuclear leukocytes. (From Pittiglio and Sacher, Fig. 25, with permission.)

Color Plate 2. Normal bone marrow showing developing white blood cells and red blood cells; leukocyte series—*A)* promyelocyte, *B)* myelocytes, *C)* metamyelocytes, *D)* bands. Developing erythroid series—*E)* polychromatophilic erythroblasts, *F)* orthochromatic erythroblasts.

Color Plate 3. *A)* Marrow showing large and small plasma cells. *B)* Megakaryocyte with platelets. (From Pittiglio and Sacher, Figs. 53 and 60, with permission.)

Color Plate 4. Peripheral blood showing normal lymphocytes, neutrophils, and platelets.

Color Plate 5. Normochromic, normocytic erythrocytes from a normal peripheral blood.

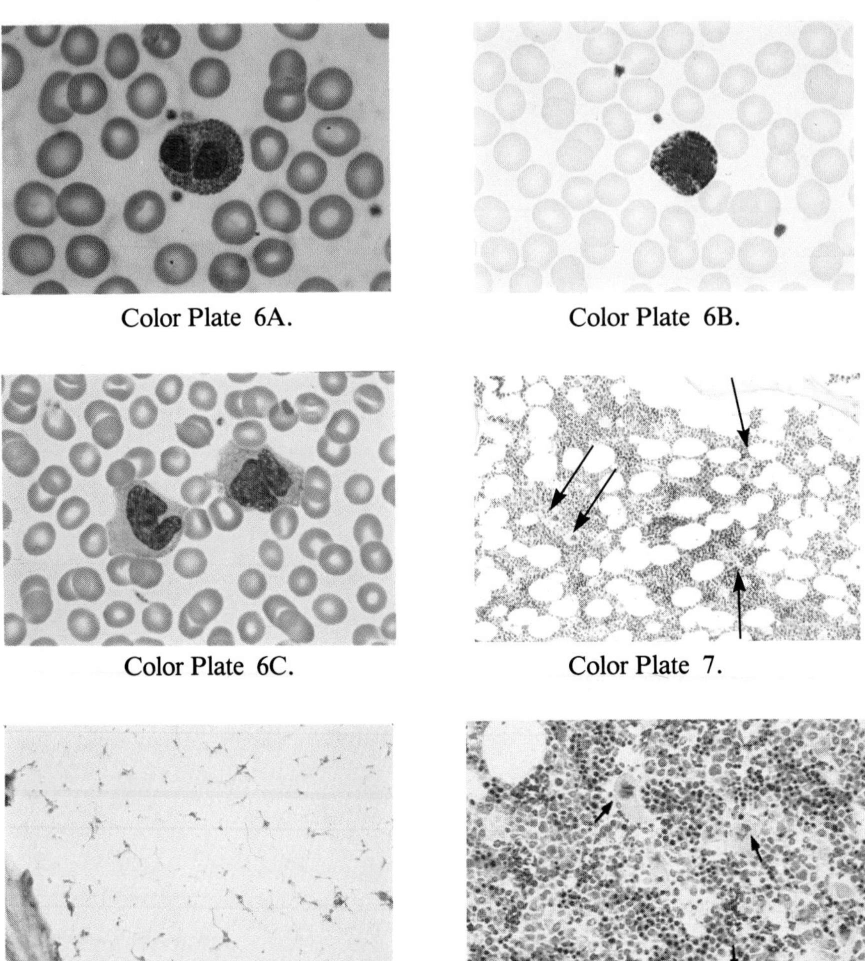

Color Plate 6A.

Color Plate 6B.

Color Plate 6C.

Color Plate 7.

Color Plate 8A.

Color Plate 8B.

Color Plate 6. *A)* Segmented eosinophil. *B)* Basophil (center). *C)* Monocytes. (From Pittiglio and Sacher, Figs. 36, 38 and 40, with permission.)

Color Plate 7. Normal bone marrow biopsy showing approximately 50% marrow cellularity. Note the megakaryocytes (low power) (arrows). (From Pittiglio and Sacher, Fig. 79, with permission.)

Color Plate 8. *A)* Hypocellular marrow biopsy from a patient with aplastic anemia. (From Pittiglio and Sacher, Fig. 80, with permission.) *B)* Hypercellular marrow biopsy taken from a patient with a megaloblastic anemia (arrows indicate megakaryocytes).

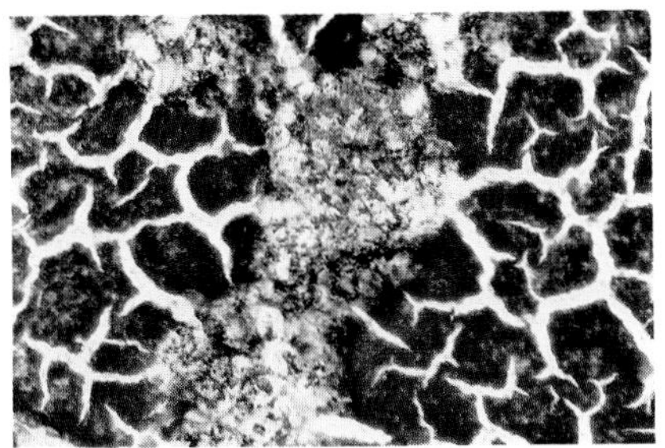

Color Plate 9A.

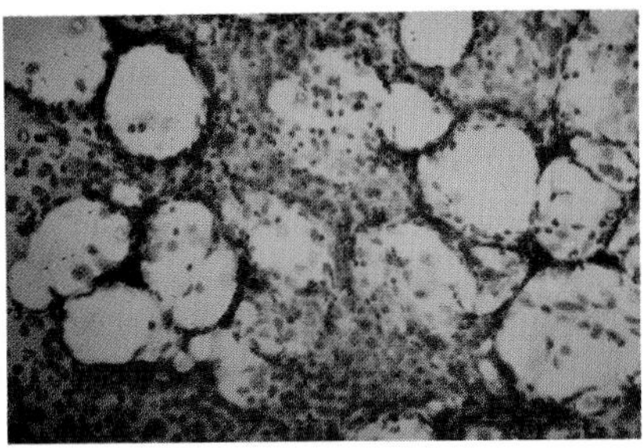

Color Plate 9B.

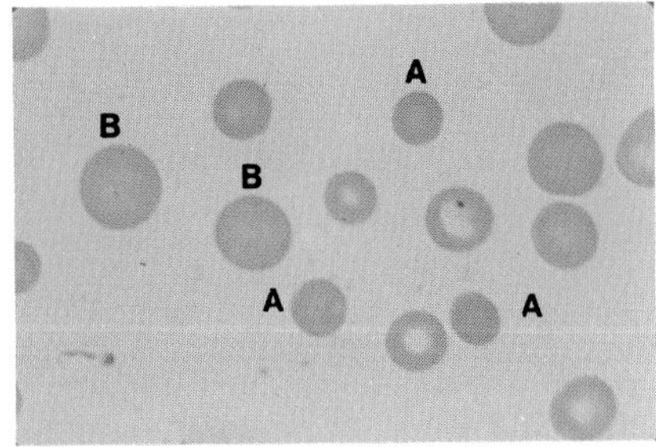

Color Plate 10.

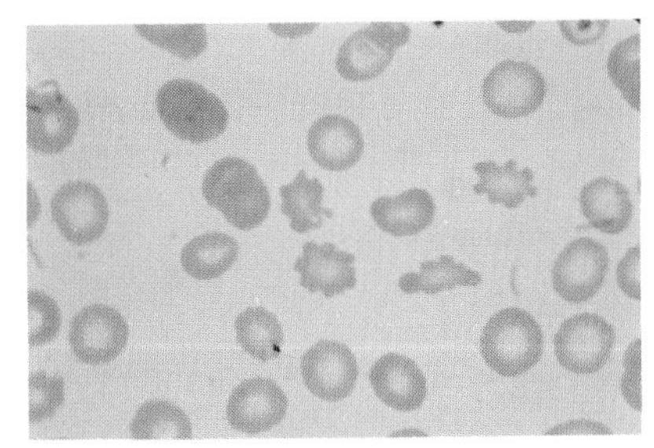

Color Plate 11.

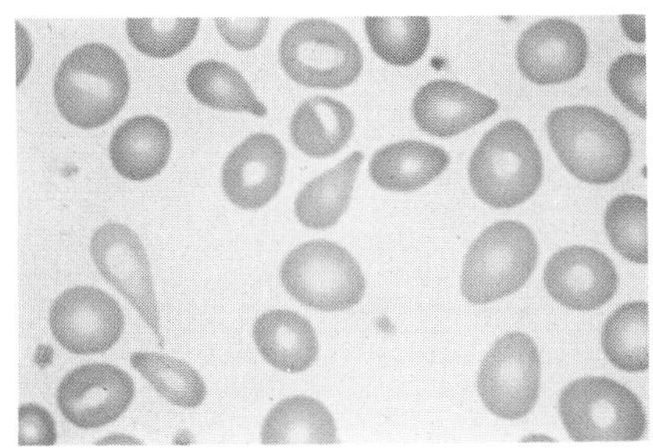

Color Plate 12.

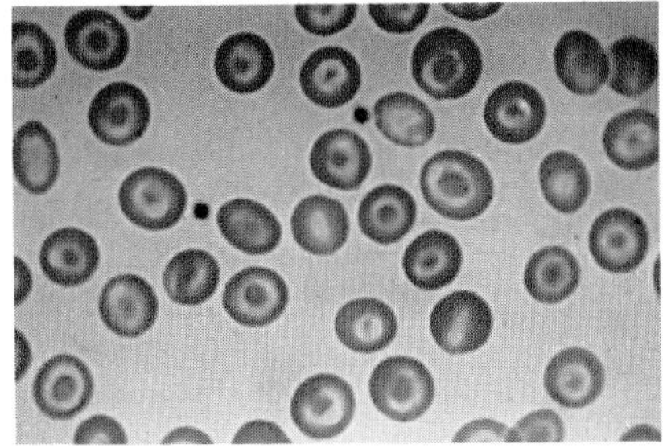

Color Plate 13.

Color Plate 9. *A)* Bone marrow showing normal iron stores; stained with Prussian blue stain, which stains iron blue. *B)* Absent iron stores from a patient with iron deficiency anemia.

Color Plate 10. Peripheral blood showing *A)* spherocytes, *B)* reticulocytes—from a patient with hereditary spherocytosis.

Color Plate 11. Peripheral blood from renal disease patient showing burr cells. (From Pittiglio and Sacher, Fig. 123, with permission.)

Color Plate 12. Peripheral blood showing tear drop poikilocytes from a patient with myelofibrosis.

Color Plate 13. Hemoglobin C disease. Peripheral blood showing numerous target cells.

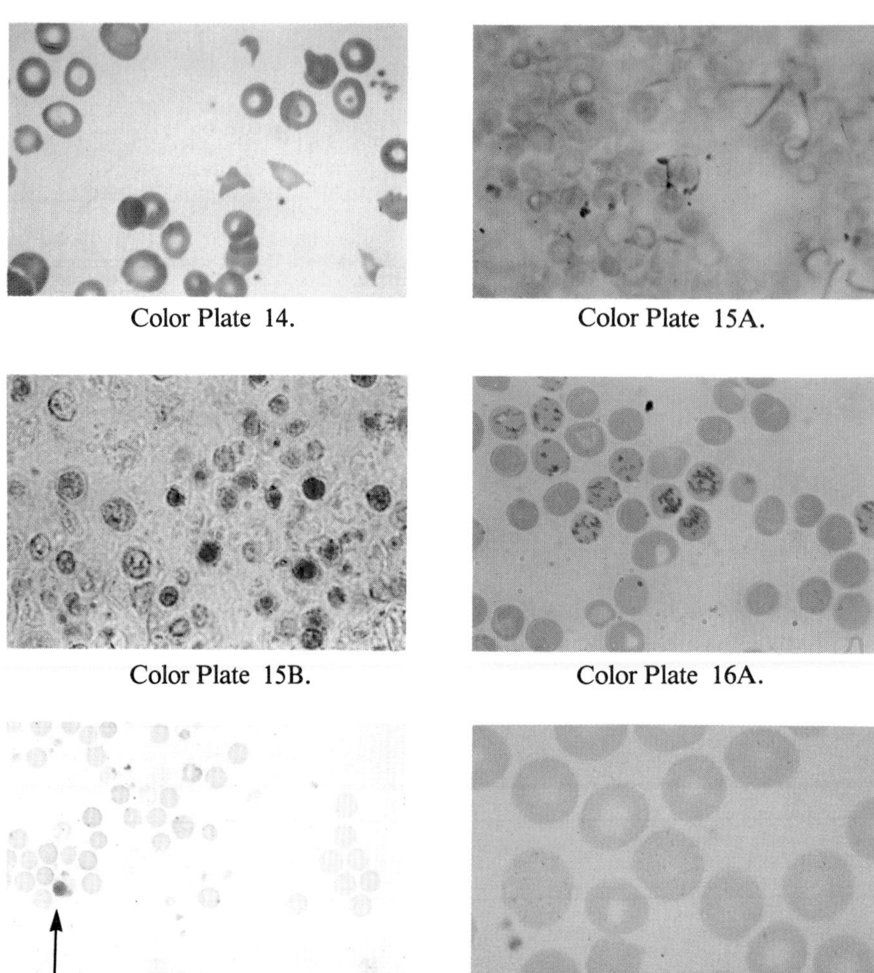

Color Plate 14.

Color Plate 15A.

Color Plate 15B.

Color Plate 16A.

Color Plate 16B.

Color Plate 16C.

Color Plate 14. Peripheral blood from a patient with cardiac valve hemolysis showing schistocytes.

Color Plate 15. *A)* Sideroblastic anemia bone marrow showing ring sideroblasts. *B)* Bone marrow showing non-ring sideroblasts in developing red blood cells from a patient with hemochromatosis.

Color Plate 16. *A)* Peripheral blood showing reticulocytes. *B)* Heinz Body preparation from a patient with glucose-6 phosphate dehydrogenase deficiency. *C)* Basophilic stippling—lead poisoning. (From Gower Medical Publishing Ltd. London, U.K.—with permission.)

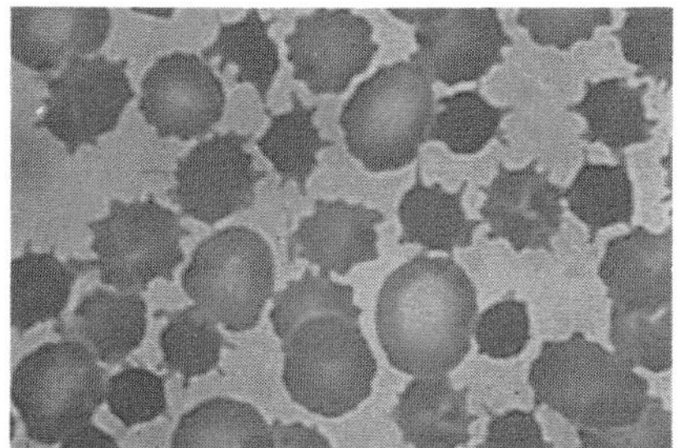

Color Plate 17.

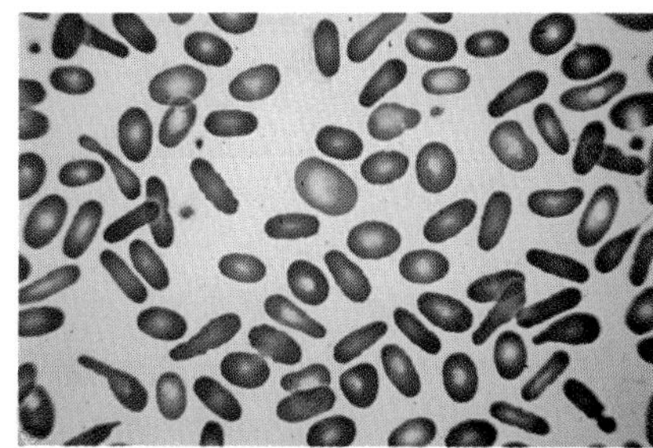

Color Plate 18.

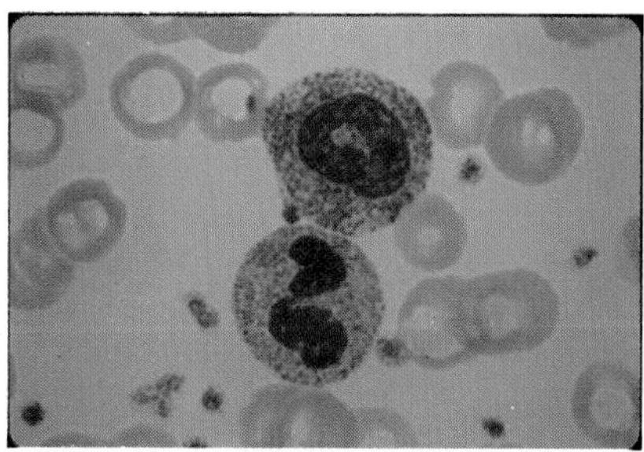

Color Plate 19.

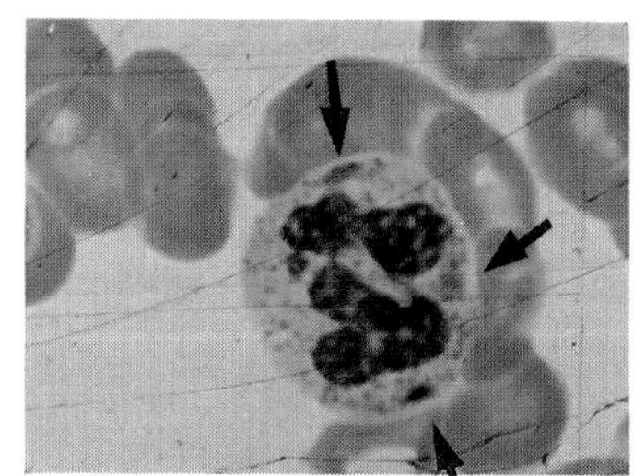

Color Plate 20.

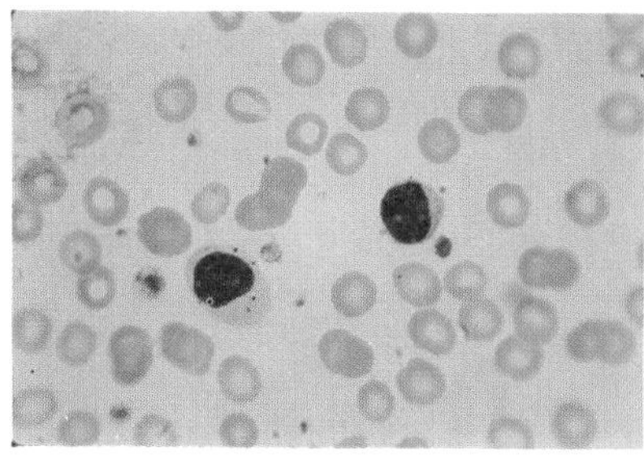

Color Plate 21.

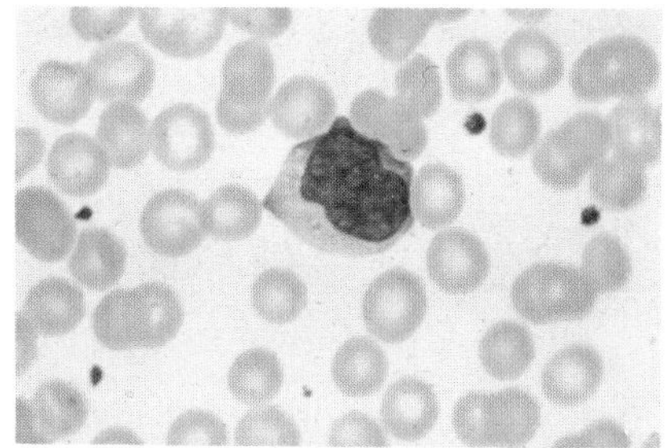

Color Plate 22A.

Color Plate 17. Acanthocytosis (patient with Abetalipoproteinemia). (From Hyun, BH, Ashton, JK, and Dolan, K, Practical Hematology. A Laboratory Guide with Accompanying Filmstrip. WB Saunders, Philadelphia, 1975, with permission.)

Color Plate 18. Hereditary elliptocytosis (peripheral blood). Note the high percentage of elliptocytes or ovalocytes. (From Pittiglio and Sacher, Fig. 88, with permission.)

Color Plate 19. Toxic granulation (peripheral blood). Note the prominent dark staining granules. (From Pittiglio and Sacher, Fig. 136, with permission.)

Color Plate 20. Döhle Bodies (arrows) note the large bluish bodies in the periphery in the cytoplasm. (From Pittiglio and Sacher, Fig. 137, with permission.)

Color Plate 21. Normal large lymphocyte with azurophilic granules (left) and normal small lymphocyte (right). (From Pittiglio and Sacher, Fig. 143, with permission.)

Color Plate 22. *A* and *B)* Peripheral blood showing atypical lymphocytes from a patient with infectious mononucleosis.

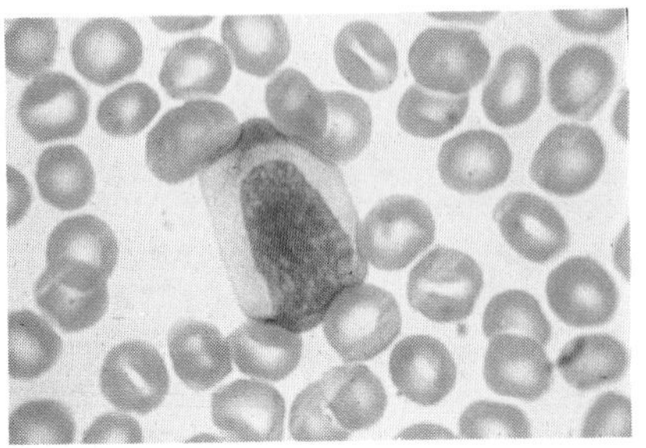

Color Plate 22B.

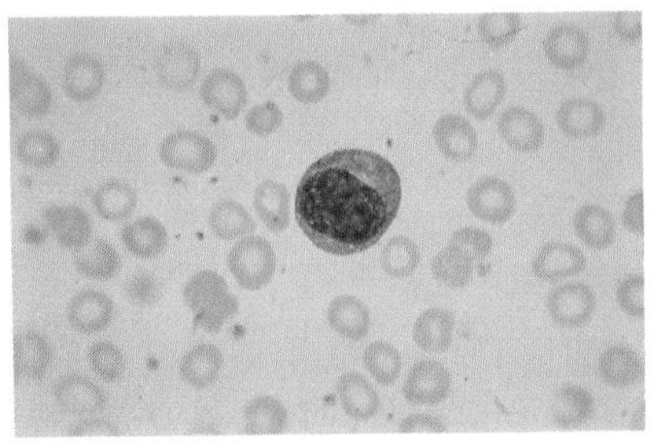

Color Plate 23.

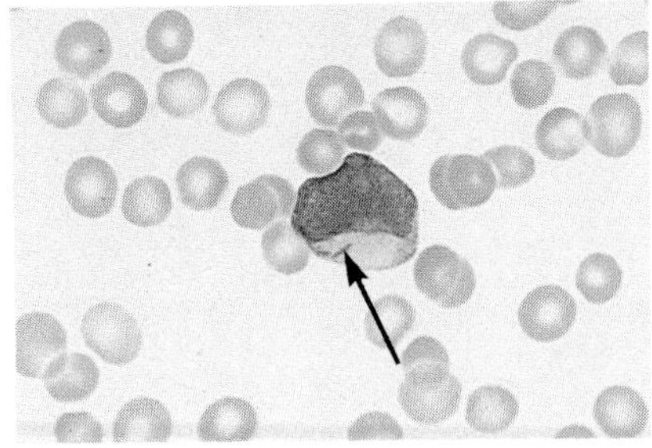

Color Plate 24.

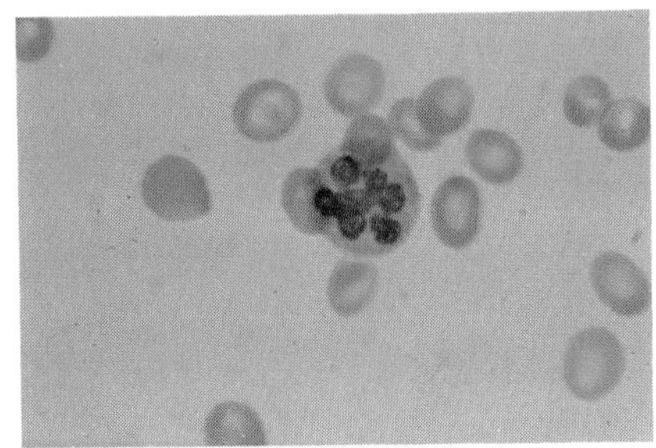

Color Plate 25.

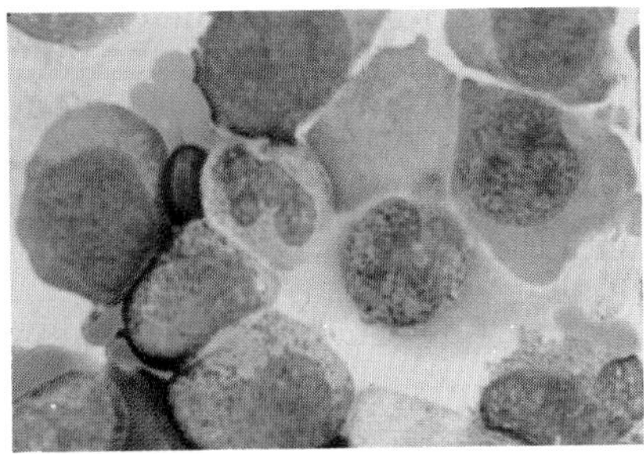

Color Plate 26.

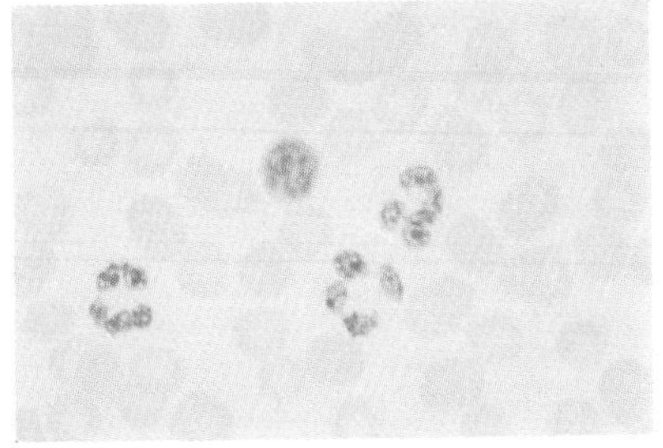

Color Plate 27A.

Color Plate 23. Plasmacytoid lymphocyte from a patient with Waldenstrom's macroglobulinemia. (From Pittiglio and Sacher, Fig. 143, with permission.)

Color Plate 24. Peripheral blood-Auer rod in myeloblast from a patient with acute myelogenous leukemia. (From Pittiglio and Sacher, Fig. 149, with permission.)

Color Plate 25. Peripheral blood showing neutrophil hypersegmentation (folic acid deficiency).

Color Plate 26. Bone marrow from pernicious anemia showing numerous megaloblastic erythroid precursors and abnormal large myeloid precursors.

Color Plate 27. Leukocyte alkaline phosphatase. *A)* Low in chronic myelogenous leukemia. *B)* Strongly positive in leukemoid reaction. (From Pittiglio and Sacher, Figs. 177 and 182, with permission.)

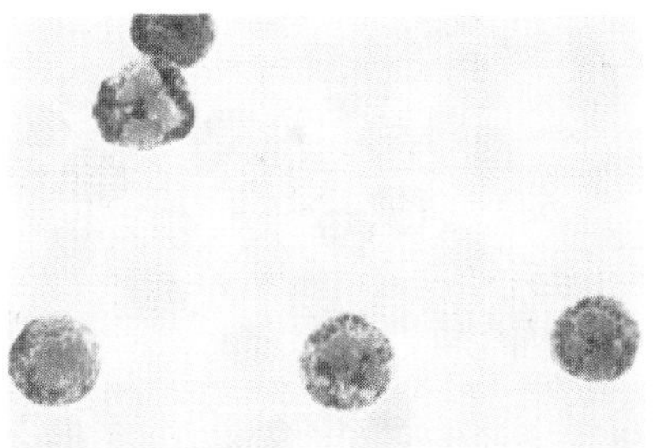

Color Plate 27B.

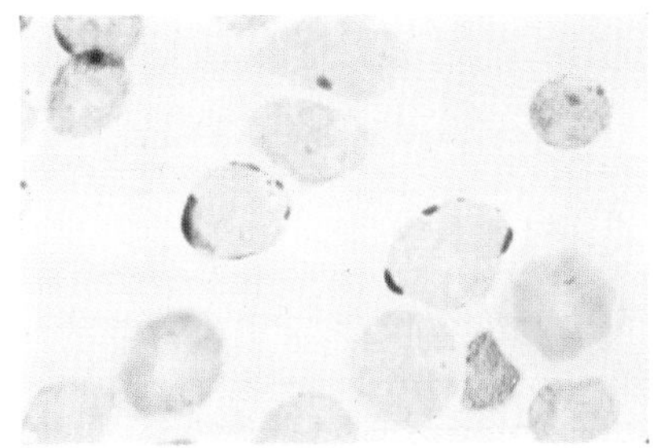

Color Plate 28.

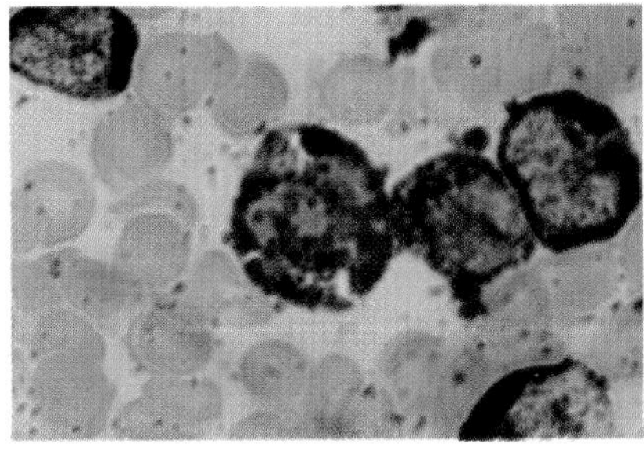

Color Plate 29.

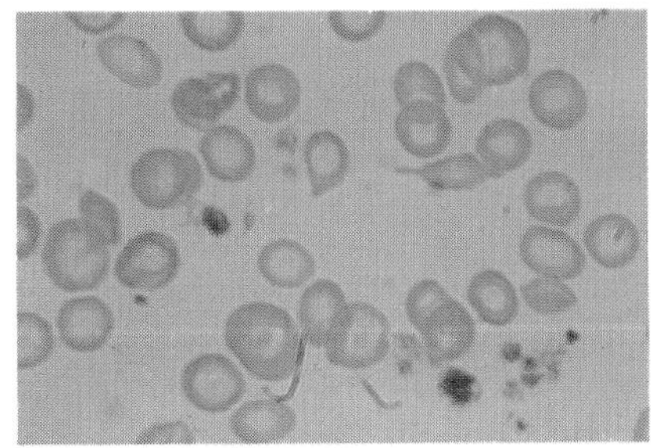

Color Plate 30A.

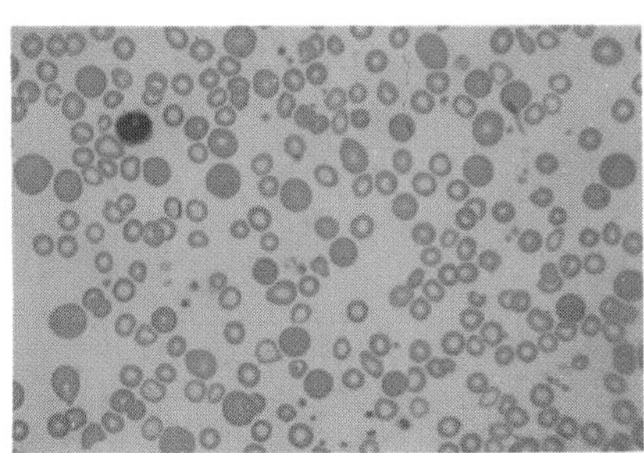

Color Plate 30B.

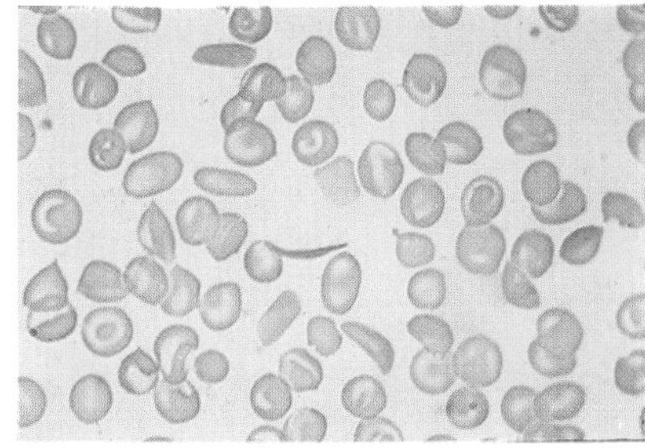

Color Plate 31.

Color Plate 28. Periodic acid-Schiff positivity in acute lymphoblastic leukemia. Note the (block) staining pattern. (From Pittiglio and Sacher, Fig. 154, with permission.)

Color Plate 29. Bone marrow myeloblasts showing Sudan black staining in acute myelogenous leukemia.

Color Plate 30. *A)* Peripheral blood-iron deficiency anemia. NOTE: Hypochromic microcytic cells with target cells and tear drop forms. *B)* Peripheral blood: Iron deficiency after iron therapy. Note numerous polychromatophilic cells (reticulocytes).

Color Plate 31. Sickle thalassemia syndrome (peripheral blood). (From Pittiglio and Sacher, Fig. 105, with permission.) NOTE: Sickle cells and target cells.

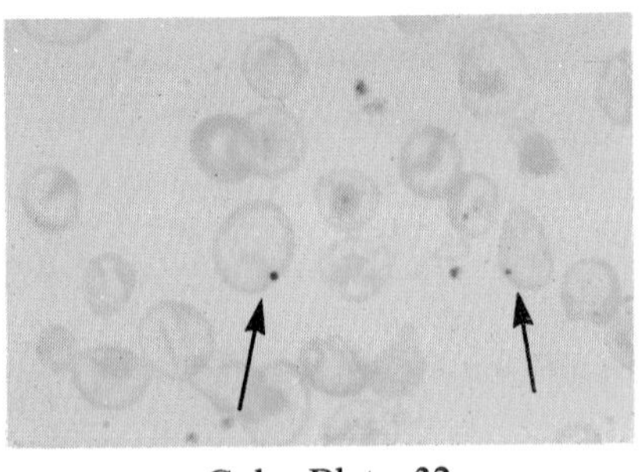

Color Plate 32.

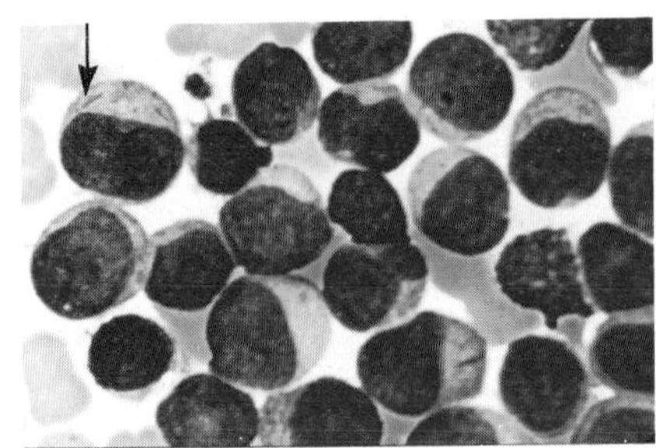

Color Plate 33.

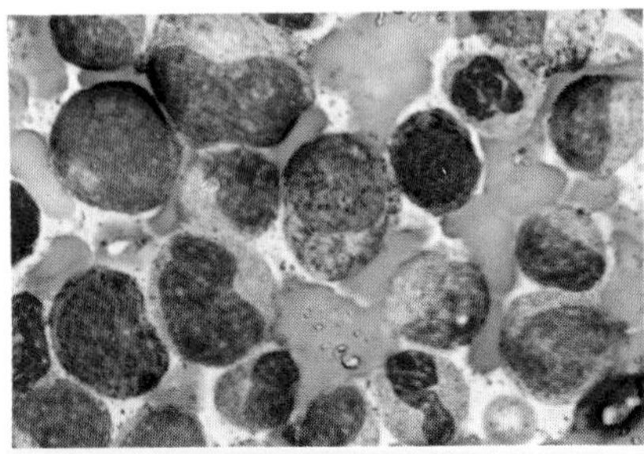

Color Plate 34.

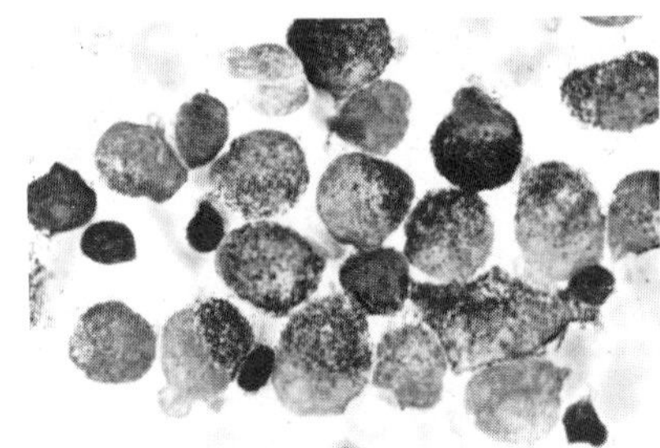

Color Plate 35.

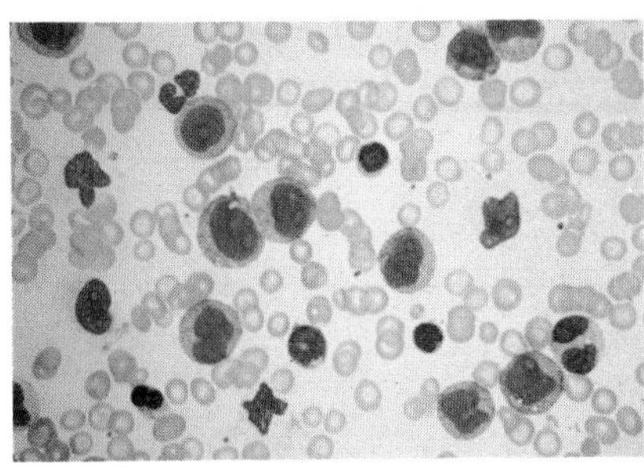

Color Plate 36.

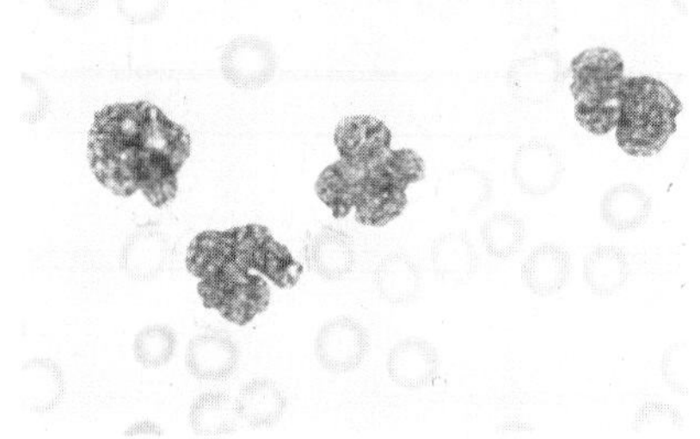

Color Plate 37.

Color Plate 32. Blood film in thalassemia—NOTE: Hypochromic microcytic RBCs and Howell Jolly bodies (arrows).

Color Plate 33. Bone marrow: Acute myeloblastic leukemia without maturation (FAB—M 1). NOTE: Auer rod (arrows).

Color Plate 34. Bone marrow: Acute myeloblastic leukemia with limited maturation (FAB—M 2).

Color Plate 35. Bone marrow: Acute promyelocytic leukemia (FAB—M 3). (From Pittiglio and Sacher, Fig. 162, with permission.)

Color Plate 36. Peripheral blood: Acute myelomonocytic leukemia. (FAB—M 4).

Color Plate 37. Peripheral blood: Acute monocytic leukemia (FAB—M 5). (From Pittiglio and Sacher, Fig. 168, with permission.)

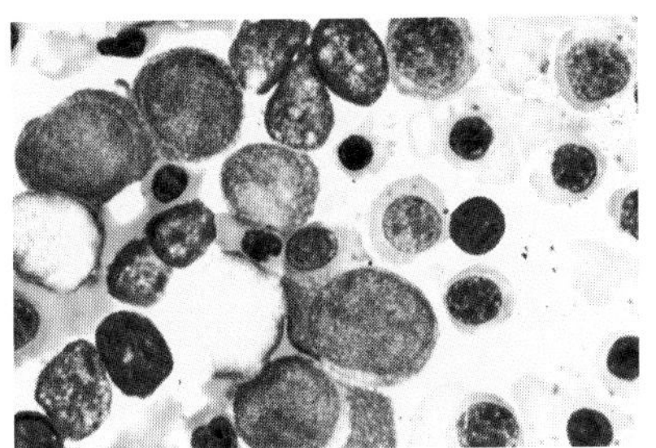

Color Plate 38A.

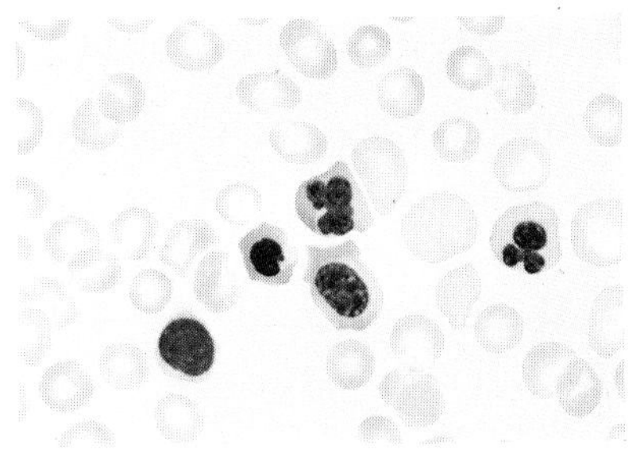

Color Plate 38B.

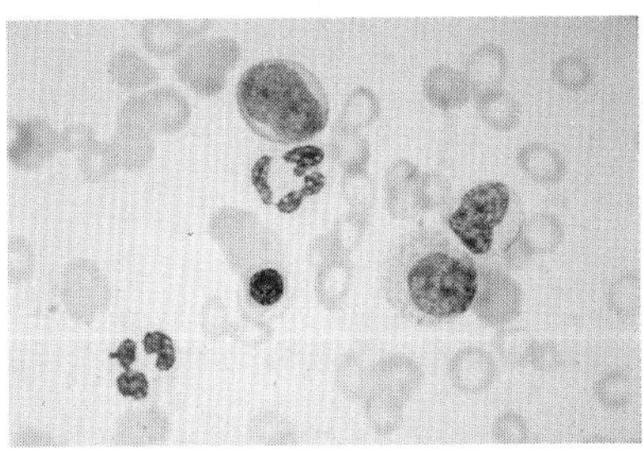

Color Plate 39A.

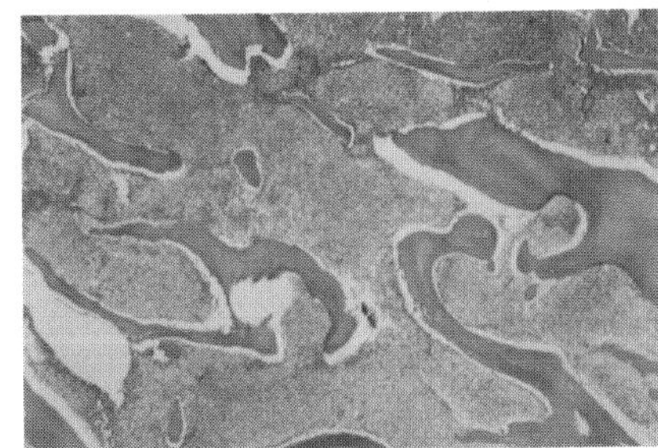

Color Plate 39B.

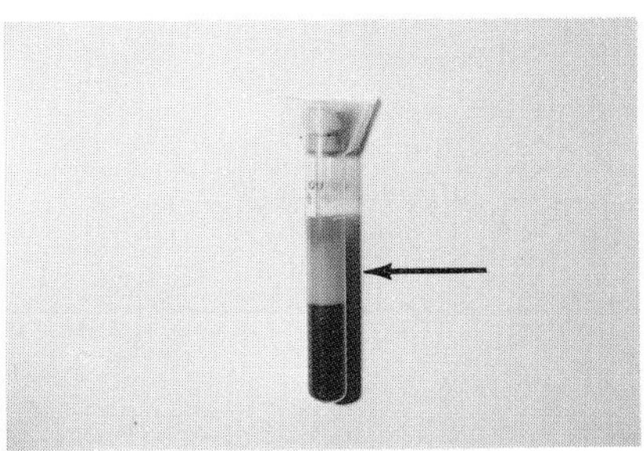

Color Plate 40A.

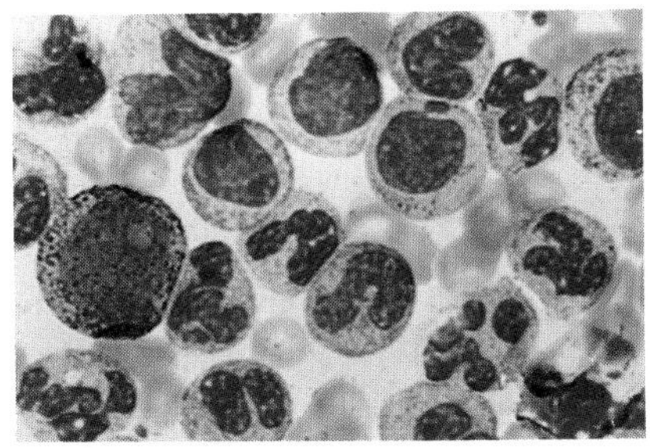

Color Plate 40B.

Color Plate 38) *A)* Bone marrow: Acute erythroleukemia (FAB—M 6). NOTE: Megaloblastoid dyserythropoiesis. *B)* Acute erythroleukemia peripheral blood. NOTE: Dysplastic nuclei in nucleated red blood cells. (From Pittiglio and Sacher, Figs. 169 and 170, with permission.)

Color Plate 39. *A)* Peripheral blood showing typical leukoerythroblastic reaction. Note immature white cells and red precursors in the peripheral blood. *B)* Bone marrow biopsy showing fibrosis replacing normal marrow elements from a patient with idiopathic myelofibrosis. (From Pittiglio and Sacher, Fig. 131, with permission.)

Color Plate 40. *A)* Blood sample from a patient with chronic myelogenous leukemia (after standing) showing exaggerated "buffy coat" (white central zone—see arrow) white cell count 300,000/μl. *B)* Bone marrow: Showing myeloid hyperplasia with all myeloid precursors present in abundance from a patient with chronic myelogenous leukemia.

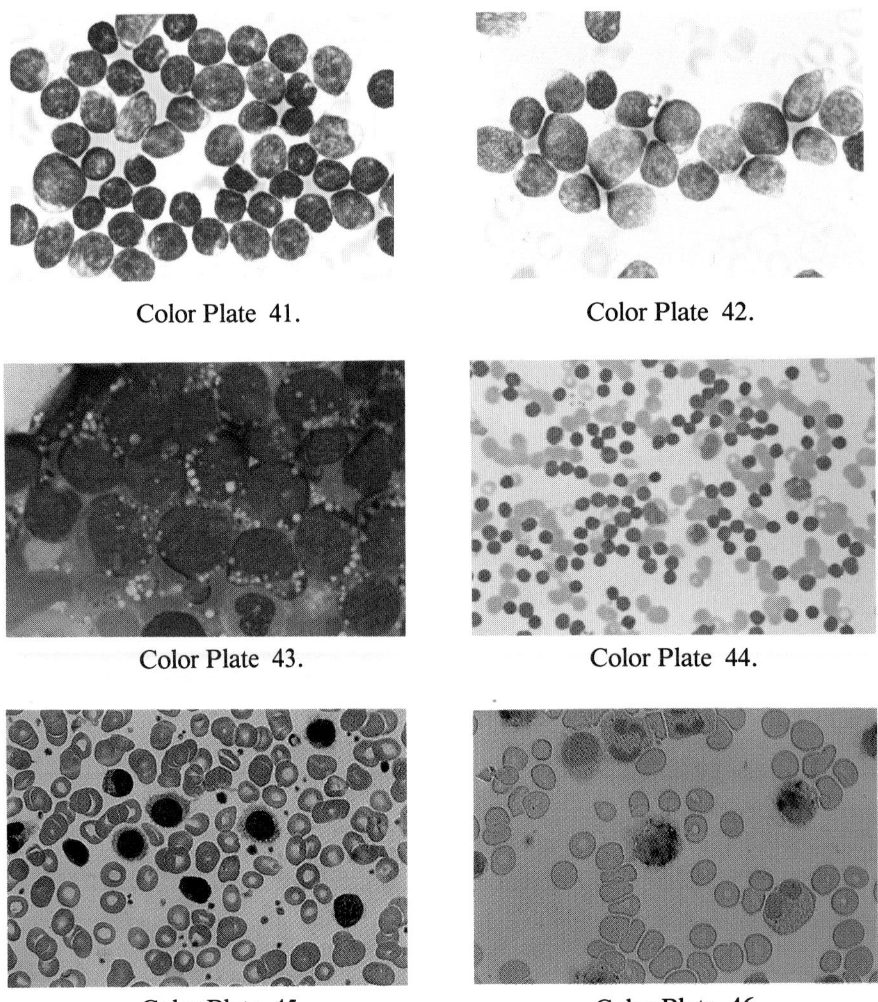

Color Plate 41.

Color Plate 42.

Color Plate 43.

Color Plate 44.

Color Plate 45.

Color Plate 46.

Color Plate 41. Acute lymphoblastic leukemia (FAB—L 1). (From Pittiglio and Sacher, Fig. 157, with permission.)

Color Plate 42. Acute lymphoblastic leukemia (FAB—L 2). (From Pittiglio and Sacher, Fig. 158, with permission.)

Color Plate 43. Acute lymphoblastic leukemia (Burkitt type—FAB L 3).

Color Plate 44. Peripheral blood: Chronic lymphocytic leukemia—small regular mature appearing lymphocytes.

Color Plate 45. Peripheral blood showing hairy cell leukemia. Note hairy projections from lymphoid cells.

Color Plate 46. Peripheral blood: positive tartrate resistant acid phosphatase (TRAP) in hairy cell leukemia.

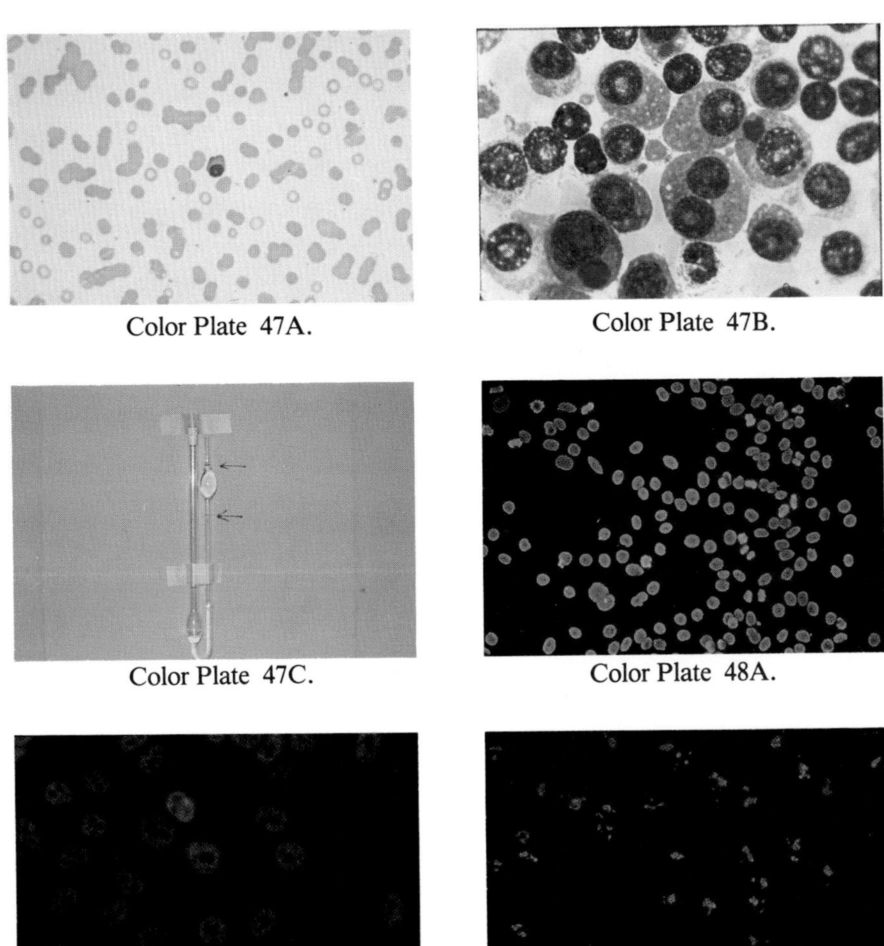

Color Plate 47A.

Color Plate 47B.

Color Plate 47C.

Color Plate 48A.

Color Plate 48B.

Color Plate 49A.

Color Plate 47. *A)* Peripheral blood from a patient with multiple myeloma showing extensive rouleaux. *B)* Bone marrow: Showing masses of large plasma cells with prominent nucleoli—including a bi-nucleated plasma cell from a patient with multiple myeloma. *C)* Viscosometer to measure serum viscosity. Arrows indicate distance of fluid flow. The time taken to measure rate of flow of serum compared to water gives the relative viscosity. (From Pittiglio and Sacher, Fig. 188, with permission.)

Color Plate 48. Fluorescent antinuclear antibody patterns: *A)* homogeneous, *B)* speckled.

Color Plate 49. FANA pattern: *A)* nucleolar, *B)* antimitochondrial (kidney).

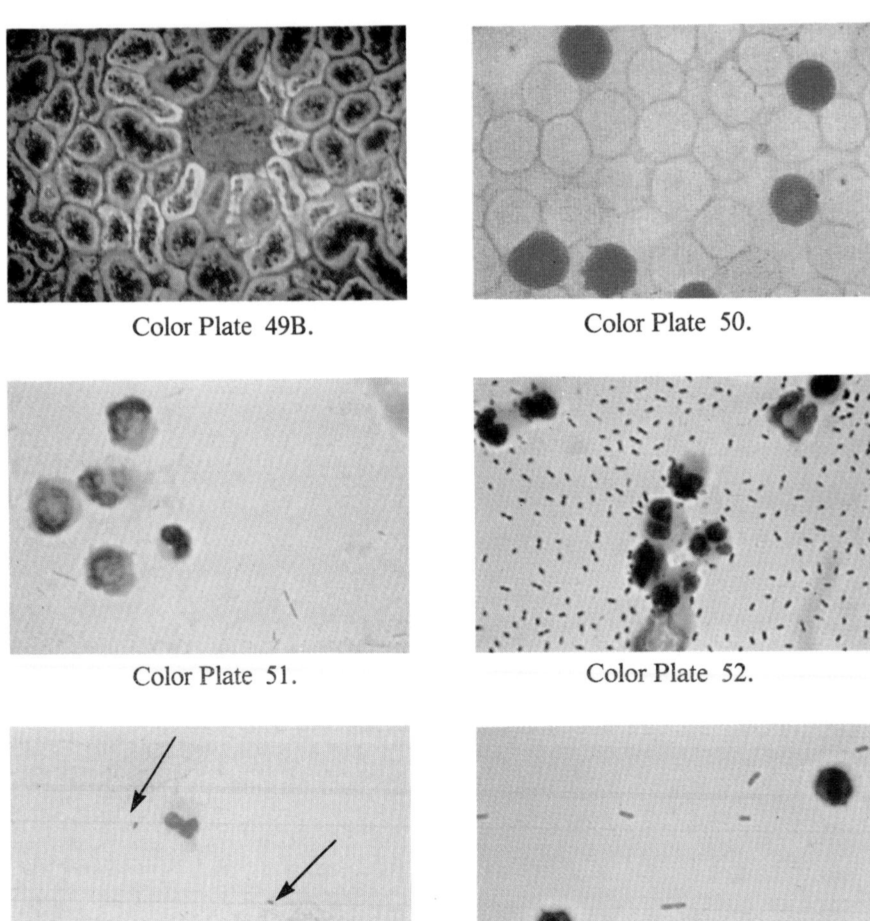

Color Plate 49B.

Color Plate 50.

Color Plate 51.

Color Plate 52.

Color Plate 53.

Color Plate 54.

Color Plate 50. Fetal hemoglobulin: Kleihauer Betke Stain of newborn blood. Red cells containing hemoglobin F maintained red staining color; clear staining cells contain hemoglobin A. (From Listen, Look and Learn. National Committee for Careers in the Medical Laboratory.)

Color Plate 51. Gram stain smear of cerebrospinal fluid (CSF) from a patient with *Hemophilus influenzae, meningitis.* (Gram negative pleomorphic bacilli) NOTE: The varied length of the bacilli.

Color Plate 52. Gram stain smear of cerebrospinal fluid from a patient with *Streptococcus pneumoniae* meningitis. (Gram positive diplococci)

Color Plate 53. Gram stain smear of CSF from a patient with *Neisseria meningitidis* meningitis. (Gram negative diplococci) (From Roche Laboratories, Nutley, N.J., with permission.) (See arrows).

Color Plate 54. Gram stain smear of urine from a patient with *Escherichia coli* urinary tract infection. (Gram negative bacilli)

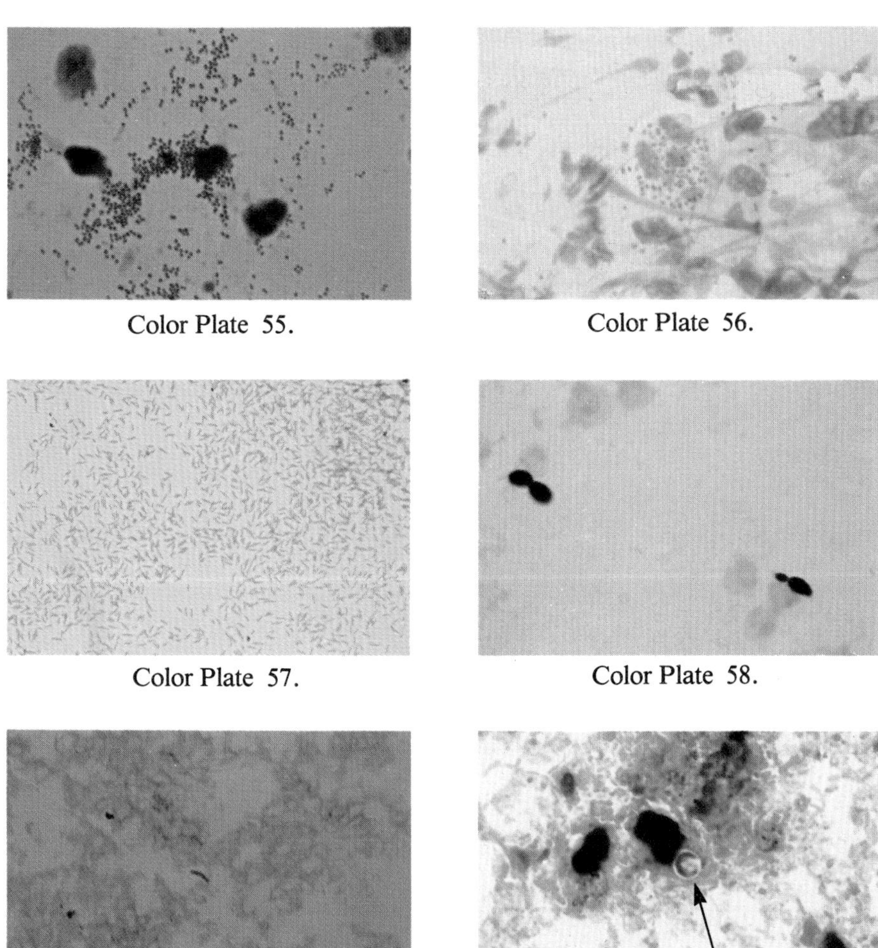

Color Plate 55.

Color Plate 56.

Color Plate 57.

Color Plate 58.

Color Plate 59.

Color Plate 60.

Color Plate 55. Gram stain smear of pus from a patient with *Staphylococcus aureus* wound infection. (Gram positive cocci in clusters)

Color Plate 56. Gram stain smear of discharge from a patient with *Neisseria gonorrhoeae* (Gram negative diplococci; NOTE: Intracellular distribution)

Color Plate 57. Gram stain smear of *Campylobacter jejuni.* NOTE: Curved gram negative bacilli.

Color Plate 58. Gram stain smear of discharge from a patient with *Candida albicans* vaginitis. (Gram positive oval budding yeast)

Color Plate 59. Kinyoun stained smear of sputum from a patient with *Mycobacterium tuberculosis* pneumonia. (acid-fast bacillus)

Color Plate 60. Modified Kinyoun stained smear of stool from a patient with *Cryptosporidium* enteritis (see arrow).

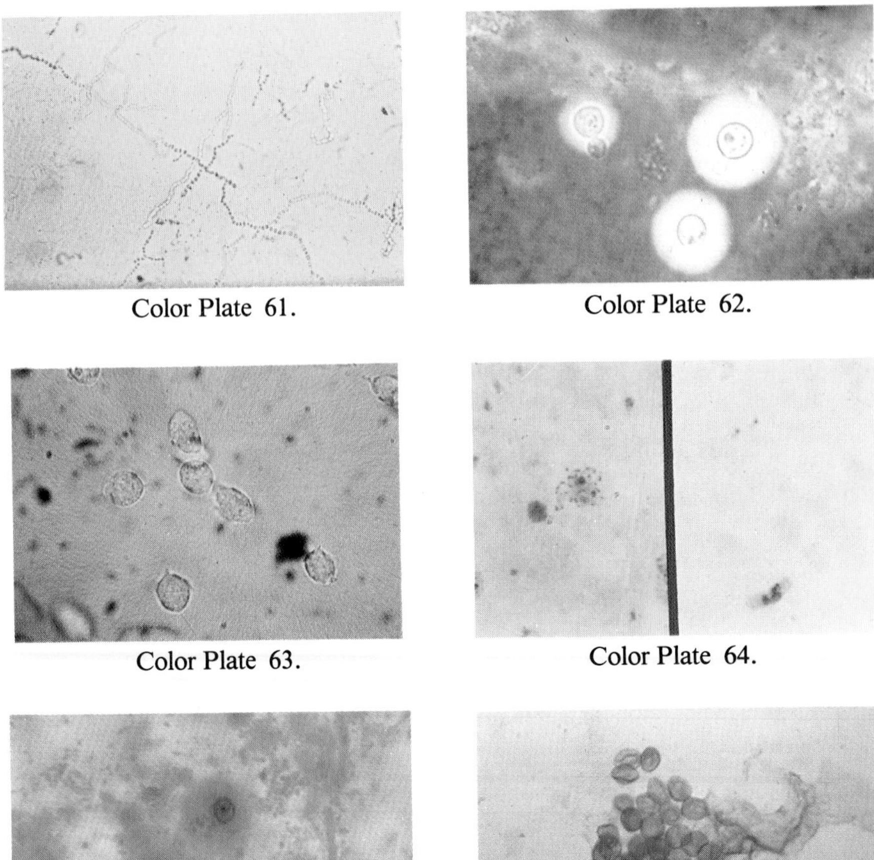

Color Plate 61.

Color Plate 62.

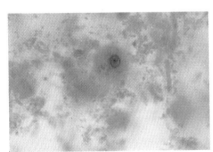

Color Plate 63.

Color Plate 64.

Color Plate 65.

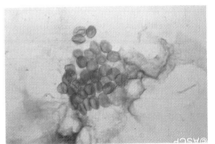

Color Plate 66.

Color Plate 61. KOH preparation of scrapings from a patient with skin ringworm. NOTE: String-like fungal hyphae. (From Gower Medical Publishing Ltd., London, UK, with permission.)

Color Plate 62. India ink preparation of CSF from a patient with *Cryptococcal* Meningitis. NOTE: Halo-like capsule. (From Gower Medical Publishing Ltd., London, UK, with permission.)

Color Plate 63. Trichrome stain of stool from a patient with *Giardia lamblia* infection.

Color Plate 64. Giemsa stained smears of peripheral blood from patients with malaria. Giemsa stain showing *Plasmodium vivax malarial trophozoites. A. Plasmodium vivax* (thick smear). *B. Plasmodium falciparum* (thin smear). (From MEDCOM, Inc., with permission.)

Color Plate 65. Trichrome stain of stool from a patient with *Entamoeba histolytica* infection. NOTE: Trophozoite with single prominent nucleus.

Color Plate 66. Toluidine blue stain of *Pneumocystis carinii* in bronchial alveolar lavage fluid. (From the American Society for Clinical Pathologists, Chicago, IL, with permission.)

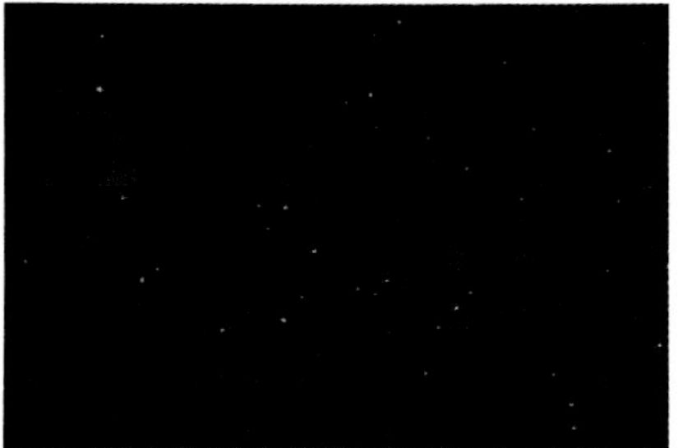

Color Plate 67.

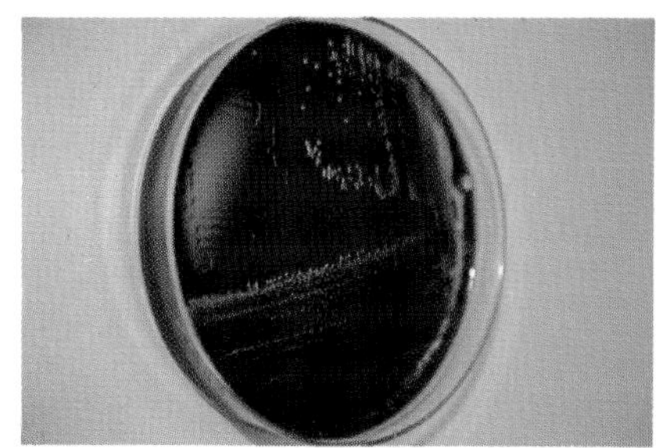

Color Plate 68.

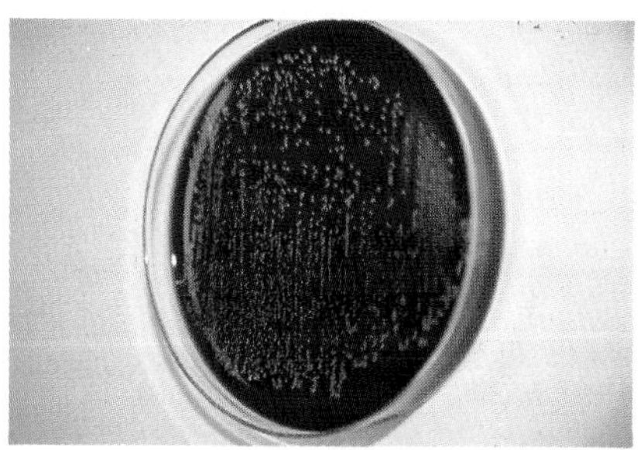

Color Plate 69.

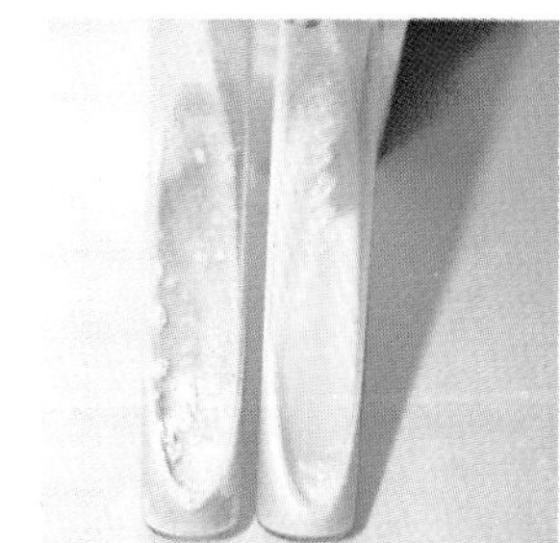

Color Plate 70.

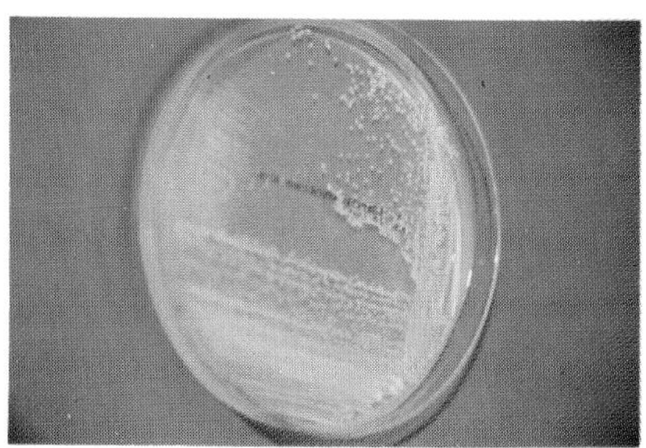

Color Plate 71A.

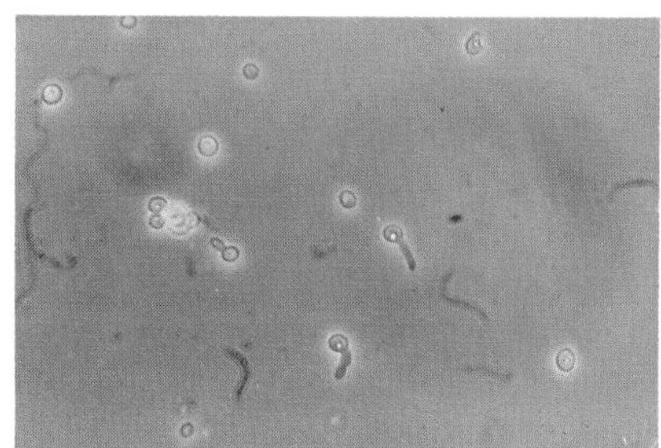

Color Plate 71B.

Color Plate 67. Positive direct immunofluorescence smear from a patient with *Chlamydia trachomatis* cervicitis. (From Syva Inc., Palo Alto, CA, with permission.)

Color Plate 68. Four quadrant streaking method for obtaining isolated colonies.

Color Plate 69. Colony count streaking method for quantitating microorganisms.

Color Plate 70. Cultures of mycobacteria growing on Lowenstein-Jensen medium.

Color Plate 71. *A)* Growth of *Candida albicans* on Sabouraud-dextrose agar. *B) Candida albicans* showing germ tube formation. (From Gower Medical Publishing, London, UK, with permission.)

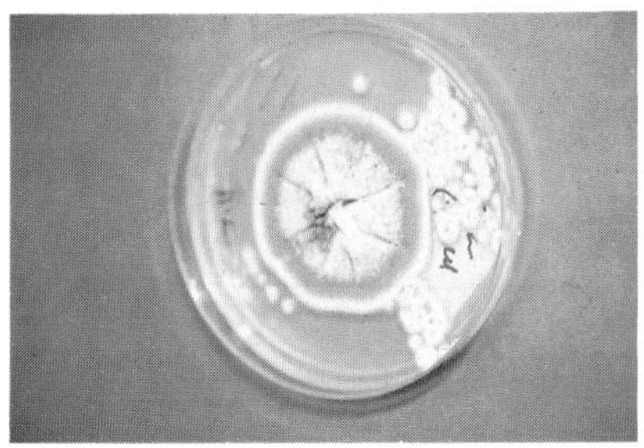

Color Plate 72.

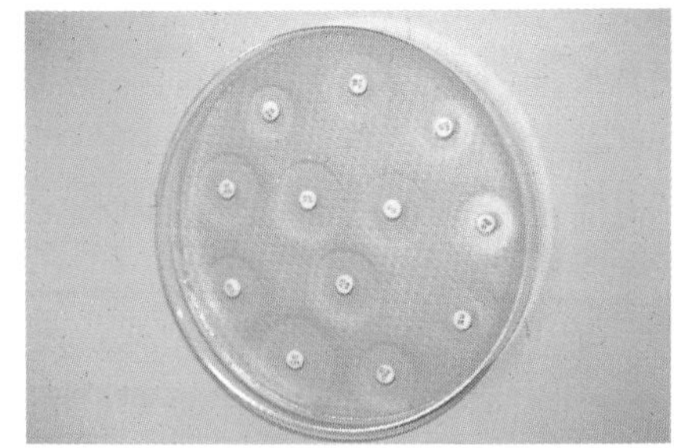

Color Plate 73A.

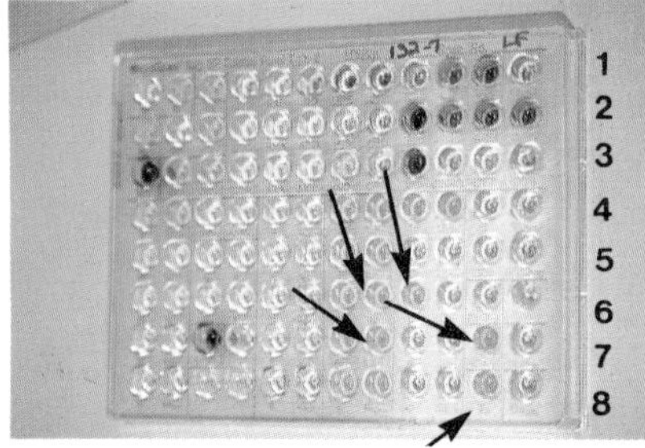

Color Plate 73B.

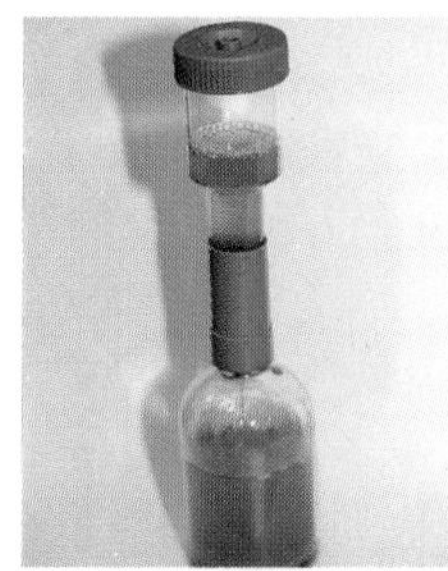

Color Plate 74.

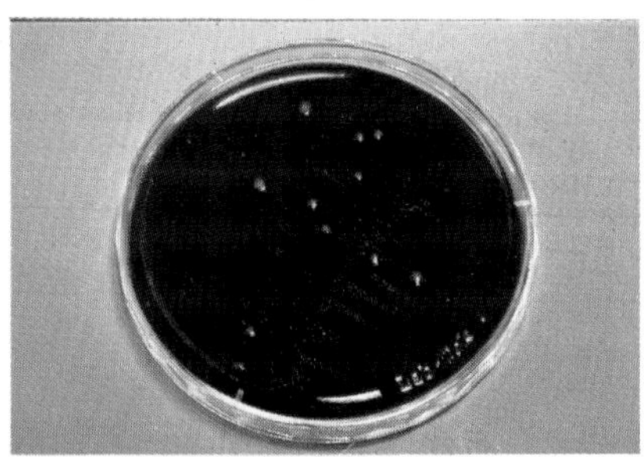

Color Plate 75.

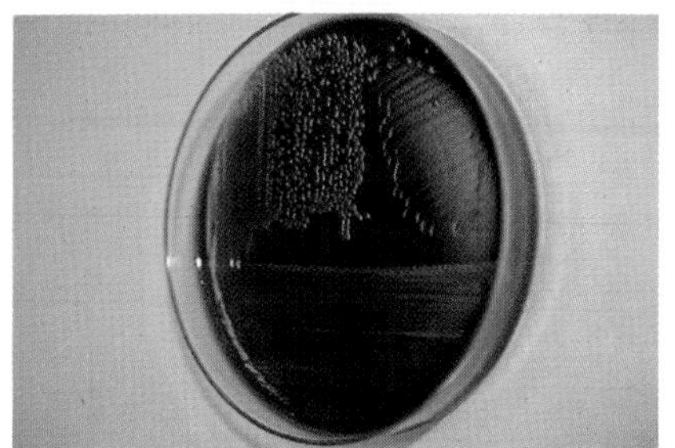

Color Plate 76.

Color Plate 72. Growth of *Aspergillus fumigatus* on Sabouraud-dextrose agar.

Color Plate 73A. Agar disk diffusion antimicrobial susceptibility test. NOTE: Circular zones of growth inhibition around antibiotic impregnated filter paper disks.

Color Plate 73B. Broth microdilution antimicrobial susceptibility test. (Combo tray) First 3 columns contain biochemical identification test wells. Remaining 5 columns contain antimicrobial dilutions. Note greenish growth in several wells (see example—arrow) indicate antimicrobial resistance.

Color Plate 74. Blood culture method showing evidence of microbial growth. Growth is evidenced by turbidity of the broth, and with this particular blood culture system, by manometric displacement of broth into the reservoir attached to the top of the bottle.

Color Plate 75. Lysis centrifugation/direct plating. Growth of bacteria following plating of lysed blood to agar. (From E. I. DuPont de Nemours and Co., Wilmington, DE, with permission.)

Color Plate 76. Growth of *Haemophilus influenzae* on chocolate agar; showing mucoid colonies.

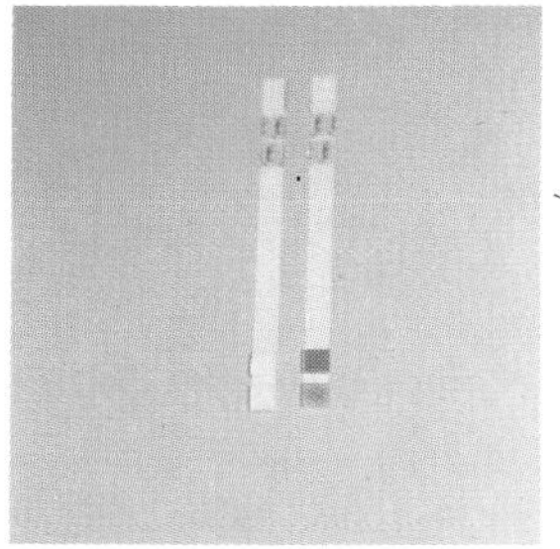

Color Plate 77.

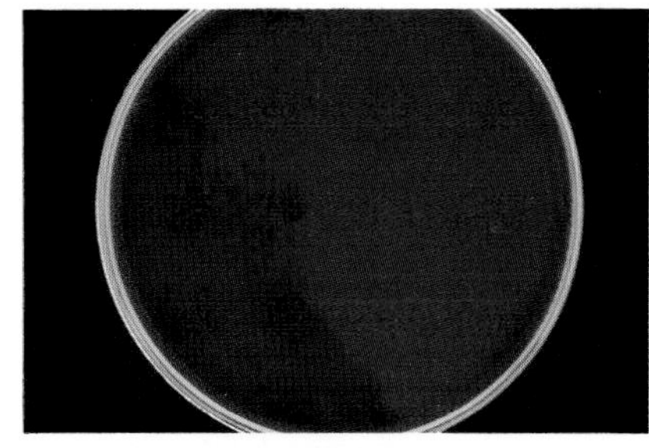

Color Plate 78.

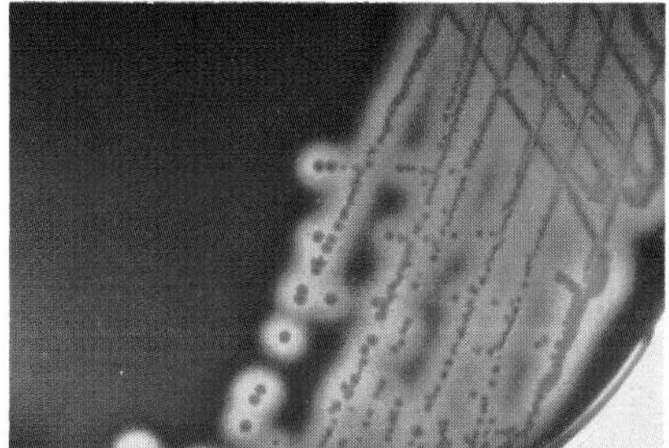

Color Plate 79.

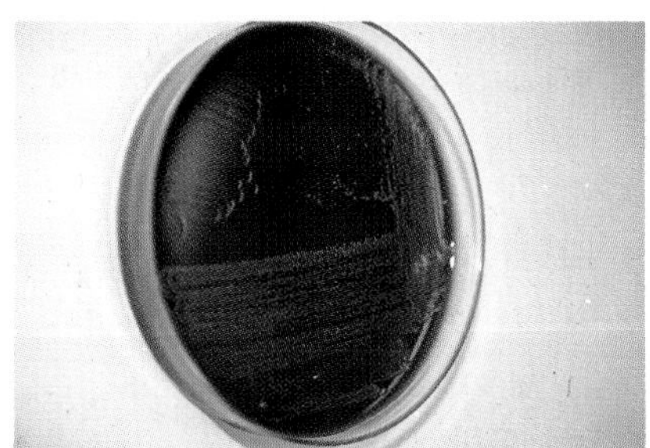

Color Plate 80.

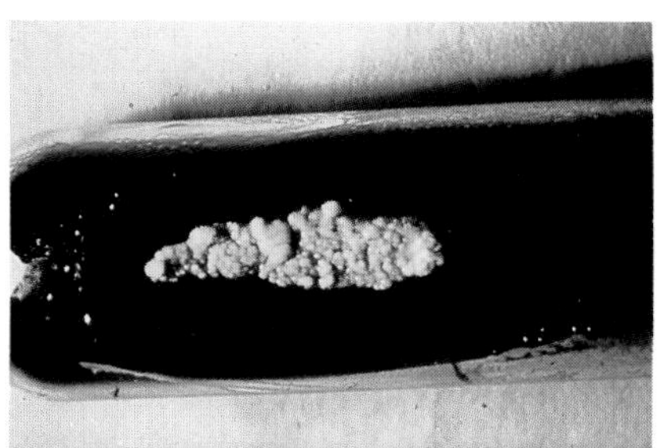

Color Plate 81A.

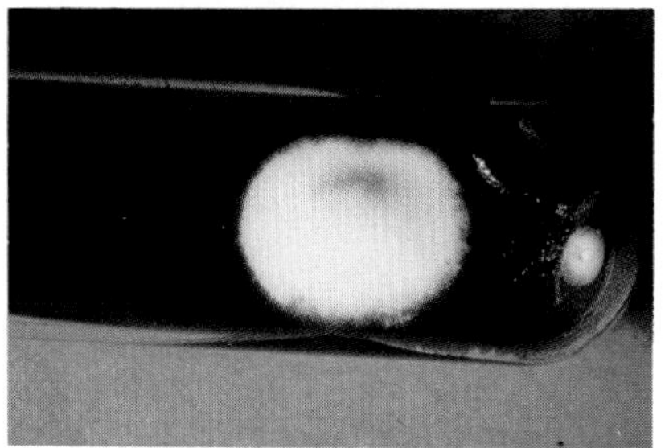

Color Plate 81B.

Color Plate 77. Leukocyte esterase and urine nitrate dipstick results showing positive and negative results. A positive leukocyte esterase result is indicated by purple color development in the filter paper pad at the bottom end of the dipstick. A positive nitrite result is indicated by red color development in the filter paper pad immediately above the leukocyte esterase test pad.

Color Plate 78. Alpha hemolysis on 5% sheep blood agar exhibited by viridans group streptococci.

Color Plate 79. Beta hemolysis on 5% sheep blood agar exhibited by group A streptococci following growth in an anaerobic environment. (From Marion Laboratories, Kansas City, MO, with permission.)

Color Plate 80. Growth of *Neisseria gonorrhoea* on modified Thayer-Martin agar.

Color Plate 81. Growth of dimorphic fungus *Histoplasma capsulatum—A)* Yeast phase. *B)* Mold phase. (From Gower Medical Publishing, Ltd., London, UK, with permission.)

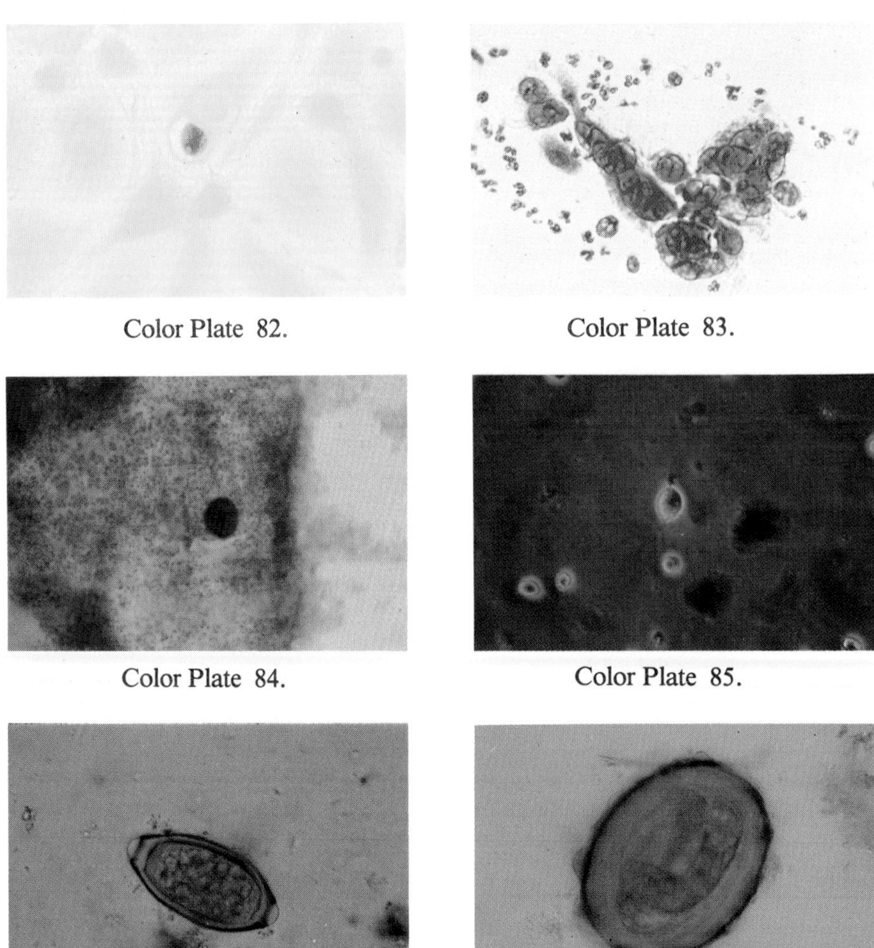

Color Plate 82.

Color Plate 83.

Color Plate 84.

Color Plate 85.

Color Plate 86A.

Color Plate 86B.

Color Plate 82. Cervical scraping showing iodine stained intracytoplasmic inclusion bodies of *C. trachomatis.* (From Gower Medical Publishing, Ltd., London, UK, with permission.)

Color Plate 83. Tzanck preparation showing multinucleate cells from a herpes simplex genital infection.

Color Plate 84. Gram stain smear of vaginal discharge showing "clue cells". Epithelial cells coated with large number of gram variable rods.

Color Plate 85. Wet mount of vaginal discharge showing a *Trichomonas vaginalis* trophozoite. (From Gower Medical Publishing, Ltd., London, UK, with permission.)

Color Plate 86. *A)* Wet mount of a *Trichuris trichiuria* egg in formalin preserved stool. *B) Ascaris lumbricoides* egg in stool.

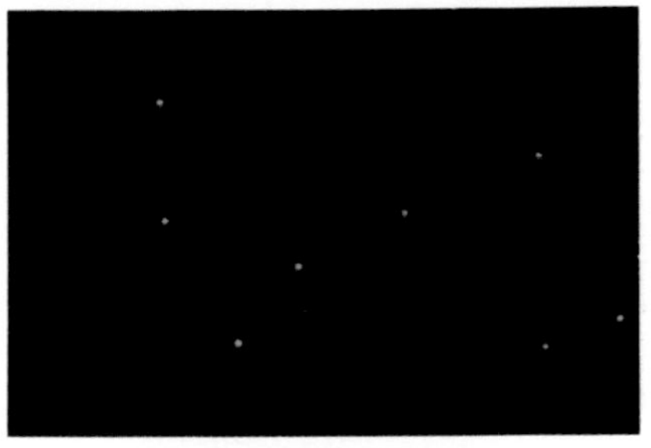

Color Plate 87.

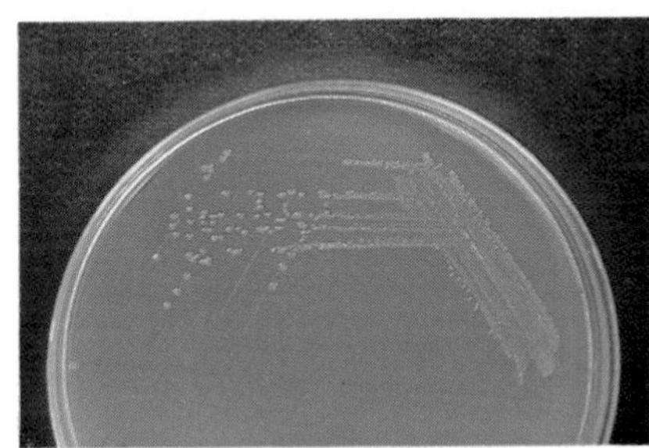

Color Plate 88.

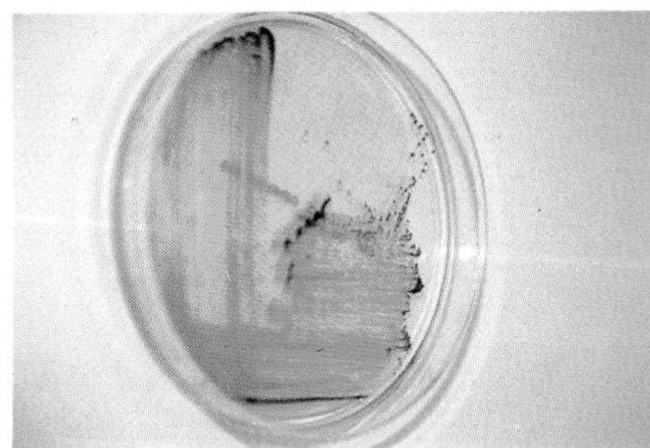

Color Plate 89.

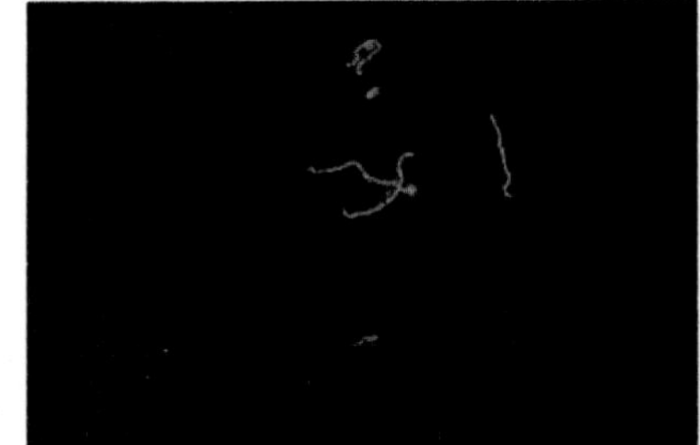

Color Plate 90.

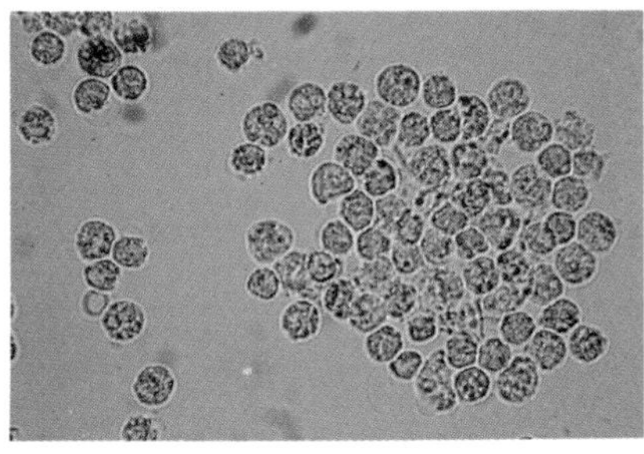

Color Plate 91.

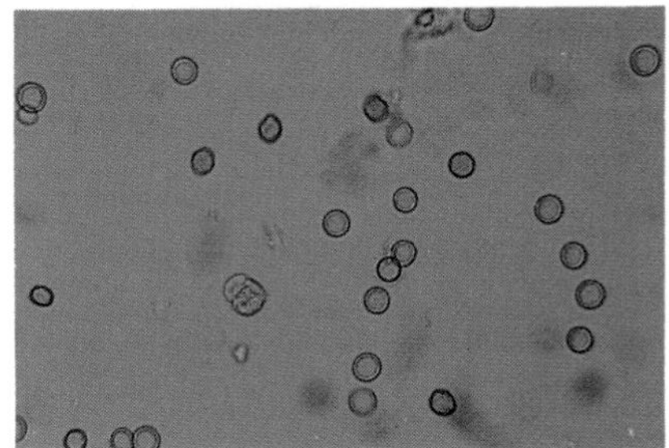

Color Plate 92.

Color Plate 87. Indirect immunofluorescence assay for *Cryptosporidium oocysts.*

Color Plate 88. Growth of *Shigella sonnei* on desoxycholate citrate agar demonstrating lack of lactose fermentation. (From Gower Medical Publishing, Ltd., UK, with permission.)

Color Plate 89. Growth of *Salmonella enteritidis* on salmonella-shigella (SS) agar. NOTE: Black colonies indicate hydrogen sulfide production.

Color Plate 90. Indirect fluorescent *Treponemal* antibody-positive result. (From Gower Medical Publishing, Ltd., London, UK, with permission.)

Color Plate 91. Urine: white blood cells (From Strasinger, Fig. 1, with permission.)

Color Plate 92. Urine: red blood cells. (From Strasinger, Fig. 2, with permission.)

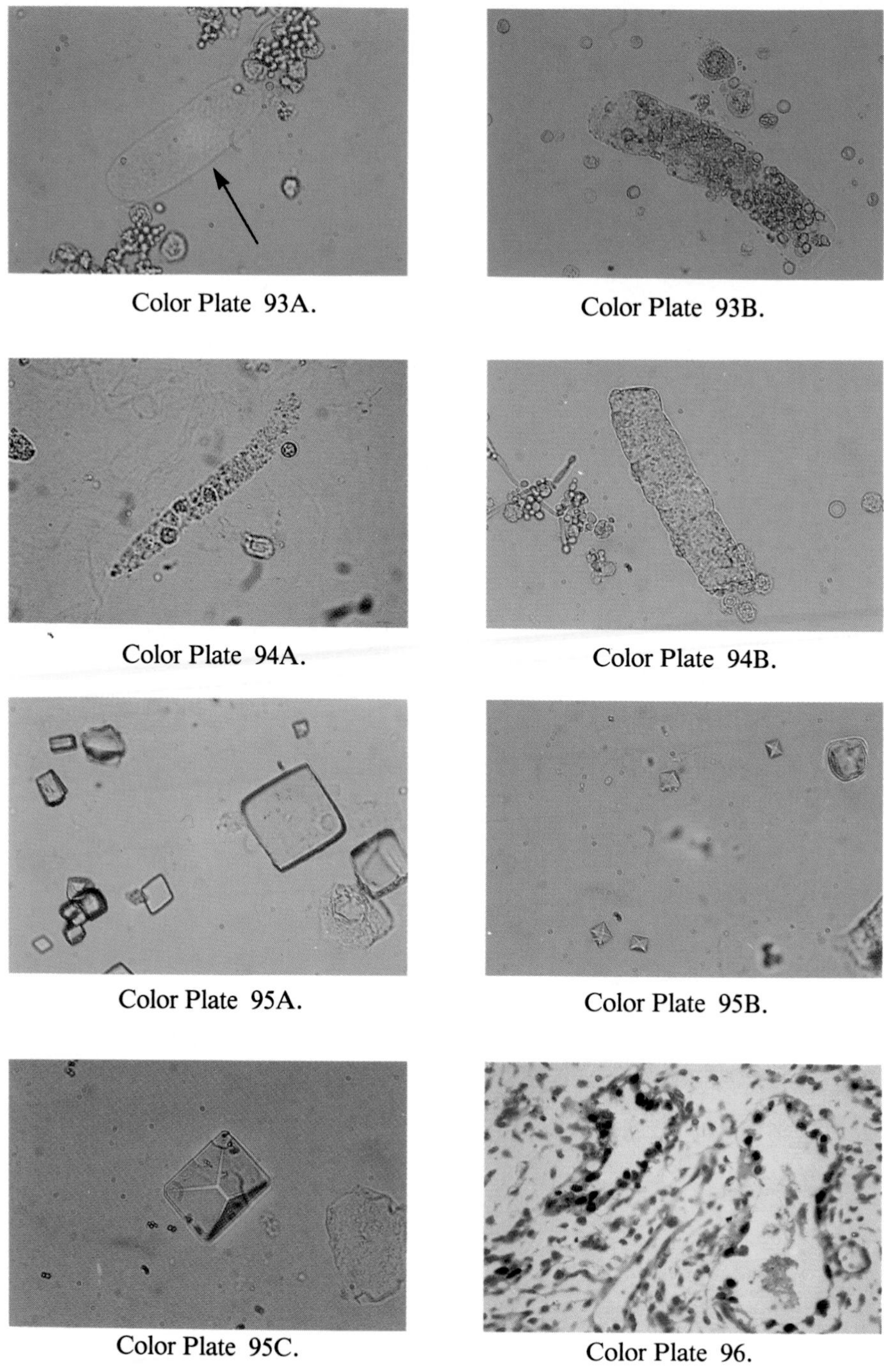

Color Plate 93A.

Color Plate 93B.

Color Plate 94A.

Color Plate 94B.

Color Plate 95A.

Color Plate 95B.

Color Plate 95C.

Color Plate 96.

Color Plate 93. *A)* Hyaline cast. *B)* Red cell cast and mucus. (From Strasinger, Figs. 9 and 11, with permission.)

Color Plate 94. *A)* White blood cell and granular cast. *B)* Coarsely granulated cast. (From Strasinger, Figs. 2 and 14, with permission.)

Color Plate 95. *A)* Uric acid crystals. *B)* Calcium oxalate crystals. (Strasinger Figure 18.) *C)* Triple phosphate crystals. (From Strasinger, Figs. 17, 18, and 20, with permission.)

Color Plate 96. In situ DNA hybridization for detection of adenovirus (blue-black inclusions) infecting the airway lining cells of human lung (red counter stain with safranin.)

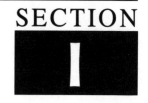

General Principles

OUTLINE

CHAPTER

1

PRINCIPLES OF INTERPRETATION OF LABORATORY TESTS

Laboratory measurements and examinations provide the hard scientific data used to deal with problems identified by the clinical evaluation, and are an essential part of the information that contributes to the patient data base. Indications for ordering laboratory tests constitute the most important considerations of laboratory medicine. Approximately 10–15% of the national health budget in the United States goes to laboratory testing, and for hospitalized patients, this constitutes 15–20% of their bill. Laboratory information can be used diagnostically or to confirm a preliminary diagnosis made during the history and physical examination. This chapter reviews how laboratory procedures are involved in the diagnostic process to define the patient's medical problem and its management.

The disciplines of laboratory medicine include several major areas:

1. *Hematology* with examination of the cellular elements of blood and also its clotting factors;
2. *Chemical Pathology,* including the measurement of over 200 substances in serum and body fluids;
3. *Blood Banking* and *Transfusion Medicine;*
4. *Medical Microbiology,* entailing diagnostic bacteriology, mycology, virology, and serology;
5. *Medical Microscopy* for the examination of urine and other body fluids;
6. *Radioimmunoassay* for endocrine and other special assays; and
7. *Immunology,* involving both immunochemistry and cellular immunity.

ACCURACY AND PRECISION

When using the data obtained through a laboratory measurement, one must be familiar with the limitations and applications of the data, in particular with the terms *accuracy* and *precision.* Accuracy refers to how closely the measurement approaches the true value of the substance being analyzed. Accuracy is synonymous with correctness. Precision describes how closely together fall repeat measurements of the same substance in the same sample. Precision is synonymous with reproducibility. Some laboratory measurements may have less than ideal accuracy, but still have very good precision. For purposes of monitoring patient care, it is probably better to have greater precision than accuracy, since this enables a good (consistent) evaluation of treatment response or changes in the course of a patient's illness. In this regard, a change in the patient is more likely to account for a variation in the laboratory measurement than is an analytic variation when using modern automated chemistry systems.

To illustrate the significance of accuracy versus precision, consider the example of repeat measurements of glucose on a single sample in which the glucose is known to be 100 mg/dl. Method A yields the following values on five separate measurements:

109, 110, 112, 108, and 111 (average 110) mg/dl.

On the same material, method B yields the values:

90, 110, 120, 80, and 110 (average 100) mg/dl.

Method A is much more reproducible (precise) than method B, but method B may have greater accuracy since the average value is closer to true glucose than with method A. However, the wide deviations of method B would make it unsuitable for clinical use. Although method A has a positive bias in its results, a physician user could easily compensate for that type of error and be comfortable in relying on method A.

SPECIFICITY AND SENSITIVITY

Appreciation and correct utilization of laboratory data require an understanding of the terms *specificity* and *sensitivity.* Specificity means how good a test is at detecting only those individuals that have a disease as opposed to falsely labeling some healthy persons as having disease. In more technical terms, the specificity of a test reflects its ability to detect true negatives with very few false positive results. It is expressed mathematically as:

$$\frac{\text{true negatives}}{\text{true negatives} + \text{false positives}} = \text{specificity}$$

where these negative and positive results refer to values obtained on individuals with a particular disease under investigation. Ideally, specificity means that only patients with that disease will demonstrate positive values by that test.

Sensitivity means how well a test detects disease without missing some diseased individuals by falsely classifying them as healthy. In technical terms, the sensitivity of a test indicates its ability to generate more true positive results and few false negative ones. Its mathematical expression is:

$$\frac{\text{true positives}}{\text{true positives} + \text{false negatives}} = \text{sensitivity}$$

Any increase in false positive results (normal people falsely testing positive for a disease) will decrease a test's specificity, whereas an increase in false negative results (sick people falsely testing negative for the disease) will diminish the test's sensitivity.

The ideal measurement or examination would have both specificity and sensitivity equal to 100%. Unfortunately, no actual laboratory test meets these criteria completely. In order to detect disease, one requires maximum sensitivity, but often at the expense of specificity. The patient therefore may be falsely labeled as having a disease when in fact the disease is not present. An example when high sensitivity is mandatory is in the screening of blood donors for hepatitis. It is much better to exclude all true carriers of the disease from donating their blood for transfusion even though some healthy individuals will be incorrectly excluded as well because of the high sensitivity of the testing for hepatitis. Conversely, when dealing with a known illness (or in situations in which there has already been made a strong presumptive diagnosis based on clinical or other status), it is preferable to have very high specificity. For example, when a patient is admitted to the hospital with chest pain and there is suspicion of myocardial infarction, it is desirable to utilize a test with very high specificity for myocardial damage (creatine kinase isoenzyme MB). A poorly specific test will indicate that a patient may not have a disease when the disease really exists, whereas a less sensitive test will indicate that the disease exists when it does not.

PREDICTIVE VALUES

The *predictive value* of a laboratory measurement is equally important and also somewhat easier to deal with in concrete terms of understanding whether or not a patient has a particular disease. The predictive value takes into account the prevalence of a disease in the population or community. Thus, the predictive value of the same test can be markedly different when applied to different geographic locations or to people of differing age, sex, or other demographics. The predictive value of a positive test result indicates the likelihood that the individual has the disease, whereas the predictive value of a negative test result reflects the likelihood that the individual is free of that disease. In general, the higher the prevalence of a disease (i.e., the percentage of people who have the disease) within the population, the greater is the predictive value of a positive test result. The mathematical expressions for predictive values are:

$$\text{predictive value (positive result)} = \frac{\text{true positives}}{\text{true positives} + \text{false positives}}$$

$$\text{predictive value (negative result)} = \frac{\text{true negatives}}{\text{true negatives} + \text{false negatives}}$$

Let us consider the application of these principles to a population of individuals who are to be screened for a disease with a test that is known to be 90% accurate in detecting the disease when it occurs and gives only 5% positive results in persons free of that disease. The following is a useful way to diagram the possible events:

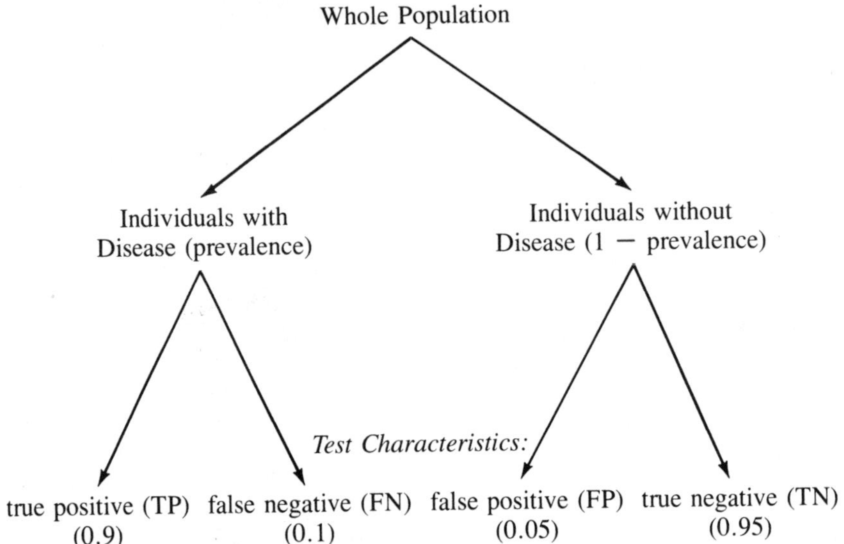

By this, it is indicated that, of all persons with the disease, 90% will give a true positive test result and 10% will give a false negative result; of all persons who do not have the disease, 5% will give a false positive result and 95% will give true negative results. These characteristics are a reflection of test sensitivity and specificity. At first glance, these numbers seem to be reasonably in favor of making a diagnosis perhaps simply on the basis of this one test. However, the prevalence of disease in the population will really establish just how useful the test will be. Let us consider three particular prevalence rates. For a prevalence of 1% (i.e., 0.01),

$$\begin{aligned} TP &= 0.01 \times 0.9 &&= 0.009 \text{ (or 0.9\% of the total results)} \\ FN &= 0.01 \times 0.1 &&= 0.001 \\ FP &= 0.99 \times 0.05 &&= 0.0495 \\ TN &= 0.99 \times 0.95 &&= 0.9405 \end{aligned}$$

At this low prevalence, most test results in the entire population will be true negatives (94.05%). However, the predictive value of a positive result is

$$0.009/(0.009 + 0.0495) = 0.154.$$

This indicates that only 15.4% of positive results occur in individuals with the disease, whereas 84.6% of positive results occur in the absence of disease. Therefore, a positive result is roughly five times more likely to be in error than it is to predict disease.

As the prevalence of disease changes, the predictive value can change quite dramatically. For a prevalence of 5%, the figures become:

$$\begin{aligned} TP &= 0.05 \times 0.9 &&= 0.045 \\ FN &= 0.05 \times 0.1 &&= 0.005 \\ FP &= 0.95 \times 0.05 &&= 0.0475 \\ TN &= 0.95 \times 0.95 &&= 0.9025 \end{aligned}$$

In this instance, most results are still true negatives, but the predictive value of a positive result becomes much better: 0.045/(0.045 + 0.0475) = 0.486 or 48.6%. If the prevalence is higher still (set to 20%), the results are:

$$\begin{aligned} TP &= 0.2 \times 0.9 &&= 0.18 \\ FN &= 0.2 \times 0.1 &&= 0.02 \end{aligned}$$

$$FP = 0.8 \times 0.05 = 0.04$$
$$TN = 0.8 \times 0.95 = 0.76$$

and the predictive value of a positive result is: 0.18/(0.18 + 0.04) = 0.818 or 81.8%. Of course, all these calculations would be modified if the test sensitivity and specificity were altered as well, and one approach to dealing with this problem of high false positives is to change the cut-off point of the reference range (see below). This maneuver of course leads to loss of sensitivity and consequent failure to detect some true positives. A more acceptable strategy is to consider results of two or more different tests that corroborate and substantiate one another. For example, the combination of isoenzyme analysis of creatine kinase and isoenzyme analysis of lactate dehydrogenase is superior to that of either isoenzyme analysis alone in the diagnosis of myocardial infarction.

There is an analogous formulation of the predictive value of a negative test result as it indicates absence of disease. However, its use is more typically confined to ruling out disease rather than to the particular diagnosis of abnormality. The power of the predictive value of a negative test result then is in its ability to exclude disease, allowing the physician to explore other more promising diagnoses.

Another test characteristic is termed the *efficiency,* or ability to detect correctly both true positives and true negatives, expressed as:

$$\text{efficiency} = \frac{TP + TN}{TP + FP + TN + FN}$$

or

$$\text{efficiency} = \frac{\text{true results}}{\text{all results}}$$

As false positive and false negative results are minimized, the efficiency of a test approaches 100%. A high efficiency indicates that a test is very good at correctly categorizing results as true positive or true negative.

REFERENCE RANGES (NORMAL VALUES)

Whenever laboratory test results are reported, there is also a notation as to the range of expected values for the substances analyzed. These ranges are values to be found in normal or healthy individuals. In order to establish such ranges characteristic of health, the laboratory measurements are performed on a large number of normal persons and the values obtained are plotted in a distribution graph. An example of this is shown in Figure 1–1 for the distribution of total protein concentration in the serum of a group of healthy medical students. In this instance, the values are centered about 7.2 g/dl with a nearly symmetrical scatter of values both above and below that central value. From inspection of this graph, we are inclined to accept the healthy range of total serum protein as 6.0 to 8.2 g/dl. However, the end results have low frequencies and could reflect overlap with values obtained on sick populations. To assist in applying specific guidelines in setting the limits of normal, we can resort to statistical analysis of these data. Since the distribution of total protein has the general configuration of a bell-shaped curve, it is convenient to apply the mathematical formulation for a Gaussian or normal distribution. It should be recognized that the word "normal" has two different meanings. In the mathe-

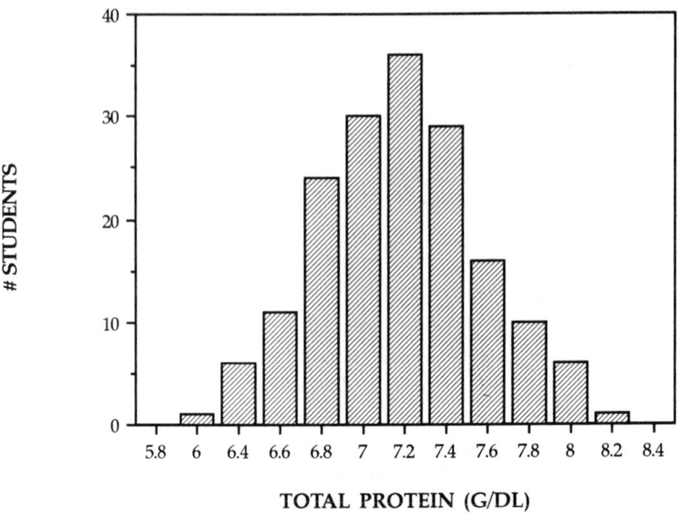

Figure 1–1. The distribution of total serum protein values in 173 healthy medical students. This plot is symmetric and appears to follow a gaussian (normal) mathematical distribution.

matical sense, it refers to a specific mathematic formula that fits data in such a bell-shaped distribution. In the medical sense, normal refers to a state of health. It is not always true that laboratory test results from a "normal" healthy population follow a "normal" Gaussian mathematical distribution. However, for convenience and for uniformity of application, the statistical values of mean and *standard deviation* (SD) of laboratory data are calculated using the formula for a normal distribution. By this convention, it is true that approximately 95% of healthy results (or normal) will fall within the range ±2 SD of the mean value (i.e., two standard deviations on either side of the mean) and 5% of healthy results will fall outside this range.

It would be scientifically incorrect to assume that this range of total protein obtained on young healthy adult medical students can be applied to all other *age groups* (newborn, children, elderly). In fact, it is most desirable to establish this range for each age group separately. We refer to these age-specific ranges as *reference ranges* or *reference intervals* to denote that they reflect more appropriately the demographic group against which a given patient should be compared. Many analytes show a great degree of variability with age. For example, the enzyme alkaline phosphatase is much higher in the blood of children who have growing bones than in adults. In fact, a normal healthy value for alkaline phosphatase in a child would be distinctly abnormal in an adult. Many other substances also show age-related differences, many of which have greatest variation during the change from childhood to adulthood.

There are also reference ranges based on other groupings, such as sex. We know that women tend to have lower levels of red blood cells and of hemoglobin than do men. Figure 1–2 is a comparison of the hemoglobin values in female versus male medical students. There is an obvious difference in hemoglobin of almost 3 g/dl lower in the women students than in the men. This difference is due in part to a

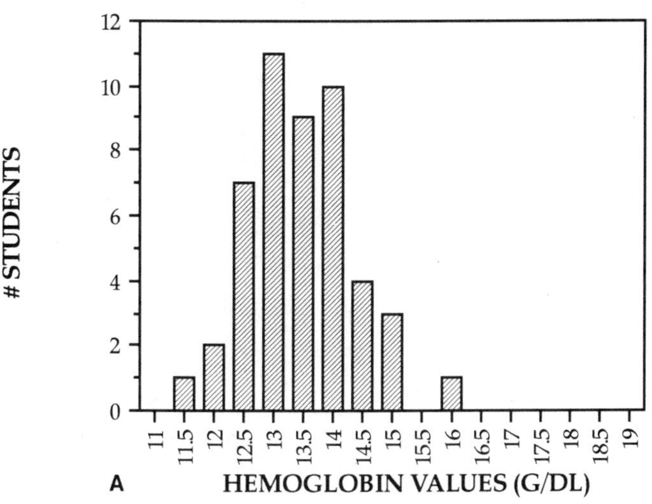

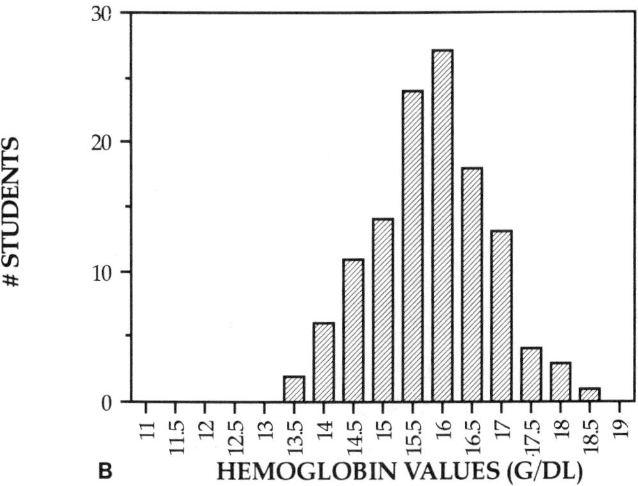

Figure 1–2. Distribution plots of hemoglobin in female (*A*) and male (*B*) medical students illustrating sex-related reference ranges.

woman's loss of blood by menstruation and also to a correlation with lean body mass, which is different between men and women. Whatever the reason, it is most appropriate to judge hemoglobin and other red blood cell measurements in terms of the age- and sex-specific reference interval.

A serum analyte that demonstrates a strong sex-related reference range is uric acid (Fig. 1–3). Men tend to have higher values than do women by almost 2 mg/dl. The

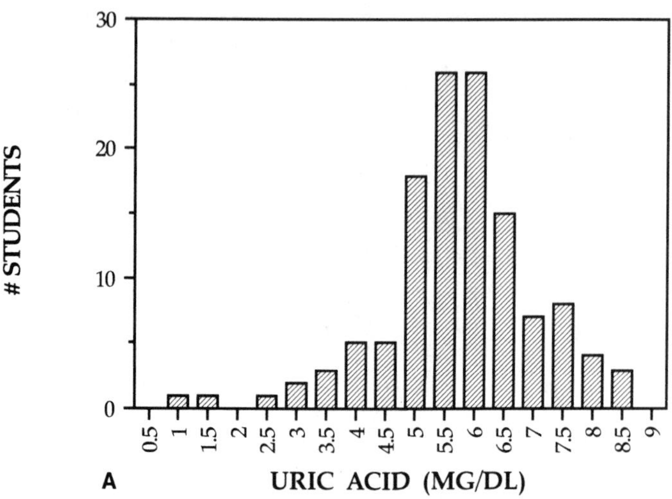

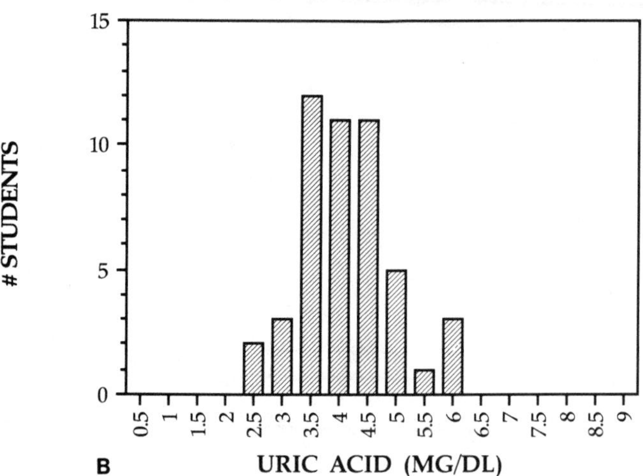

Figure 1–3. Distribution plots of serum uric acid in male (*A*) and female (*B*) medical students illustrating sex-related reference ranges.

distribution of uric acid in male medical students (Fig. 1–3) also illustrates the interesting point of some very low values (1.0 and 1.5 mg/dl) that do not occur in the women studied. These very low values appear to be separate from the bulk of the distribution and are termed "outliers." They are probably due to some inherent differences in the way those two individuals' kidneys excreted uric acid when compared with excretion plus reabsorption of uric acid in most normal people. Although there is no real clinical significance to these very low values, they would be excluded from consideration in establishing the statistics for a reference range because they are obvious outliers.

Other factors can lead to alteration of the expected values in healthy individuals. These include degree of exercise, pregnancy, diet (vegetarian versus meat-eating), tobacco use, and many other subcategories that could even be based on occupation, altitude, distance from an ocean, medications, etc. For practical purposes, all of these additional factors cannot be accounted for by the laboratory. It is common laboratory practice to report reference ranges that are specific for age and sex and to let the physician interpret the results further in light of other specific factors.

SOURCES OF ERROR

In addition to physiologic and population-based variations in the levels of analytes, there must also be considered the potential for analytic variation due to methodology. This type of variability is relatively easy to quantify by performing multiple repeat measurements of the same substance on the same sample. For example, repeat measurements of serum creatinine may give the values 1.3, 1.4, 1.5, 1.4, 1.3, and 1.4. This level of variability is acceptable since it does not alter clinical assessment. If the variability were 1.0, 1.5, 2.0, 1.7, and 2.1, it would be unacceptable for the practice of monitoring changes in renal function, since significant pathologic changes could be smaller than the analytic ones. In order to compare methods and establish their validity, we calculate the *coefficient of variation* (CV) of a method as the standard deviation obtained from multiple measurements on the same sample divided by the mean value. Modern instrumentation has become so reproducible in performance due to standardized equipment and reagents that most automated methods can be expected to have CVs in the range of only a few percent, whereas methods with manual pipetting steps usually have CVs of 10–15% or greater.

Other factors that can affect the quality and variation of laboratory tests are outlined in Table 1–1. For substances that fluctuate in the circulation with a *diurnal variation,* timing of collection can be very important so as not to be measuring a valley when you think you are measuring a peak (e.g., cortisol, iron). Recent ingestion of food is also very important for evaluating glucose and triglycerides and for lipid fractionation. In addition, other substances can have minor alterations after food ingestion (phosphorus, uric acid, alkaline phosphatase). The technique of venipuncture is also critical in obtaining good quality specimens. Too long an application of the tourniquet will result in acidosis in the specimen and also hemoconcentration. The proper sequence of tubes must be maintained with serum clot tubes drawn before those with additives so that no anticoagulant (e.g., with high potassium) may accidently contaminate the serum. Care must also be exercised to prevent hemolysis of the sample and to obtain whole blood samples free of minor clots for performance of the complete blood count and of plasma clotting studies. In addition, blood samples should be transported promptly and handled appropriately to prevent deterioration of some constituents.

Human error can also account for laboratory variation. This includes errors in the performance of testing (usually minimized by the use of automated equipment), selecting a specimen to analyze from the wrong patient, transcriptional mistakes, and virtually any action along the whole chain of collecting, processing, analyzing,

Table 1–1. FACTORS AFFECTING THE QUALITY OF LABORATORY DATA

I. *Patient preparation*
   a. Time of day
   b. Fasting/nonfasting
II. *Specimen collection*
   a. Venipuncture technique
   b. Proper tube for blood, plasma, or serum
   c. Labeling of correct sample
III. *Specimen handling*
   a. Transport
   b. Processing
   c. Storage
IV. *Analysis*
   a. Method precision (coefficient of variation)
   b. Method accuracy (calibration)
   c. Manual versus automated method
V. *Reporting*
   a. Calculation
   b. Transcription
   c. Hard copy versus verbal report

and reporting. Laboratories that put forth the effort to track down errors of this nature can generally eliminate or minimize systematic problems. However, it is a common experience in many institutions that the incidence of mislabeling patient specimens frequently exceeds the rate of errors actually occurring in the laboratory in the analytic phase. Therefore, it is essential that the medical personnel obtaining blood and other samples correctly label those specimens, preferably at the side of the patient so that no confusion will later arise as to the correct identity of the sample. Many laboratories perform quality control checks on serial samples to ensure that they are from the correct patient. Automation and computerization have made this procedure (called a *delta check*) both practical and efficient. For example, hematology samples from a single patient should have roughly the same red cell mean cell volume (MCV) from day to day. If the MCV suddenly shifts from one day to the next, it is likely that the patient's label was placed on a tube of blood from another patient. This suspicion can be confirmed by typing the red cells in both the old and new samples. Similar checks are prompted by abrupt changes in chemical parameters as well (e.g., glucose, creatinine, enzymes).

INDICATIONS FOR ORDERING LABORATORY MEASUREMENTS AND EXAMINATIONS

There are five major reasons for ordering a laboratory measurement:

1. to confirm a clinical impression or to make a diagnosis (e.g., blood glucose for diabetes mellitus, hemoglobin for anemia);
2. to rule out a disease or diagnosis (e.g., pregnancy test to rule out an ectopic pregnancy in a case of acute abdominal pain);

3. to provide prognostic information (e.g., serum levels of aspartate amino transferase and alanine amino transferase to determine the severity of hepatitis);
4. to provide therapeutic guidelines (e.g., prolongation of the prothrombin time in anticoagulant therapy); and
5. to screen for disease.

Laboratory screening is perhaps the least valid reason to perform measurements widely and with no previous clinical suspicion or indications. However, there are some important applications of screening, including the premarital test for syphilis (Venereal Disease Research Laboratory [VDRL] or rapid plasma reagin [RPR]) and the assessment of newborns for phenylketonuria and for hypothyroidism as mandated by law. In addition, it is standard practice to screen donated blood units prior to transfusion for the presence of potential transfusion-transmitted infections such as hepatitis and the human immunodeficiency virus of acquired immune deficiency syndrome (AIDS).

PROFILE OR PANEL TESTING

A collection of different measurements related to a particular organ, organ system, or disease is referred to as a profile or panel grouping. A "health profile" refers to general measurements of multiple substances that reflect the function of several organ systems (i.e., SMAC-type profiling, Chem 20, etc.). These profiles are facilitated by performance on a single instrument that is capable of doing all the measurements. An organ panel need not be limited to a particular instrument for analysis since it may reflect many different functions of the organ. The design of an organ panel should take into account the needs of the medical staff of a hospital for maximizing both sensitivity and specificity by use of appropriate combinations of determinations. One potential bad aspect of these panels is that after a correct diagnosis is made, the panel is ordered routinely as a standing order without consideration as to whether monitoring of the disease state requires all the repetition of confirmatory data on a daily basis. Although a single instrument may be capable of performing all or the bulk of those determinations, there is nevertheless a sizeable cost to continue to perform all of those repeat tests, some of which may not be useful at all in the making of further clinical decisions. Examples of organ panels are liver function tests that include several enzymes and bilirubin and also the complete blood count, both of which have been widely used for years.

The large profile of roughly 20 tests can be thought of as an amalgam of several different but overlapping organ panels. Thus, the screening of many organs can be done by reviewing all of these results collectively, as indicated in Table 1–2. In addition to the organ associations noted in that table, there are many others with highly specific connections such as high calcium and hyperparathyroidism, electrolyte abnormalities and endocrine disease, enzyme elevations and malignancy. With experience, a physician becomes accustomed to recognizing patterns of abnormalities that are very useful in directing the diagnostic work-up toward more conclusive procedures based on these screening tests. This practice can be very useful in the initial evaluation of a new patient when there is not a large data base on which to make clinical judgment.

There are also arguments against extensive use of profile and panel testing; in particular, the mere use of the profile might (falsely) identify laboratory values that are outside of the reference range in a normal individual. The more laboratory

Table 1–2. CHEM 20 HEALTH PROFILE WITH SOME ORGAN ASSOCIATIONS OF EACH ANALYTE

Glucose *F,R**	Bilirubin, direct *L*
BUN *K,L,F*	Bilirubin, total *L*
Creatinine *K,F*	LDH *L,M*
Uric acid *K*	SGOT (AST) *L,M*
Sodium *K,F*	SGPT (ALT) *L*
Potassium *K,F*	Alkaline phosphatase *L,B*
Chloride *K,F*	Albumin *N,L,K*
Bicarbonate *K,F*	Total protein *N,L*
Calcium *B,F*	Cholesterol *N,R*
Phosphorus *K,B*	Triglycerides *N,R*

**K* = kidneys, *L* = liver, *B* = bone, *N* = nutrition, *M* = muscle, *R* = cardiac risk assessment, *F* = fluid and electrolyte balance.

parameters performed, the more likely that one or more results will be outside the reference range. As an example, let us assume that the reference range for each analyte of a Chem 20 is set to include 95% of a healthy population. Then the probability of a healthy person having a normal result on any one test is 95% or 0.95 and the probability of having an abnormal result is $1 - 0.95 = 0.05$. The probability of that person having normal results on two tests is $0.95 \times 0.95 = 0.9025$ and the probability of having one or two abnormal results is $1 - 0.9025 = 0.0975$. This mathematical progression continues as illustrated in Table 1–3. The probability that a person will have normal results on all 20 tests is $0.95^{20} = 0.3585$. Thus, the probability that the healthy will have one or more out-of-range results is $1 - 0.3585 = 0.6415$. This is a fairly high probability of falsely calling someone abnormal and is the major theoretical limitation of widespread profile testing, because of the extremely high likelihood of incidental out-of-range results.

Table 1–3. PROBABILITIES OF NORMAL AND ABNORMAL RESULTS ON MULTITEST PANELS

Number of Tests	Probability of Being within Reference Range	Probability of at Least 1 Result Being out of Range
1	$0.95^1 = 0.95$	$1 - 0.95 = 0.05$
2	$0.95^2 = 0.9025$	$1 - 0.9025 = 0.0975$
3	$0.95^3 = 0.8574$	$1 - 0.8574 = 0.1426$
4	$0.95^4 = 0.8145$	$1 - 0.8145 = 0.1855$
.	.	.
.	.	.
.	.	.
10	$0.95^{10} = 0.5987$	$1 - 0.5987 = 0.4013$
.	.	.
.	.	.
.	.	.
20	$0.95^{20} = 0.3585$	$1 - 0.3585 = 0.6415$

Table 1–4. CRITICAL VALUES THAT REQUIRE IMMEDIATE COMMUNICATIONS

Test	Critical Value
Hematology	
Hct	<14% >60%
WBC	<2000/μl on a new patient or a 1000 difference from previous, if less than 4000/μl >50,000/μl on a new patient
Smear	Shows leukemic cells (progranulocytic or blast) Shows abnormal leukemoid reaction Positive for malaria or other parasites
Platelets	<20,000/μl and not previously reported >1 million/μl
Reticulocyte	>20%
Prothrombin time	>40 seconds
Chemistry	
Serum bilirubin	>18 mg/dl (newborn)
Serum calcium	<6 mg/dl >13 mg/dl
Serum glucose	<40 mg/dl >500 mg/dl
Serum phosphate	<1 mg/dl
Serum potassium	<2.5 mEq/liter >6.5 mEq/liter
Serum sodium	<120 mEq/liter >160 mEq/liter
Serum bicarbonate	<10 mEq/liter >40 mEq/liter
Arterial or capillary PO_2	<40 mmHg
Arterial or capillary pH	<7.2 >7.6
Arterial or capillary PCO_2	<20 mmHg >70 mmHg
Microbiology	
Blood culture	Positive
Gram stain on CSF and any body fluids (pleural, synovial, peritoneal, etc.)	Positive

This argument is not valid for test strategies in the monitoring of disease processes or effects of diseases by means of organ panels. An argument against organ panels is that they take away from the physician the decision-making as to which laboratory tests to order. It is important that the selection of the specific organ panels be made in conjunction with the practicing clinicians who are most familiar with the organ and disease entities. Additional arguments for the use of these *laboratory diagnosis related groups (LDRG)* are that they may reduce duration of hospital stay for some patients and that they use the resources of the laboratory more efficiently.

PRIORITY REPORTING: STAT AND PANIC VALUES

In the setting of acute care medicine in hospitals, there is frequently need for immediate turnaround of laboratory results to the physician within one hour or less of drawing the specimen in order to modify therapy. This type of priority is designated *stat* for the Latin word *statim* meaning "immediately." Tests that fall into this category include glucose in diabetic ketoacidosis, some drug levels such as theophylline, amylase in suspected pancreatitis, creatine kinase in suspected myocardial infarction, hematocrit, blood gases, and potassium. In fact, there may be a need for many other determinations under a variety of clinical situations in which a clinical decision of medical management will be made.

Sometimes the results of a test are so far out of expected range that it may be life-threatening. In that situation, it should be the responsibility of the laboratory to contact the physician or other medical personnel to communicate that result immediately. This should be done whether the test was ordered stat or not. To comply with this policy, each laboratory should establish a procedure to include the threshold levels that mandate this action. These levels are termed *critical values* or *panic values* and are confined to a list of analytes that truely do have the potential to be lethal if left unchecked for a short period. Examples of critical values are listed in Table 1–4. As a matter of good medical practice, the laboratory should keep a log of each critical value call, to include the doctor or other person contacted, the patient's name, the value of the analyte, the time and date called, and the name of the caller.

In summary, in order to utilize laboratory measurements properly, it is necessary to have an appreciation of the technical validity (accuracy and precision) of a test, its diagnostic value (sensitivity, specificity, predictive value), optimal specimen collection, potential sources of error, and the ultimate clinical usefulness of tests for screening, diagnosing, and monitoring disease.

REFERENCES

1. Galen, S and Gambino, SR: Beyond Normality: The Predictive Value and Efficiency of Medical Diagnosis. John Wiley and Sons, Inc., New York, 1975.
2. Murphy, J and Henry, JB: Effective utilization of clinical laboratories. Hum Pathol 9:625, 1978.
3. Pauker, SG and Kassirer JP: The threshold approach to clinical decision making. N Engl J Med 302:1109, 1980.
4. Lundberg, GD: Using the Clinical Laboratory in Medical Decision-Making. American Society of Clinical Pathologists Press, Chicago, 1983.
5. Winkel, P and Statland BE: The theory of reference values. In Henry, JB (ed): Clinical Diagnosis and Management by Laboratory Methods, ed 17. WB Saunders, Philadelphia, 1984, p 51.
6. Statland, BE and Winkel P: Pre-instrumental sources of variation. In Henry, JB (ed): Clinical Diagnosis and Management by Laboratory Methods, ed 17. WB Saunders, Philadelphia, 1984, p 61.

HEMATOLOGY

OUTLINE

CHAPTER 2

TESTS

CHAPTER

2

HEMATOLOGIC METHODS

Hematology is the study of the blood and the blood-forming tissues that comprise one of the largest organ systems of the body. Blood constitutes 6–8% of the total body weight, and consists of blood cells suspended in a fluid called plasma. The three main blood cells are the red blood cells (erythrocytes), white blood cells (leukocytes), and platelets (thrombocytes). The fluid plasma forms 45–60% of the total blood volume; the red blood cells (RBC) occupy most of the remaining volume. White blood cells and platelets, although functionally essential, occupy a relatively small proportion of the total blood mass. The proportion of cells and plasma is regulated and is kept relatively constant.

The principal function of circulating blood is transportation; red blood cells remain within the circulatory system and contain the oxygen-transporting pigment hemoglobin. White blood cells are responsible for the body's defenses and are transported by the blood to the various tissues where they perform their physiologic roles. Platelets are responsible for preventing blood loss from hemorrhage, and exert their main effects at the blood vessel wall. The plasma proteins are important transporters of nutrients and metabolic byproducts to the respective organs for storage and excretion. Many of the large proteins suspended in plasma are also of interest to the hematologist, in particular, those proteins concerned with the prevention of hemorrhage by coagulation. The hematology laboratory is concerned with defining normal and abnormal blood cells or blood pigments and determining the nature of the abnormalities. The coagulation laboratory is concerned with evaluating people in whom there is abnormal hemostasis, either by excessive bleeding or abnormalities in coagulation or thrombosis. Hematology laboratory studies are often extremely important in appreciating the overall well-being of the patient, and are frequently used in health screening tests.

HEMATOPOIESIS

Hematopoiesis refers to the formation and development of all types of blood cells from their parental precursors. Blood cells in normal adults are manufactured in the marrow of the bones forming the axial skeleton. From infancy to adulthood there is a progressive change of productive marrow to occupy the central skeleton, especially the sternum, ribs, vertebral bodies, pelvic bones, and the proximal portions of the long bones. During fetal development, hematopoiesis is first established in the yolk sac, later transfers to the liver and spleen, and finally to the bony skeleton (Fig. 2–1). Hematopoiesis gradually decreases in the shafts of the long bones, and after the age of four years, fat cells begin to appear. Generally, hematopoiesis is regulated by both cell-to-cell regulation and humoral regulation, and also according to the demands of the body. Therefore, blood cell production is kept relatively constant, but has the capacity to increase with increasing demand. Organs that were capable of sustaining hematopoiesis in fetal life always retain this ability should the demand arise.

The marrow is a special environment for hematopoietic growth and development. In the bone marrow, hematopoiesis occurs in the extravascular part of the red marrow, which consists of a fine supporting reticulin framework interspersed with vascular channels and developing marrow cells. A single layer of endothelial cells separates the extravascular marrow compartment from the intravascular compartment. When the hematopoietic marrow cells are mature and ready to circulate in the peripheral blood, the cells leave the marrow parenchyma by passing through fine "windows" in the endothelial cells, and emerge into the venous sinuses.

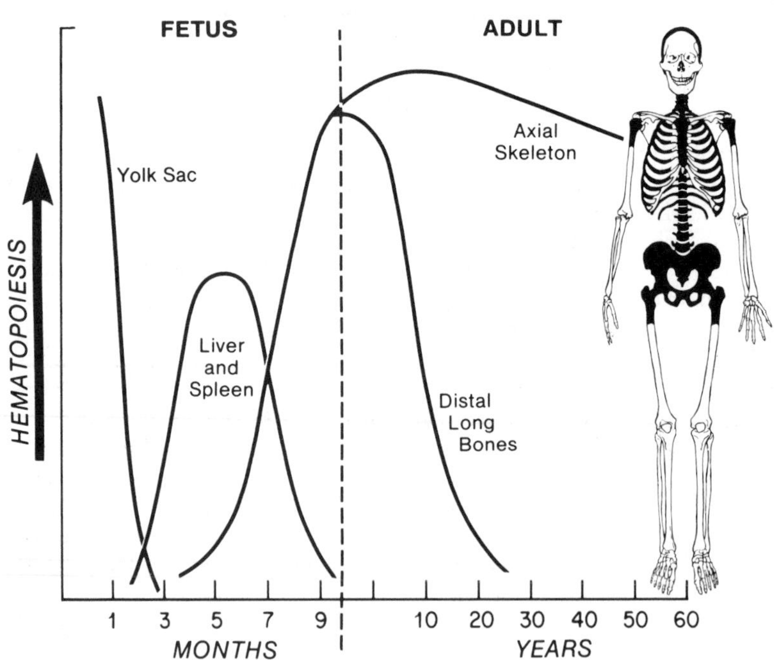

Figure 2–1. Location of active marrow growth in the fetus and adult. During fetal development, hematopoiesis is first established in the yolk sac mesenchyme, later moves to the liver and spleen, and finally is limited to the bony skeleton. From infancy to adulthood, there is a progressive restriction of productive marrow to the axial skeleton and proximal ends of the long bones, shown as the shaded areas on the drawing of the skeleton. (From Hillman and Finch,[4] p 2, with permission.)

Most of the cells in the circulating blood are incapable of further division, are relatively short-lived, and are replaced constantly from the bone marrow. The main blood cell groups, including the red blood cells, white blood cells, and platelets, are derived from a pleuripotent hematopoietic stem cell. This stem cell is the first in a sequence of regular and orderly steps of cell growth and maturation (Fig. 2–2). The pleuripotent stem cell may mature along morphologically and functionally diverse lines, depending on conditioning stimuli and mediators, and may either produce other stem cells and self-regenerate or mature in two main directions. Stem cells may become committed to the lymphoid cell line for lymphopoiesis, or toward the development of a multipotent stem cell capable of sustaining myelopoiesis, erythropoiesis, and platelet production *(CFU-GEMM)* (see Fig. 2–2). Morphologically, these multipotent and pleuripotent stem cells appear as small cells with an appearance similar to a mature lymphocyte.

The majority of stem cells remain in a resting (G_0) state from which they can be recruited to meet an emergency situation such as hemorrhage, infection, or bone marrow injury. The hematopoietic stem cells evolve as *growth units* under the influence of *growth factors.* Red cell development, or erythropoiesis, is sustained by the multipotent stem cell maturing into a *burst-forming unit—erythroid* (BFU—E), controlled by a *burst-promoting activity (BPA).* A single burst-forming unit—erythroid is capable of producing a colony of more than 1,000 developing red cells. This now constitutes a *colony-forming unit—erythroid,* or CFU—E. Growth and maturation of the BFU—E is under the influence of hormonal factors, especially the hormone *erythropoietin.* The hematopoietic stem cell may also give rise to other colony-forming units (CFU), which grow and mature to granulocytes, monocytes, eosinophils, basophils, and megakaryocytes under the influence of specific *colony-stimulating factors (CSF)* (see Fig. 2–2). Bone marrow growth may be studied in the laboratory using *in vitro* culture methods. Colonies may be formed on culture media containing the specific growth factors derived from extracts of supporting marrow cells, or purified by recombinant DNA technology, and their effects in sustaining marrow cell growth may be analyzed in culture.

Erythropoiesis

Erythrocytes are derived from the committed erythroid precursor cells, as described above, through a process of mitotic growth and maturation. The level of tissue oxygenation regulates the production of red cells that transport oxygen to the tissues (effective erythropoiesis). *Erythropoietin* is a hormone produced largely by the kidney that stimulates the CFU—E stem cells to speed up growth and enhance maturation. The specific pathways regulating tissue oxygen fluctuations with changes in erythropoietin levels are not understood. Although erythropoietin is neither synthesized nor stored in the kidneys, renal function and oxygen levels are the main factors controlling erythropoietin release. It appears that tissue hypoxia elicits renal secretion of an enzyme—renal erythropoietic factor—that interacts with a circulating protein to produce active erythropoietin.

Anything that lowers tissue oxygen delivery increases erythropoietin levels, provided the individual has adequately functioning kidneys. Low blood hemoglobin levels, impaired oxygen release from hemoglobin, impaired respiratory oxygen exchange, and poor blood flow are common causes of tissue hypoxia (see Polycythemia). Erythropoietin concentration is therefore high in most anemias, hemoglobin disorders, pulmonary disease and severe circulatory defects.

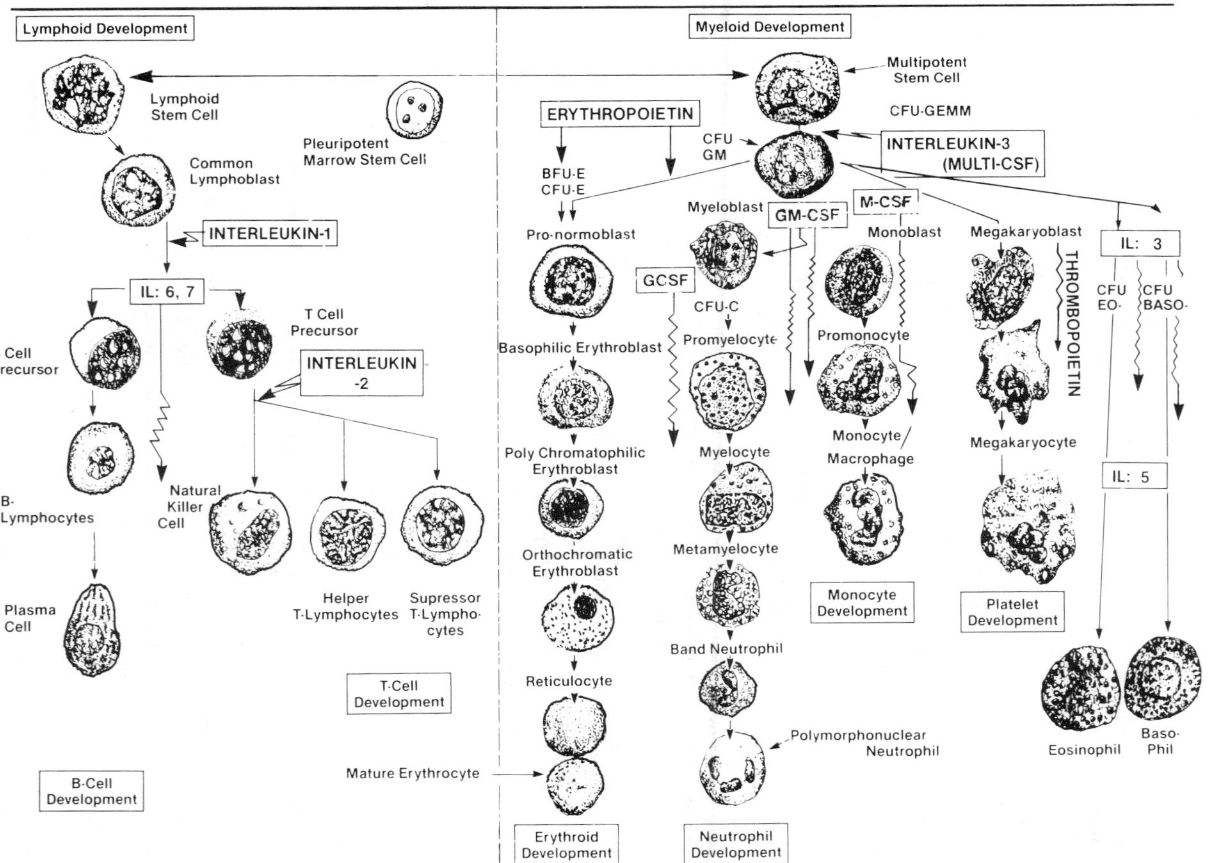

Figure 2–2. Sequence of marrow cell growth and maturation.

The capacity of erythropoietin to produce erythropoiesis is dependent on an adequate supply of nutrients and minerals, in particular iron, folic acid, and vitamin B_{12}, to the marrow. If the marrow has the capacity to respond, red cell production increases. In many anemias and hemoglobin disorders, the nature of the disease limits an appropriate erythropoietic response. Patients without kidneys do produce red cells, but at a lower than normal rate. In severe renal failure, or in people who have had both kidneys surgically removed, a stable but severely anemic state exists that is limited in its response to hypoxic stimuli. The liver produces whatever erythropoietic factor is functioning in this case.

Erythropoietin accelerates nearly every stage of red cell production. The rate at which the committed stem cells (BFU—E and CFU—E) divide and differentiate toward red cell production is especially increased. Erythropoietin also increases the rate of cell division, speeds the incorporation of iron into the developing red cells, shortens the time of cell maturation, and hastens (and increases) entry of immature red cells (reticulocytes) into the circulation (see Color Plates 1, 2, and 16A). This capacity may be measured in the laboratory by a *reticulocyte count.* The *erythron* is the term used to describe the total population of mature erythrocytes and their precursors in the blood and bone marrow. Normally, 10–15% of developing red cells die within the marrow. This phenomenon, called ineffective erythropoiesis, may be increased in certain disease states.

Granulopoiesis

The whole blood concentration of circulating white blood cells (leukocytes) is kept relatively constant, despite a large number that die every day. These leukocytes are replaced by cell division and the production of new white cells in the marrow is termed *granulopoiesis.* Amplification of leukocytes occurs by mitosis, a process of sequential cell growth and division. The stem cells are capable of self-reproduction and development into mature white cells in an orderly sequence of maturation, and are then released from the bone marrow into the circulation. A process of *differentiation* occurs, whereby the immature white cells gradually develop and exhibit characteristics of mature functional leukocytes.

Developing white cells may be divided into various physiologic compartments: 1) the *proliferating pool,* 2) the *maturation pool* and *storage pools,* 3) the *circulating pool,* and 4) the *marginating pool* (Fig. 2–3). Under certain physiologic and pathologic stimuli, granulocytes may be released from the storage and marginating pools within minutes, followed somewhat later by enhanced granulocyte production. Unlike erythropoiesis, no substance comparable to erythropoietin has been found, although total granulocyte mass seems to influence leukocyte production. Nevertheless, cell–cell interaction and the release of the humoral factors (CSFs) described below do control both the production and maturation of white cells.

GROWTH FACTORS

The factor that can influence maturation of a stem cell to granulocyte, monocyte, and megakaryocyte production is called *colony-stimulating factor for granulocytes and monocytes* (GM—CSF). This is a differentiation-promoting growth factor that allows and stimulates production of granulocytes and monocytes. The process of differentiation represents a process of repression or expression of genetic material. Therefore, granulocytes share with the monocytes a common progenitor cell that is termed the CFU—GM, or colony-forming unit—granulocyte, monocyte. Exposure

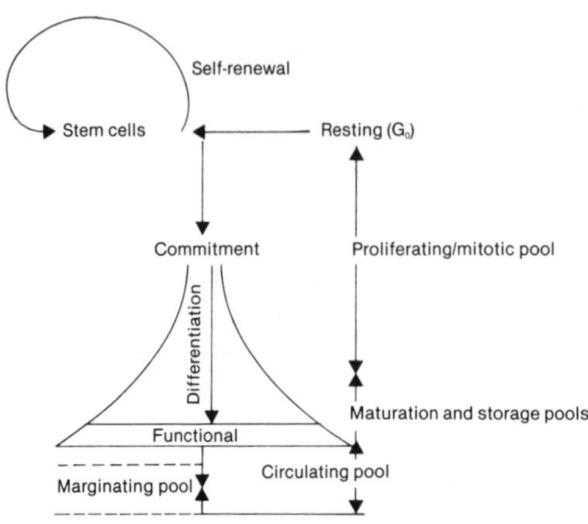

Figure 2–3. Granulocytic compartments.

of this unit to colony-stimulating factor from monocytes and macrophages will facilitate the growth of granulocyte and monocyte colonies. Another factor G—CSF promotes differentiation more preferentially to granulocytes. The intermediate cells during this process of differentiation are also shown in Figure 2–2 (once the granulocytes are mature, they are released into the peripheral blood and subsequently circulate and leave the blood to enter the tissues). Under normal conditions, the rate of production of granulocytes and their rate of egress from the marrow is constant.

Myeloid Growth and Distribution

Granulopoiesis is a continuous evolution from the earliest myeloid precursor to the myeloblast and finally to the most mature cell, the neutrophil (see Color Plates 2 and 4). This process requires 7–11 days. Myeloblasts, promyelocytes, and myelocytes all are capable of division and comprise the *proliferating or mitotic pool.* Beyond this stage no mitosis occurs, and the cells mature through several phases. This phase is now termed the *maturation pool.* It comprises metamyelocytes, bands, and segmented neutrophils. An excess of these cells may remain in the marrow for release when needed. This population constitutes the *storage pool.* The storage pool cells may remain in the marrow for approximately 10 days, and serve as a reservoir when needed. The peripheral blood granulocytes are distributed in two main phases termed the *circulating pool* (approximately 50%) and cells that are closely aligned to the blood vessel wall termed the *marginating pool.* Cells may distribute between the circulating and the marginating pool in response to various inflammatory, infectious, or drug stimuli. The granulocytic compartments are diagrammatically represented in Figure 2–3.

The major functions of neutrophils are 1) host defense involving migration to areas of infection and inflammation, 2) recognition and processing of foreign antigens, 3) phagocytosis and killing, and 4) digestion of tissue debris and microorganisms. Phagocytosis is enhanced by processing, opsonization, or preparation of the antigen or microorganism (see Leukocyte Function). There are three main types of mature granulocytes termed *neutrophils, eosinophils,* and *basophils* (see Color Plates 4 and 6). The process of production is similar, except toward the later maturation phases where typical intracellular granules become evident. The staining characteristics of these granules define the cell types (see staining of peripheral blood). Eosinophils contain red-pink granules, basophils contain blue-black granules, and neutrophils have a less pronounced neutral staining. Each of these cells has specific functions that will be discussed later. The major thrust of myelopoiesis is, however, directed toward the neutrophil series.

Neutrophils remain in the circulation approximately 7–10 hours, and as these cells migrate to the tissues they are replenished in the blood by cells released from the bone marrow. Release from the bone marrow into the venous sinuses occurs through similar fine endothelial pores, as described in erythropoiesis. Neutrophils exit the circulation in between the blood vessel endothelial cells into the tissues. Their ability to focus in at a site of infection or inflammation is governed by attracting stimuli called *chemotactic factors,* which are released from damaged tissue or bacteria. The neutrophil cell membrane has receptors for these factors, which evoke metabolic changes within the neutrophil. Neutrophil degradation products, microbial products, and cellular breakdown products all seem to influence granulocyte kinetics. As a result of these various stimuli, the numbers of circulating granulocytes rise and immature granulocytes may be released into the peripheral blood. Normally, no more than 5% of the circulating granulocytes are immature, and by far the majority of these are at the band stage (see Fig. 2–2 and Color Plate 2D). Under intense granulocytic stimulation, large numbers of band cells, some metamyelocytes, and occasionally even myelocytes find their way into the circulation.

The other major direction of differentiation of the CFU—GM is toward monocyte production. *Monocytes* are actively phagocytic leukocytes that also play a major role in defense from pathogenic organisms and forming antigens. The earliest cell produced, termed the monoblast, matures through the *promonocyte* to the mature monocyte (see Color Plate 6C). The monocytic precursors are usually inconspicuous in normal marrow. Monocytes leave the marrow when mature and enter the venous sinusoids to circulate in the peripheral blood. They circulate for approximately 12–14 hours before migrating to the tissue sites.

Lymphopoiesis

Lymphopoiesis is the term used to describe the growth and maturation of lymphocytes (see Fig. 2–2 and Color Plate 4). The *lymphocyte* is the second most abundant white cell circulating in the peripheral blood. Lymphocytes are primarily concerned with the immune defense system. Normal marrow may be composed of up to 20% developing lymphocytes. Lymphocytes are also derived from the marrow stem cell, but the control of lymphocyte production within the marrow is not well understood. Following maturation, the lymphocytes enter the peripheral blood, circulate for a variable length of time depending on the nature of the cell, and subsequently repopulate the lymph nodes or lymphatic organs. The earliest lymphoid cell is a *lymphoblast,* which is generally indistinct and inconspicuous in normal marrow. Lymphocytes are conditioned by two main organ systems, the thymus (T-lymphocytes) or the bone marrow (B-lymphocytes). Morphologic criteria are not useful in determining the subtype or functional characteristics of lymphocytes. B-lymphocytes may differentiate further to produce plasma cells, which comprise less than 4.5% of the normal marrow differential count. Plasma cells have a characteristic morphology with an eccentric cell nucleus, a juxtanuclear halo, and a chromatin pattern described as a cartwheel (see Color Plate 3A). Plasma cells manufacture antibody (immunoglobulin) (see also Chapter 7).

Megakaryopoiesis

The characteristic giant cells, the *megakaryocytes,* are precursors of the blood platelets. Platelets prevent bleeding by forming small platelet plugs into defects in capillary walls, and also facilitate blood coagulation. The process of platelet development from megakaryocytes is termed *megakaryopoiesis.* The *megakaryocyte* is the largest cell in the bone marrow and also arises from the multipotent stem cell (see Fig. 2–2 and Color Plates 3B and 7). It is believed that a hormone similar to erythropoietin, termed *thrombopoietin,* may control proliferation and maturation of megakaryocytes. The earliest precursor of the megakaryocyte is termed a *megakaryoblast*. During the stage of megakaryocyte maturation, the nucleus undergoes multiple divisions without corresponding divisions in the cell. Therefore, a multinucleate cell is formed (see Color Plate 3B). As the cell matures, abundant cytoplasm accumulates. Platelets are formed by the development of demarcation membranes within the cytoplasm, and individual platelets are extruded through the endothelial cells of the marrow sinusoids into the venous sinuses. Mature circulating platelets, like mature red cells, have no nucleus. A single megakaryocyte can release several thousand platelets. Following platelet release, the bare nucleus of the megakaryocyte is sometimes seen in marrow preparations. Platelets vary in size from 1 to about 4 μm in diameter, but may occasionally be larger. They stain light blue and have multiple cytoplasmic granules (see Color Plates 3 and 4). These granules contain functional constituents that are important in the control of bleeding (see Chapter 5). The circulating platelet count is kept within a narrow range and appears to be controlled by factors including absolute platelet mass within the body and the release of thrombopoietin.

LABORATORY EVALUATION OF HEMATOPOIESIS

Direct Marrow Sampling

The elements of hemopoietic activity can be evaluated both quantitatively and qualitatively. The amount of functional bone marrow can be most simply determined by direct microscopic evaluation. Bone marrow function can also be determined by cell labeling with specific radioisotopic tracer elements, which are incorporated within the developing erythroid precursors. In this manner, the use of radioactive iron can be used to evaluate hemoglobin production and sites of erythropoiesis. Other tracer elements can be used to determine the quantity and distribution of bone marrow activity (indium or technetium) or the survival of red blood cells (chromium).

BONE MARROW ASPIRATION AND BIOPSY

Microscopic examination of aspirated bone marrow tissue is usually the simplest method of assessing both the amount of bone marrow and the nature of cell growth and maturation.

A bone marrow aspirate is performed by the introduction of a needle through the outer bony layers into the marrow cavity and the withdrawal of a sample of marrow "juice" for examination. Sites for bone marrow *aspiration* are the posterior iliac crest of the pelvis, the sternum, and the anterior iliac crest. In young children, the proximal portion of the tibia may be used.

The detail and relationship of the developing marrow cells to one another, as well as the pattern of maturation, is best assessed by microscopic examination of the aspirated marrow tissue. Hematopoietic bone marrow contains fat and other connective tissue as well as the blood-forming cells. It is fluid enough to be aspirated through the needle, but only the first few drops should be used for examination because in the later aliquots, peripheral blood dilutes the marrow material. Tiny fragments of connective tissue as well as free-floating cells will be withdrawn. The morphology of these free cells provides the information on the maturation sequence of the cells (see Color Plates 1–3).

Bone Marrow Biopsy. In this test, a trephine needle is inserted through the outer portion of the bone (cortex) and the internal trochar is removed, producing a hollow bore. A small portion of the bone is beveled by cutting and rotating into the bone tissue. The specimen then is broken off and removed. It is placed in histologic fixative and submitted to the histology laboratory. Bone marrow biopsies are usually performed from the iliac crests since these provide a large area of bone from which a core biopsy can be removed.

In general, the bone marrow aspirate provides valuable information about the cytologic and morphologic detail, whereas the bone marrow biopsy provides important information regarding the bony structures and the relationship of the cells to one another and to other connective tissue elements. In particular, cellularity of the marrow, abnormal cellular elements, metastatic cancer, and fibrous tisue scarring can best be assessed by the bone marrow biopsy (see Color Plate 8).

For both aspiration and biopsy, a meticulous aseptic technique is necessary since infectious material can be introduced into the bone marrow, and can then rapidly reach the entire circulation. The skin and subcutaneous tissues are anesthetized by local injection, which is also infiltrated into the periosteal bone. Despite adequate local anesthetic infiltration, pain is usually elicited following aspiration since the interstices of the bone marrow cannot be anesthetized. These areas are exquisitely sensitive to pressure, and suction similarly elicits pain. Suction or aspiration pain is a normal phenomenon, and its absence on occasion is indicative of infiltrative bone marrow disease.

Following removal of the tissue, an antibiotic-impregnated dressing is applied with pressure over the area for approximately five minutes. With attention to aseptic detail, as well as care and local pressure dressing application, bone marrow aspirates and biopsies can be performed even in patients with bleeding disorders. The technique provides very useful information for understanding the nature of many hematologic diseases, as well as metastatic malignancy.

BONE MARROW CELLULARITY AND MYELOID: ERYTHROID RATIO

Bone marrow cellularity, the relationship of developing hematopoietic cells to the fat spaces within the marrow, is present as a relatively fixed proportion. Normally, a 1:1–2:1 ratio of marrow cells to marrow fat is present (see Color Plates 7 and 8). Greater than a 2.1 cell-to-fat ratio constitutes *hypercellularity.* This may occur when any or all of the marrow elements are present in abundance. The nature of the cell line that is more abundant can give important clues as to mechanisms of anemia or leukocyte abnormalities. Table 2–1 lists the normal values of bone marrow precursor cells.

Although circulating blood contains 500–1,000 times as many red cells as white cells (5 million red cells per microliter as compared with 5–10,000 white cells per

Table 2–1. DIFFERENTIAL COUNTS OF NUCLEATED BONE MARROW CELLS*

	Range of Mean Values†
Myeloblast	0.3–2.0
Promyelocyte	1.4–5.0
Myelocyte	4.2–8.9
Metamyelocyte	6.5–22.0
Band	13.0–24.0
Mature granulocyte	
Neutrophil	15.0–20.0
Eosinophil	0.5–2.0
Basophil	0.0–0.2
Lymphocyte	14.0–16.0
Monocyte	0.3–2.4
Plasma cell	0.3–1.3
Pronormoblast	0.2–0.6
Basophilic normoblast	1.4–2.0
Polychromatophilic normoblast	6.0–21.0
Orthochromic normoblast	1.0–3.0
M:E ratio	2.3–3.5 to 1.0

*Figures are for adults and are taken from several series as reported in Williams, et al (eds): Hematology, McGraw-Hill, New York, 1983, and in Wintrobe, et al: Clinical Hematology, ed 8, Lea and Febiger, Philadelphia, 1981.

†Values are expressed as percent of nucleated cells present.

microliter), nucleated white cells in the bone marrow outnumber the nucleated erythrocytic cells by 3:1. This is called the myeloid: erythroid ratio or M:E. Many factors contribute to this disproportion:

- Red cells require 5–6 days for bone marrow development, but the nucleus disappears after 2–3 days. Maturing red cells enter the circulating blood very promptly, even before the last maturational events have occurred. Red cells remain in the circulation for about 120 days before senescence and destruction.
- Nucleated granulocytic cells are numerous in the marrow because granulocytes have conspicuous nuclei throughout the 5–7 days of marrow development, and large numbers of mature cells remain within the marrow as a storage pool.
- On the average, granulocytes spend between 7–24 hours in the circulating blood and have a total lifespan of only 9–15 days.

The combination of massive granulocyte turnover, persistence of the nucleus, and marrow retention of mature cells makes the myeloid series the predominant nucleated form when marrow is examined. The normal M:E is 2:1 to 4:1.

Cytologic Evaluation of Bone Marrow

The aspirated marrow is smeared onto a cover slip or glass slide and evenly spread. Hematopoietic cells form trails or spreads amongst the marrow spicules. Cellularity is evaluated within the spicules, whereas the cytologic detail is determined in the spread marrow trails (see Color Plates 1, 2, 7, and 8).

- The orderly sequence of erythropoiesis is determined, as is the orderly sequence of myelopoiesis. In this manner, a bone marrow differential count can be obtained and the maturation is appreciated.
- The quantity of cells (activity), as well as the presence of all maturation elements, is evaluated.
- The relationship of the myeloid to the erythroid cells is determined as indicated above.
- Any abnormal non-hematopoietic cells are noted.
- Some of the less abundant marrow elements, such as lymphocytes and plasma cells, are assessed.
- Special stains may be performed on the marrow to determine iron status (discussed in the chapter on anemias).

Table 2–1 indicates the range of normal values for cells in aspirated marrow. Paraffin-embedded tissue biopsy sections are unsuitable for detailed morphologic differential counts. The number of megakaryocytes or platelet precursors can be evaluated both within marrow aspirates and marrow biopsies quite easily (see Color Plate 7). On occasion, aspirated material cannot be obtained despite adequate technique. This condition is termed a "dry tap" and occurs:

- when the hemopoietic activity is so sparse that virtually no marrow cells exist to be withdrawn, with severe hypocellularity or marrow aplasia present;
- when the marrow contains tightly packed, sticky, highly immature cells that cannot be aspirated, which occurs in some cases of acute leukemia; and
- when marrow fibrosis (scar tissue) or metastatic cancer are present.

Under these circumstances, the marrow biopsy is much more helpful because it determines the absence of marrow cells or the nature of the infiltrating cellular elements.

LABORATORY EVALUATION OF ERYTHROPOIESIS

Marrow Cytology

Color Plates 1, 2E, and 2F show the developmental morphology of erythrocyte precursor cells. The earliest precursor is the *proerythroblast,* which is a large, immature cell with multiple nucleoli and a deeply basophilic cytoplasm. This cell matures into the *basophilic erythroblast.* With increasing synthesis of hemoglobin, the cytoplasm of the cell takes on a pinkish hue (on Giemsa stains) and the nucleus becomes more pyknotic and clumped, producing a *polychromatophilic erythroblast.* Further maturation is associated with more nuclear clumping and continued cytoplasmic hemoglobinization in the *orthochromatic erythroblast.* Finally, the nucleus is extruded, leaving the cell with residual cytoplasmic RNA producing polychromasia and the morphologic appearance of a *reticulocyte.*

Reticulocyte Count

As red cells mature, several days are needed for the hemoglobin-containing cells to rid themselves of residual cytoplasmic ribonucleic acid after the nucleus has been expelled. Part of this process occurs in the bone marrow and part in the circulation. During this last phase of maturation, the RNA-containing cell is slightly larger than the mature cell; it contains miscellaneous fragments of mitochondria and other organelles as well as ribosomal RNA. These cells, called *reticulocytes,* can often be distinguished on Wright-stained peripheral blood smears by their larger size and slightly gray or purple appearance. The reticulofilamentous material that gives these cells their name is seen only after supravital staining, but it is also responsible for several staining abnormalities seen on routine smears. *Polychromasia* is diffuse grayish or blue discoloration, and *basophilic stippling* is the punctate form of blue discoloration mentioned above (see Color Plates 10B, 16A, and 16C).

Normal cells spend 1–2 days circulating as reticulocytes and 120 days circulating in the mature form, and approximately 0.5–2.5% of circulating red cells are reticulocytes. A reticulocyte count of 0.5–2.5% indicates normal marrow activity if the hemoglobin level is normal. An elevated reticulocyte count in the presence of normal hemoglobin levels indicates that the red cells are being lost or destroyed, but the marrow has increased erythrocyte production to compensate. With low hemoglobin levels, a reticulocyte count of 0.5–2.5% indicates that the response to anemia is inadequate. This can result from defective or decreased bone marrow production or a reduced amount of erythropoietin. The reticulocyte count is usually reported as a percentage of circulating erythrocytes. If an individual has anemia, the number of circulating erythrocytes fall and therefore a "normal" reticulocyte percentage (0.5–2.5%) will increase. The reticulocyte count is therefore corrected for the anemia by multiplying the measured percentage (reticulocyte count) by the ratio of the patient's hematocrit against a normal hematocrit. The reticulocyte count may then be corrected for anemia as follows:

$$\text{CR} = \frac{\text{OR} \times \text{Patient's Hematocrit}}{\text{Mean Normal Hematocrit (45)}}$$

where:

CR = Corrected Reticulocyte Count
OR = Observed Reticulocyte Count

When the marrow is healthy and has adequate stores of iron and other precursors, the degree of reticulocytosis parallels the degree of blood loss or red cell destruction. Patients with defects of cellular maturation or hemoglobin production sometimes have *ineffective erythropoiesis.* In these conditions, erythroid production is greatly increased (hyperplastic), but the reticulocyte count is disproportionately low because many cells never mature sufficiently to enter the peripheral blood. Pernicious anemia and thalassemia are prime examples of ineffective erythropoiesis (see Color Plate 8B).

After blood loss or effective therapy for certain anemias such as iron deficiency anemia, a rising reticulocyte count indicates that the marrow is responding by making more erythrocytes. A single hemorrhagic episode causes reticulocytosis, beginning within 24–48 hours and reaching a peak at 4–7 days. Normal levels resume when the hemoglobin concentration stabilizes. Persistent reticulocytosis or a second rise in the reticulocyte count indicates continuing or recurrent blood loss.

In iron deficiency, and especially in anemia resulting from prolonged blood loss, therapeutic iron administration produces a reticulocyte response within 4–7 days. The reticulocyte count remains elevated until normal hemoglobin values are achieved. Vitamin B_{12} replacement therapy for pernicious anemia also causes a prompt, continuing reticulocytosis. This is often used as a challenge test when physiologic doses of vitamin B_{12} are given to people suspected of having vitamin B_{12}

deficiency. If reticulocytosis fails to occur, the diagnosis should be suspect (see p 84).

The reticulocyte count is commonly used as a measure of marrow erythroid production. This is only valid if the reticulocyte maturation time is known, and some laboratories report a reticulocyte production index per day. Often the absolute reticulocyte count is expressed in reticulocytes per microliter.

Erythropoietin Assay

As already mentioned, *erythropoietin* is the hormone that preferentially increases erythrocyte-committed progenitors and decreases the maturation time of erythrocytes within the marrow (see Fig. 2–2). Erythropoietin also increases the absolute reticulocyte count, which, to some extent, is a reflection of erythropoietin production. Erythropoietin can, however, be measured, and current assay systems use either radioimmunoassays or enzyme-linked immunoassay techniques. Formerly, erythropoietin was only measured by a bioassay that is now outmoded. Erythropoietin values can be extremely helpful in differentiating primary polycythemia where there is an uncontrolled marrow production (unregulated by erythropoietin) and erythropoietin levels are low, from secondary erythrocytosis, where there is a controlled excess of erythroid production stimulated by tissue hypoxia and mediated through erythropoietin. In these latter conditions, erythropoietin values are high (see Diseases of Red Blood Cells).

HEMOGLOBIN PRODUCTION AND CONTROL

As was outlined above, the erythron, which comprises developing red cell precursors as well as circulating mature erythrocytes, is regulated by erythropoietin and oxygen tension. The major function of the erythrocytes is to transport oxygen to the tissues, and to do so the red cell must be deformable enough to negotiate the small capillaries in the microcirculation. In addition, the red cell must contain adequate amounts of the oxygen-binding pigment *heme,* which is neatly packaged within a protein envelope called *globin.* The delicate structure of the erythrocyte, therefore, is geared to the transport of oxygen and the maintenance of hemoglobin in a functional state. The synthesis of both heme and globin is also finely controlled. The heme portion of hemoglobin consists of a porphyrin ring structure into which iron is precisely suspended (Fig. 2–4). The globin portion is a protein comprising two pairs of amino acid chains termed alpha and non-alpha (beta, gamma, delta, etc.). Adult hemoglobin A consists of 2 alpha chains and 2 beta chains. Raw materials necessary for the production of hemoglobin, and indeed red cells, must be in constant supply because there are a large number of erythrocytes synthesized daily. Vitamins and minerals as well as amino acids need to be provided. Deficiencies of these components can lead to a reduced number of erythrocytes or decreased amounts of hemoglobin pigment. This state is termed *anemia* (see Diseases of Red Blood Cells).

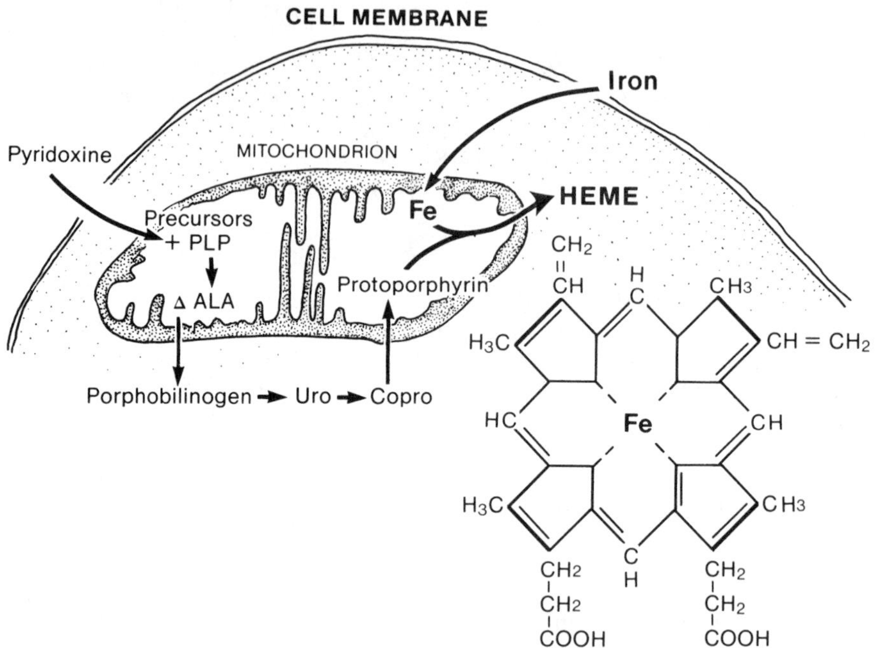

Figure 2–4. Heme formation. The mitochondrion is responsible for the synthesis of protoporphyrin, a stepwise process beginning with the formation of delta aminolevulinic acid from glycine and succinyl-CoA, with pyridoxal-5-phosphate (PLP) as an essential cofactor. The sequence of porphobilinogen, uroporphyrin, and coproporphyrin formation then occurs in the cytoplasm, followed by an intramitochondrial assembly of protoporphyrin and iron to form heme. The structure of the final product, the heme molecule, is shown. It consists of four porphyrin moieties assembled in a ring structure around a central iron molecule. (From Hillman and Finch,[4] p 8, with permission.)

Heme Synthesis

The two parts of the hemoglobin molecule (*heme* and *globin*) have very different synthetic pathways. Each hemoglobin molecule has four identical heme moieties attached to the four globin protein chains. The heme moieties consist of four symmetrically ringed 4-carbon structures called pyrrole rings, which constitute a molecule of *porphyrin.* This porphyrin ring is also seen in other proteins in addition to hemoglobin, including myoglobin and other enzymes (catalase, cytochromes, and peroxidase). Biosynthesis of heme involves stepwise production of a porphyrin framework, followed by the insertion of iron into each of the four heme groups (see Fig. 2–4).

Synthesis of the porphyrin requires construction of a straight line chain of carbon-containing groups that is closed into a single pyrrole ring. Four pyrroles linked together, after several changes and exchanges of substituent groups, form the final iron-free compound *protoporphyrin.*

The constitutent carbon groups constituting this chain are derived from the amino acid glycine and a coenzyme, succinyl coenzyme A.

- These two compounds are initially condensed to form the compound *aminolevulinic acid (ALA)*. This straight line compound is the first precursor distinctively associated with heme synthesis. The enzyme catalyzing this reaction, *ALA-synthetase,* appears to be a rate-limiting enzyme in this metabolic pathway. *Pyridoxal phosphate* (vitamin B_6) is also a coenzyme for this reaction, which is stimulated by the presence of the hormone erythropoietin and inhibited by the manufacturing of heme (negative feedback control). This pathway is initiated in the mitochondria and cytoplasm of the developing cell.
- Two molecules of ALA combine to form *porphobilinogen,* a single-ring molecule.
- Subsequently, four molecules of this compound condense to form a four-ringed (tetrapyrrole) compound, *uroporphyrinogen.*
- Subsequent steps in this synthesis include conversion of this compound to *coproporphyrinogen.*
- Coproporphyrinogen is converted to *protoporphyrin.*
- Finally, protoporphyrin is coupled with iron in the presence of another rate-limiting enzyme, *ferrochelatase* (heme synthetase), to form the oxygen-carrying pigment heme. Unused coproporphyrin and uroporphyrin are excreted in the urine and feces. If heme synthesis is impaired, abnormal quantities of these compounds and other precursors may be excreted. Identification and measurement will be discussed in later sections (see Porphyrias in Chapter 3).

Therefore, the clinical states associated with abnormal heme production may include anemia and the genetic or acquired enzyme disorders that produce abnormal accumulation of the porphyrins (porphyria).

The insertion of four heme molecules into the four globin molecules constitutes the final synthesis of hemoglobin. Heme is synthesized in the mitochondria, and globin incorporation occurs in the cytoplasm of the developing erythrocyte.

Globin Synthesis

Globin synthesis is also discussed under Diseases of Globin Production (thalassemias and hemoglobinopathies). Normal adult hemoglobin (HbA—95% of adult hemoglobin) consists of four polypeptide chains comprising two alpha chains and two beta chains (α_2, β_2), each with its own attached heme group. Normally, alpha and beta chains are produced in equal proportions. Other minor chains are also synthesized in the adult and include a delta (δ) chain and a fetal gamma (γ) chain, which constitute the two minor adult hemoglobins.

- $\alpha_2\gamma_2$ constitutes Hemoglobin F or fetal hemoglobin (<2.5%).
- $\alpha_2\delta_2$ constitutes the other minor hemoglobin, hemoglobin A_2 (<2.5%).

Presumably the synthesis of globin is also under the control of erythropoietin, although its site of action is uncertain. Globin synthesis is also induced by free heme. Globin synthesis occurs, particularly in the early, or basophilic, erythroblast, and continues to a limited extent even in the anucleate reticulocyte. It has been estimated that as much as 15–20% of hemoglobin is synthesized during this later stage. The genes for globin synthesis are located on chromosomes 11 (gamma, delta, and beta chains) and 16 (alpha)(see Fig. 3–2). Some embryonic hemoglobins are also encoded on these respective chromosomes. The regulation of DNA expression with subsequent formation of RNA (ribonucleic acid) and protein synthesis is now well elucidated. Anemias may occur because of abnormalities at the DNA level, defects in interpreting the template RNA, or because nonsense messenger codes are not translated or expressed during protein synthesis. These will be discussed in the respective sections dealing with thalassemias and hemoglobinopathies (see Chapter 3). Since each individual chromosome is inherited from each parent, genetic expression is clearly dependent on which gene is transferred to the offspring. Inherited disorders of hemoglobin production may cause serious anemias. Globin messenger RNA, harvested from reticulocytes, forms a suitable *in vitro* cell system in which to study globin synthesis in the research laboratory. These genetic codes have been elucidated, and direct the assembly of 141 amino acids into the alpha chain and 146 amino acids into the non-alpha chains.

During fetal life, embryonic chains subsequently switch over to the major fetal hemoglobin ($\alpha_2\gamma_2$, hemoglobin F). This represents the dominant hemoglobin in late fetal and early neonatal life. Conversion of fetal hemoglobin to adult hemoglobin ($\alpha_2\beta_2$) is completed by 3–6 months of age. The actual mechanisms controlling the switch are as yet undetermined (see also Fig. 3–4).

ADDITIONAL FACTORS ESSENTIAL FOR HEMOGLOBIN SYNTHESIS

Vitamin B_{12} and Folic Acid

Vitamin B_{12} consists of a porphyrin ring attached to a nucleotide base (Fig. 2–5A). The porphyrin ring is very similar to heme, except that cobalt is substituted for iron. The metabolism of vitamin B_{12} (cyanocobalamin) and folic acid (pteroylmonoglutamic acid) is vitally involved in the synthesis and intermolecular exchanges of 1- and 2-carbon fragments. These reactions affect the synthesis of purines and pyrimidines, and thus influence DNA synthesis (Fig. 2–6). Deficiency states cause defective DNA production, abnormal nuclear and cytoplasmic development, and the production of large, dysmature, megaloblastic cells (see Vitamin B_{12} and Folic Acid Deficiency, p. 83).

Metabolism of Vitamin B_{12} and Folic Acid

Vitamin B_{12} is synthesized in nature by microorganisms. Humans cannot synthesize vitamin B_{12} and acquire their supplies by eating animal tissues. The normal human diet consists of 5–30 μg of vitamin B_{12} daily, of which 1–5 μg are absorbed. Normal body stores consist of 3000–5000 μg of which 1000 μg are stored in the liver. Absorption of vitamin B_{12} occurs in the terminal ileum under the influence of a substance produced in the parietal cells of the stomach called *intrinsic factor.* Intrinsic factor is essential for the absorption of vitamin B_{12} in the terminal ileum. Intrinsic factor is a bivalent glycoprotein that preferentially binds to B_{12} and to receptors on the terminal ileum cells. Since vitamin B_{12} is abundant in nature, deficiencies are mostly the result of malabsorption or a deficiency of intrinsic factor. Following absorption, vitamin B_{12} is transported by plasma proteins termed *transcobalamins* (Fig. 2–7). There are three types of transcobalamins, termed transcobalamin I, II, and III. Transcobalamins I and III are storage proteins for vitamin B_{12}, and transcobalamin II is the transport protein. The storage transcobalamins are synthesized in granulocytes and tend to increase in instances where the granulocyte mass is exaggerated, such as myeloproliferative diseases or leukocytosis (see Chapter 3).

There are two major natural forms of vitamin B_{12}—*cyanocobalamin* and *hydroxy-*

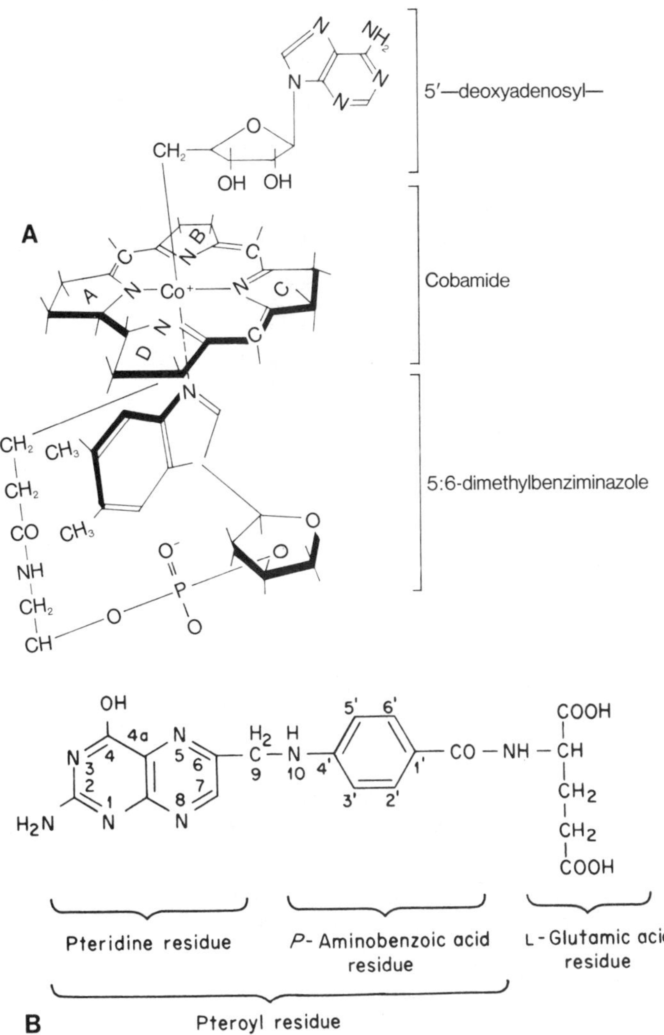

Figure 2–5. (A) Structure of vitamin B_{12} (5′ deoxyadenosyl cobalamin). (Redrawn from Chanarin, I: The Megaloblastic Anemias. Blackwell Scientific Publications, Boston, with permission.) (*B*) Structure of folic acid (pteroylglutamic acid). (From Williams, WJ, et al: Hematology, ed 3. McGraw-Hill, New York, 1983, p 320, with permission.)

cobalamin. In the body, these are converted into the functional cobalamins methylcobalamin and 5′-deoxyadenosylcobalamin. Normal body stores are sufficient to withstand a year or more of zero intake; however, states of rapid growth or cell turnover increase vitamin B_{12} requirements. Although an obligate substance for normal human metabolism, vitamin B_{12} is unequivocally required for relatively few reactions. One important reaction is the *methylation of the amino acid homocysteine to the amino acid methionine,* a conversion that not only generates methionine but also the functional folate cofactor *tetrahydrofolate.*

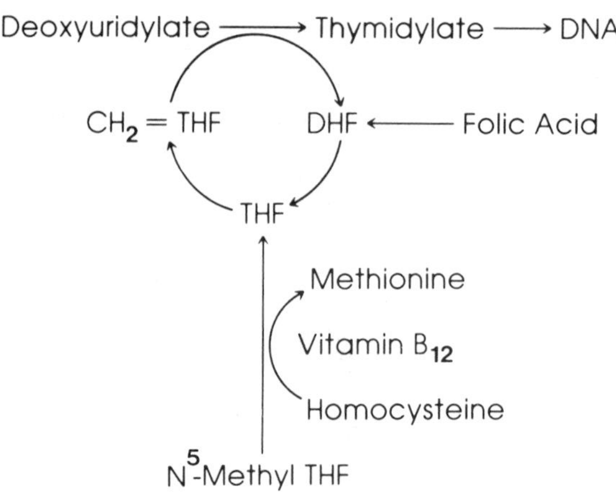

Figure 2–6. The roles of vitamin B_{12} and folic acid in DNA synthesis. THF = tetrahydrofolate; DHF = dihydrofolate; CH_2 = THF = methylene tetrahydrofolate. (From Pittiglio, DH and Sacher, RA: Clinical Hematology and Fundamentals of Hemostasis. FA Davis, Philadelphia, 1987, p 62, with permission.)

A deficiency of vitamin B_{12} produces failure to regenerate tetrahydrofolic acid from N^5-methyltetrahydrofolic acid, and may lead to megaloblastic anemia.

The key reaction may be represented by the equation:

$$\text{homocysteine} + N^5\text{-methyl-}FH_4 \xleftrightarrow[\text{methylcobalamin}]{\text{methyltransferase}} \text{tetrahydrofolic acid} + \text{methionine}$$

Folic acid is a collective term for a group of compounds derived from green, leafy foliage. These compounds consist of three moieties (see Fig. 2–5B):

- a *pteridine ring,*
- *para-amino-benzoic acid,* and
- one of a number of *glutamic acid* units.

The first two moieties are collectively termed *pteroyls,* and are further named according to the number of glutamic acid residues that are present; e.g., pteroyl monoglutamate or pteroyl polyglutamates. A normal diet consists of 500–700 μg of folate, of which 50 μg per day are absorbed, and the body has one month's supply of storage folate. Folates are absorbed throughout the small intestine, and a deficiency of folic acid usually occurs in situations of excess demand and poor dietary supply.

Metabolically active folate is derived by the reduction of the pteroyl group to dihydrofolate, and subsequently to *tetrahydrofolate,* in the presence of the enzyme *dihydrofolate reductase.* Tetrahydrofolic acid is the reduced form of folic acid and is the catalytic, self-regenerating compound that mediates 1-carbon transfers. One-carbon fragments can be bound to the pteroyl groups and transferred in intermediary metabolism involving DNA synthesis. Like vitamin B_{12}, folic acid cannot be synthesized by mammals. The major effect of folic acid deficiency is impairment of thymidine synthesis. Thymidine is part of DNA but not RNA; thus, altered *thymidine metabolism* specifically affects DNA and leaves RNA production unaffected (see Fig. 2–6). In the presence of folic acid, 1-carbon fragments are transferred from

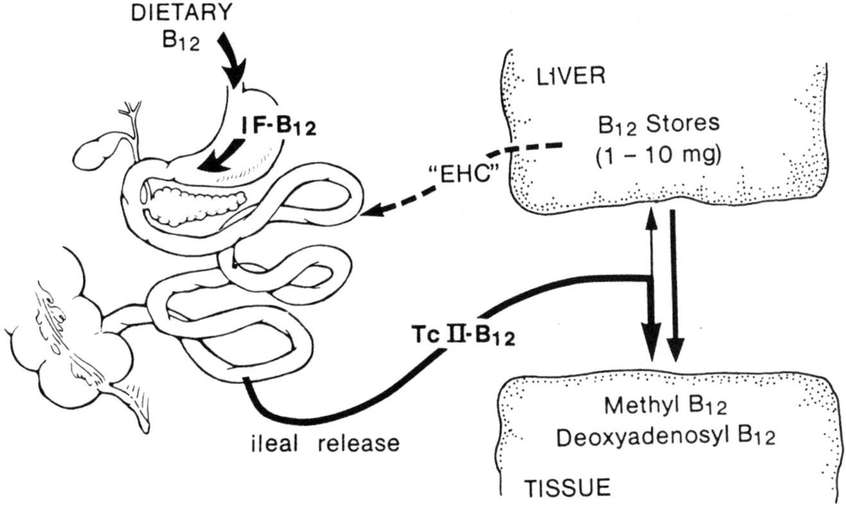

Figure 2–7. The absorption, transport, and storage of vitamin B_{12}. Dietary vitamin B_{12} is liberated by peptic acid digestion and then bound to intrinsic factor (IF-B_{12}) produced by the gastric parietal cells. This protects the vitamin B_{12} until it reaches the terminal ileum, where it is released from the intrinsic factor and bound to transcobalamin II (Tc II) for transport to liver and tissues. In normal individuals, 1–10 mg of vitamin B_{12} is stored in the liver. These B_{12} stores may be released and transported directly to tissues or to a lesser extent secreted into bile for reabsorption, an enterohepatic cycle (EHC). (From Hillman and Finch,[4] p 79, with permission.)

deoxyuridine to deoxythymidine on the pteroyl group. Folic acid is also involved in other pathways involving 1-carbon transfers, and its deficiency also impairs *histidine catabolism.* This abnormality produces no clinical disability, but does cause large quantities of the metabolite *formiminoglutamic acid (FIGLU)* to accumulate after a histidine load is given to a folate-deficient subject. This previously formed the basis for documenting folic acid deficiency. Normal values for Vitamin B_{12} and folate metabolism are shown in Table 2–2.

Laboratory Determinations of Vitamin B_{12} and Folic Acid

Serum vitamin B_{12} and serum folate may be assayed by several techniques that are discussed in Chapter 3. The usual assay system is radioimmunoassay. The normal ranges for vitamin B_{12} are 200–900 pg/ml, and for folate are 3–20 ng/ml.

Cobalamin deficiency is almost always due to vitamin B_{12} malabsorption. Pernicious anemia is the commonest cause, and is due to a lack of *intrinsic factor.* Intrinsic factor is normally produced by the parietal cells of the gastric mucosa and is deficient in any condition depleting this production, such as atrophic gastritis or gastrectomy. Intestinal malabsorption syndromes, veganism, or intestinal bacterial overgrowth with organisms requiring vitamin B_{12} may also produce deficiency.

Vitamin B_{12} and folic acid deficiency may be differentiated by measuring serum levels. Vitamin B_{12} deficiency is confirmed by testing B_{12} absorption using the uri-

Table 2–2. NORMAL VALUES FOR VITAMIN B_{12} AND FOLATE METABOLISM

Folic Acid	
Serum:	3–20 ng/ml
Red cells:	165–600 ng/ml
FIGLU:	Urinary excretion up to 17 ng/day
Methylmalonate:	Urinary excretion up to 10 mg/day
Schilling Test:	15–40% of 0.5-μg dose
	5–40% of 1.0-μg dose
Vitamin B_{12} (serum):	200–900 pg/ml

nary excretion of *radiolabeled B_{12}* after an oral dose given with or without intrinsic factor *(Schilling Test).*

Laboratory Determination of B_{12} Absorption (Schilling Test)

The Schilling Test is used to establish:

- whether the vitamin B_{12} absorption is defective and if so,
- whether the etiology is intrinsic factor deficiency.

With normal absorption, the body receives far more vitamin B_{12} than it needs, and the excess is excreted in the urine. Urinary excretion increases if vitamin B_{12} requirements have already been met. In impaired absorption, the orally administered vitamin does not reach the circulation and therefore does not appear in the urine. Vitamin B_{12} labeled with ^{57}Co is used to follow the absorption and excretion in the urine of the orally administered (0.5–1.0 μg) vitamin B_{12}. Initially, a parenteral loading dose of unlabeled vitamin B_{12} (1000 μg) is administered to saturate the body stores so that when labeled B_{12} is absorbed, a significant amount is subsequently excreted in the urine. Normal subjects will excrete 7% or more of the radioactivity taken orally in their urine, whereas patients with pernicious anemia or other causes of vitamin B_{12} malabsorption will excrete less than 5%. Complete collection of the urine is extremely important, for the test depends on measuring the absolute amount of radioactivity excreted. Since this test depends on urinary excretion, its interpretation in renal insufficiency may be impaired because of reduced urinary output. In this case, the test may be prolonged to a 48–72-hour collection.

The *second part of the Schilling Test* is performed with the addition of *intrinsic factor.* The test is repeated with 60 μg of intrinsic factor administered orally along with cyanocobalamin. If the megaloblastic anemia is due to lack of vitamin B_{12} from intrinsic factor deficiency (pernicious anemia), malabsorption will be corrected by the oral administration of vitamin B_{12} coupled to intrinsic factor. The labeled vitamin B_{12}-bound intrinsic factor will be received by the terminal ileal cells and will be absorbed, and the labeled B_{12} will be excreted in the urine. The second phase of the test assesses the functional integrity of the terminal ileum, or whether there are blocking factors within the lumen of the intestine, preventing vitamin B_{12} absorption. Therefore, if urinary ^{57}Co excretion rises to normal when intrinsic factor is added, the diagnosis of intrinsic factor deficiency is established. A second low excretion indicates some other malabsorptive state.

Before performing the Schilling Test, it is imperative that other causes of megaloblastosis, such as folic acid deficiency (by serum folate determination), have been investigated, since the parenteral loading dose of vitamin B_{12} may confuse this investigation (see Chapter 3).

Iron Metabolism

Iron is the most abundant trace element in the body. About 65% of the body's normal 4000 mg of iron (60 mg/kg in men and 50 mg/kg in women) is bound to heme. One milligram of iron is required for each milliliter of red cells produced. Each day, 20–25 mg of iron are needed for erythropoiesis. Ninety-five percent of this required iron is recycled iron salvaged from normal red blood cell turnover and hemoglobin catabolism. Only 1 mg/day (representing 5% of the iron turnover) is newly absorbed to balance minimal iron loss incurred by fecal and urinary excretion. Figure 2–8 illustrates the continuous process of *daily iron turnover.* The remaining body iron, representing one third of total iron content, is stored within the liver, spleen, and bone marrow, or is carried in myoglobin and coenzymes of the

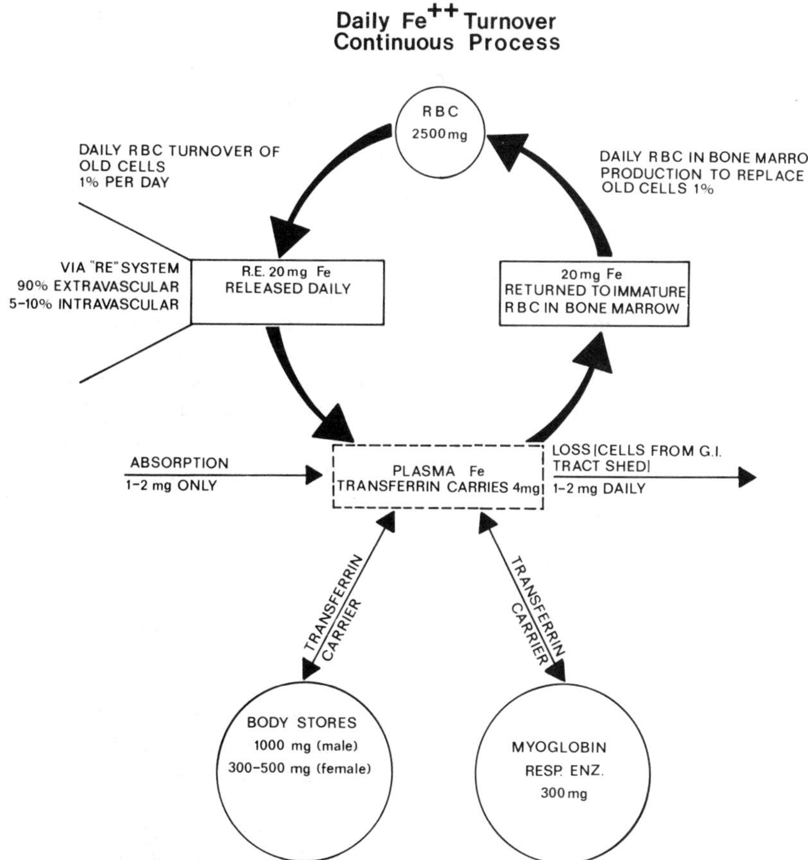

Figure 2–8. Diagram illustrating normal daily iron turnover and pathways of internal iron exchanges. (From Pittiglio, DH and Sacher, RA: Clinical Hematology and Fundamentals of Hemostasis. FA Davis, Philadelphia, 1987, p 42, with permission.)

Table 2–3. NORMAL VALUES FOR IRON METABOLISM

Serum iron (Fe): 50–150 μg/dl
Total iron-binding capacity (TIBC): 240–360 μg/dl
Percent saturation: 20–45%
Serum ferritin: 12–300 μg/liter

cytochrome electron transport proteins. Storage iron exists in the form of hemosiderin or ferritin. Normal values for iron metabolism are shown in Table 2–3.

Iron Absorption

Absorption of iron is regulated by the intestines, which admit just enough iron to cover losses without permitting excessive absorption. Normal dietary iron intake is 10–20 mg/day. The amount of iron absorbed from the diet varies greatly, depending on several factors including the amount and type of iron ingested, gastric acidity, the activity of the bone marrow, and the state of the body iron stores. Although the entire small intestine has the capacity to absorb iron, maximal absorption occurs in the duodenum and upper jejunum, owing to the presence of optimum conditions of pH. In the state of severe iron deficiency, the body can increase absorption to up to 30% of the dietary intake to compensate for the depletion.

Elemental iron is biologically active in the ferrous (Fe^{2+}) and ferric (Fe^{3+}) states. In general, an acidic or lower pH favors the ferrous state and iron absorption, whereas a neutral or alkaline pH favors the ferric state and decreased iron absorption.

Iron Transport and Storage

Iron is transported from the mucosal cells of the intestine to the blood, where it is then bound to a specific iron transport protein, *transferrin,* a plasma beta-globulin. Transferrin's capacity to bind iron in normal plasma is 240–360 μg/dl. Transferrin attaches to the receptors of the developing erythrocyte membrane and releases free iron into the erythrocyte for incorporation into heme within the mitochondria. Approximately 10–20% of the total body iron is stored as *ferritin,* constituting 0.3–1.0 g. When iron is absorbed in excess of the ferritin storage, iron is deposited in lysosomal membranes as a pseudocrystalline complex. This amorphous iron is termed *hemosiderin,* and is readily visible on light microscopy by Prussian Blue staining.

Laboratory Evaluation of Iron Status

Peripheral Blood Smear. Examination of a stained peripheral smear is the most simple, cost-effective method of characterizing iron status and getting qualitative information on the degree of hemoglobinization. Iron-deficient cells are characterized by less hemoglobin, termed *hypochromia,* and a smaller cell size, termed *microcytosis* (see Red Blood Cell Morphology and Diseases of Red Blood Cells) (see also Color Plate 30).

Serum Iron. Iron is usually measured colorimetrically following the development of a complex with a color-producing compound (chromogen). Blood levels for iron estimation should routinely be drawn in the morning after a 12-hour fast with the exclusion of all iron supplements for 12–24 hours. The normal range for serum iron is 50–150 μg/dl, averaging 125 μg/dl in men and 100 μg/dl in women. In the elderly, the serum iron levels decrease to 40–80 μg/dl. Serum iron levels vary in response to various physiologic disorders: they decrease in iron deficiency, chronic infections, and malignancy; and increase in iron poisoning, intravascular hemolysis, hepatic necrosis, pernicious anemia, and hemochromatosis.

Total Iron-Binding Capacity (TIBC). The capacity of serum *transferrin* to bind to iron is obtained by this test. The test is performed in the same way as serum iron, except that excess iron is added to the sample to saturate all *transferrin-binding sites,* and the unbound iron is removed prior to assay. Therefore, the total ability of transferrin to bind iron is assessed by the determination of the total iron bound. This assay does not measure the serum transferrin (protein) level directly, but measures the amount of Fe bound to this protein. The normal range for TIBC in adults is 240–360 μg/dl, and tends to decrease with age to approximately 250 μg/dl in people older than 70 years. Total iron-binding capacity is increased in the presence of iron deficiency, but may be normal or low in chronic disease states and malnutrition.

Transferrin Saturation. *Transferrin saturation* is not directly measured, but is obtained as a ratio:

$$\text{Percentage Saturation} = \frac{\text{Serum Iron}}{\text{TIBC}} \times 100$$

With normal iron stores and protein metabolism, *transferrin* is usually 30–35% saturated. The normal range is between 20–45% saturation. Saturation levels follow a diurnal pattern, being highest in the morning and lowest in the late afternoon and early evening. Percentage saturation is low in iron deficiency and chronic disease states, and high in sideroblastic anemia, iron poisoning, and intravascular hemolysis (see Table 3–4).

Serum Ferritin. Ferritin is present in the plasma and serum and is in equilibrium with virtually all ferritin-producing tissues. Serum ferritin is a protein devoid of iron, and is in a low concentration relative to tissue ferritin. Since it is in equilibrium with tissue ferritin, it can be a very good indicator of iron stores. Serum ferritin is measured by a radioimmunoassay, and normal ranges are 20–250 μg/ml in men and 10–200 μg/ml in children and premenopausal women. Each 1 mg/liter of ferritin represents 8–10 mg of storage iron. The measurement of serum ferritin can be particularly useful in distinguishing iron deficiency from other causes of hypochromic microcytic anemia (see Chapter 3 and Table 3–4). Serum ferritins are generally below 10 μg/ml in iron deficiency. Serum ferritin levels are elevated in inflammation, liver disease, malignancy, and other chronic diseases. In iron overload, serum ferritin may increase to as much as several thousand μg/ml.

Free Erythrocyte Protoporphyrin (FEP). As was discussed under Heme Synthesis (see Fig. 2–4), the enzyme ferrochelatase inserts ferrous iron into protoporphyrin IX in the final step of heme synthesis. *Protoporphyrin* without iron is not incorporated into hemoglobin. Erythrocytes normally produce a slight excess of protoporphyrin over what is needed for heme synthesis, but when iron is deficient, protoporphyrin increases several-fold. Ferrochelatase is a rate-limiting enzyme step in heme synthesis, and the insertion of iron into protoporphyrin facilitates a negative feedback (see Fig. 2–4). Measurement of FEP provides a sensitive early indicator of iron deficiency. It is also elevated in chronic disease states and lead poisoning, both of which produce disturbances in iron metabolism. Free erythrocyte protoporphyrin is usually measured by direct fluorescence. Normal values depend on the method and laboratory, but range from 15–18 μg/liter of RBCs. This test is useful in diagnosing iron deficiency, even after iron therapy has been instituted.

Tissue Iron Determination. Direct estimation of iron stores must occasionally be obtained for diagnosis. This may be achieved by biopsy of the liver, or more commonly of the bone marrow. Bone marrow iron can be appreciated directly in unstained preparations of aspirates as the golden refractile granule of *hemosiderin.* Generally, however, bone marrow iron stores are assessed by a reaction with Prussian Blue, which renders the hemosiderin deep blue (see Color Plate 9). Histologic grading correlates reasonably well with the iron content of the sample. This estimation of iron stores represents the most accurate determination of the body content of iron; however, information can usually be obtained using the other tests listed above.

Morphologically, hemosiderin in small granules reflects intracytoplasmic aggregates of ferritin. Erythroblasts (normoblasts) containing such granules are termed *sideroblasts* (Color Plate 15). In normal marrow, approximately 30% of the erythroblasts contain such granules, and the percentage of sideroblasts in the marrow corresponds closely to the percentage saturation of transferrin. Normally, only two small granules are found per erythroblast. These granules may become more numerous in iron overload states. Occasionally the granules may be arranged in a ring around the nucleus, and these sideroblasts are termed *ring sideroblasts* (see Color Plate 15A). Defects in heme biosynthesis in the mitochondria appear to be responsible for this distribution.

Marrow evaluation of iron stores can yield falsely normal iron estimates in patients who have recently received parenteral iron therapy or blood transfusions, since the iron is immediately taken up by macrophages (reticulo-endothelial cells), which are major sites of tissue storage iron.

RED BLOOD CELL AND HEMOGLOBIN CONCENTRATION

The factors responsible for red blood cell production (erythropoiesis) and hemoglobin synthesis have been discussed earlier in the chapter. For development of the functional mature erythrocyte, which circulates in the peripheral blood and delivers oxygen to the tissues, an intricate balance of porphyrin synthesis, iron supply, and globin synthesis neatly packaged in a deformable red cell membrane must be achieved so that the erythrocyte can traverse tiny capillaries within the tissues. Defects in any of these stages may be responsible for deficient oxygen supply to the tissues. Tests are available for quantitation of erythrocytes and for evaluating their oxygen-carrying capacity. The morphologic appearance of the red cell may also give clues about erythrocyte membrane defects. Laboratory evaluation of these parameters is useful in assessing erythrocyte structure and function, and gives an appreciation of red blood cell diseases, which will be covered in the next chapter.

The three primary variables are the amount of *hemoglobin* present in whole blood (in grams per deciliter); the proportion of red cells in whole blood, expressed as *packed cell volume* or *hematocrit,* and the *absolute number* of red cells in whole blood, usually expressed as millions of cells per microliter. *Corpuscular indices,* also called *red cell indices,* are calculations that allow the characterization of *average size* and hemoglobin content in individual erythrocytes (see also Table 2–4).

Table 2–4. NORMAL VALUES FOR COMPLETE BLOOD COUNT IN ADULTS

	Men	Women
Hematocrit	40–54%	38–47%
Hemoglobin	13.5–18 g/dl	12–16 g/dl
Red cells/μl	$4.6–6.2 \times 10^6$	$4.2–5.4 \times 10^6$
White cells/μl	$4.5–11 \times 10^3$	$4.5–11 \times 10^3$
Platelets/μl	$150–450 \times 10^3$	$150–450 \times 10^3$
Mean corpuscular volume (MCV)	80–98 fl	81–99 fl
Mean corpuscular hemoglobin (MCH)	26–32 pg	26–32 pg
Mean corpuscular hemoglobin concentration (MCHC)	32–36%	32–36%
Red cell distribution width (RDW)	11.6–14.6%	11.6–14.6%
Reticulocyte count	0.5–2.5%	0.5–2.5%

Direct Measurement of Red Cell and Hemoglobin Concentration

Hemoglobin is the main oxygen-carrying pigment and is distributed in erythrocytes. Hemoglobin is a red pigment and maximally absorbs light at a wavelength of 540 nm. If a fixed concentration of red cells is lysed, hemoglobin is liberated and can be determined spectrophotometrically at this wavelength, with the concentration being proportional to the optical density. All forms of hemoglobin, including *oxyhemoglobin, deoxyhemoglobin, methemoglobin,* and *carboxyhemoglobin,* are converted into a single stable form. Conversion to *cyanmethemoglobin* is the method most widely used because reagents and instruments can be controlled most easily against stable and reliable standards. Limitations of this technique lie in accurate sample dilution and reagent preparation, as well as careful calibration of instruments. For adult men, normal levels are 13.5—18.0 g/dl. The normal range for women is 12—16 g/dl. Hemoglobin may be measured using spectrophotometers available in physicians' offices or in most general laboratories; however, the most widely practiced method employs automated cell counters that directly measure hemoglobin in the red cell channel.

A qualitative estimation of hemoglobin concentration may be obtained by assessing the specific gravity of whole blood. This method is used as a screening technique to determine whether a person can safely donate blood. In this way a minimum safe level can be ascertained. These levels are 1.053 for women (corresponding to a hemoglobin level of approximately 12.5 g/dl) and 1.055 for men (corresponding to 13.5 g/dl). The test consists of allowing a drop of whole blood to fall through a copper sulfate solution made up to a specific gravity of 1.053 or 1.055. If the drop sinks, its specific gravity equals or exceeds that of the copper sulfate solution; if the drop rises to the top, its specific gravity is less. Inaccuracies arise if the copper sulfate solution changes its specific gravity, either through contamination or evaporation, or if there is anything besides hemoglobin in the blood that significantly affects specific gravity. Myeloma proteins, other abnormal globulins, and roentgenogram contrast materials are the most likely offenders.

Hematocrit (Packed Red Cell Volume)

Packed red cell volumes can be measured on venous or capillary blood with a macro or micro capillary technique. In the macro capillary technique, venous blood is sampled into a 100-mm-long graduated tube and centrifuged at 2260 *g* for 30 minutes. The volume of packed red cells and plasma is read directly from the millimeter marks along the sides of the tube. This method is no longer commonly employed.

The *microhematocrit* method uses either venous or capillary blood to fill a capillary tube approximately seven centimeters long and one millimeter in diameter. The filled tube is centrifuged from 4–5 minutes at 10,000 *g*, and the proportions of plasma and red cells are determined by means of a calibrated reading device. This method is rapid and simple; however, the centrifuge must be controlled for optimal centrifugal force and the tube must be carefully positioned and read out against the read-out scale. These techniques allow visual estimation of the volume of white cells and platelets that constitute the buffy coat between the red cells and the plasma (see also Color Plate 40A). The supernatant plasma should also be observed for jaundice or hemolysis. The hematocrit can also be determined using the automated electronic instruments, where it is calculated from the mean cell volume and red cell count.

Red Cell Count

Counting the red cells in a small volume of enormously diluted blood is inaccurate and rarely performed. Red cell counts are directly and accurately measured by electronic counters to give reliable and reproducible results. These instruments are programmed to give rapid computation of the corpuscular indices, which have now become a routine part of the complete blood count.

Corpuscular Indices (Red Cell Absolute Values)

The mean cell volume (MCV), mean cell hemoglobin (MCH) and mean cell hemoglobin concentration (MCHC) are sometimes referred to as the absolute red cell values and are calculated from the hematocrit (PCV), hemoglobin estimation, and red cell count. These values have been widely used in the classification of anemia and will be discussed in this context in the section on red cell diseases. Using the automated methods, the absolute values are calculated simultaneously with measured values, with the exception of the hematocrit, which is also a calculated value in the automated instruments. Hemoglobin or hematocrit values are commonly used to express the degree of anemia. These two determinations usually have a constant relationship—one hemoglobin unit in grams per deciliter is equivalent to three hematocrit units in percentage points. If, however, the erythrocyte is abnormal in size or shape or if hemoglobin manufacture is defective, there may be a disproportionate ratio.

The Mean Corpuscular Volume (MCV)

This represents the average volume of the red cells. With electronic counters the MCV is measured directly, but it may be calculated by dividing the hematocrit by the red cell count expressed in millions per microliter and multiplied by 1000. The answer is expressed in femtoliters (fl) per red cell (fl = 10^{-15} liters). The normal range is 80–100 fl.

Mean Corpuscular Hemoglobin (MCH)

This is automatically calculated in electronic counters, but may also be determined if the hemoglobin and red cell count are known. It is expressed in picograms, and may be calculated by dividing the amount of hemoglobin per liter of blood by the number of red cells per liter. The normal range is 26–32 picograms (pg = 10^{-12} grams, or micromicrograms).

Mean Corpuscular Hemoglobin Concentration (MCHC)

This is also calculated by the electronic counters following measurement of the hemoglobin and calculation of the hematocrit. It may be manually determined by dividing hemoglobin per deciliter of blood by the hematocrit. Reference values are 32–36%.

The size (MCV) and hemoglobin content (MCH) of individual cells are important in evaluating anemias and other hematologic abnormalities. Cell size may be described as *normocytic* with a normal MCV, *microcytic* with a less than normal MCV, or *macrocytic* with a greater than normal MCV. The degree of hemoglobinization of the cells can be appreciated by measuring the MCH and may be described as having normal mean hemoglobin *(normochromic)* or less than normal mean amounts of hemoglobin *(hypochromic)*.

Certain disorders are associated with an abnormally wide variation in red cell size, but an unremarkable *average* size. The resulting normal MCV may be misleading. Examination of the blood smear will detect this, but it can be electronically quantitated as the *red cell distribution width, or RDW.* The normal range is 11.6–14.6, with higher values indicating greater size variability (anisocytosis).

There is considerable variation in the hemoglobin content of the red cells at different periods of life. At birth, the hemoglobin value is higher than at any other time and falls in the immediate postnatal period. A value of 10–11 g/dl is normal for an infant of 3 months of age (see also Appendix C, Tables C2, C3).

Red Blood Cell Morphology on the Peripheral Blood Smear

Much diagnostic information can be gained by examining red cells on a well-prepared Wright-Giemsa-stained peripheral blood film. The best area is where the cells just touch without overlapping. The normal red cell is a biconcave disc, 6–8 μm in diameter. Hemoglobin imparts a reddish-orange appearance to the stained cell. The staining is deeper at the periphery of the cell, and gradually lessens as the center of the cell is approached (see Color Plate 5). The pale central area of the cell is normal and occupies approximately one third of the diameter. Cells that have a normal concentration of hemoglobin are described as *normochromic*. The outer portions of the cell stain more deeply than the center because there is a greater depth of hemoglobin solution around the periphery than in the flattened center. In the normal smear there is very little variation in size, shape, and staining characteristics *(normocytosis)*. A variation in the size of the cells is referred to as *anisocytosis*. This may occur if there is an increase in the number of small or large cells or a mixture of both. A variation in the shape of the cell is called *poikilocytosis*. Different shape variations may be important in the differential diagnosis of disease states. These will be discussed in the section on red cell diseases; however, alterations in the shape include those that are listed in Table 2–5 (see also Color Plates 10–14).

The term *hypochromia* is used to describe a decrease in the intensity of the hemoglobin staining. Hypochromia occurs when the area of central pallor occupies more than one third of the diameter of the cell (see Color Plate 30). Hypochromia, when seen in the blood film, is nearly always associated with a decrease in the MCHC. Red cells with a diffuse light blue or grayish tint in the cytoplasm are described as having *diffuse basophilia* (polychromasia) (see Color Plate 10B). These cells are young erythrocytes (reticulocytes) that have not yet completely lost their ribonucleic acid. These cells may be stained by supravital stains in reticulocyte preparations (see Color Plate 16A). They normally constitute less than 2% of the red cell population. Reticulocyte counts should be performed in any patient who has a prominent diffuse polychromasia. These cells are larger than normal and may raise the mean cell volume, producing an apparent *macrocytosis* (see also Reticulocyte Count, p. 31).

Red Blood Cell Inclusions and Stained Fragments

Basophilic Stippling

Basophilic RNA may also occur as fine stippling. This can occur in association with extensive diffuse polychromasia, but also occurs in toxic states such as lead poisoning and disorders of hemoglobin production (megaloblastic anemia and thalassemia) (see Color Plate 16C).

Howell-Jolly Bodies

These are fragments of nuclear DNA and appear as circumscribed, densely staining purple particles near the periphery of the cell (see Color Plate 10C and 32). The spleen normally removes inclusions of this sort. Cells containing *Howell-Jolly bodies* are almost always present after splenectomy, but may also occur with intense or abnormal erythrocyte production resulting from hemolysis or ineffective erythropoiesis.

Siderotic Granules

These are iron-containing granules not normally seen in *mature* erythrocytes; however, they can be present in situations associated with iron overload syndromes or after splenectomy. Special staining of these cells with Prussian Blue stain for iron may demonstrate these siderotic granules. When they are visible on Wright-Giemsa-stained smears they are called *Pappenheimer bodies.*

Heinz Bodies

These are masses of denatured hemoglobin invisible on Wright-Giemsa-stained smears, but easily seen with phase microscopy or supravital staining (see Color Plate 16B). They represent denatured hemoglobin precipitates occurring with severe oxidative stress (especially in patients with glucose 6-phosphate dehydrogenase deficiency) (see Chapter 3), or with the excess globin chain production that may occur

Table 2–5. RED BLOOD CELL ABNORMALITIES SEEN ON STAINED SMEAR

Descriptive Term	Observation	Significance
Macrocytosis	Cell diameter >8 μm MCV >100 fl	Megaloblastic anemias Severe liver disease Hypothyroidism
Microcytosis	Cell diameter <6 MCV <80 fl MCHC <27%	Iron deficiency anemia Thalassemias Anemia of chronic disease
Hypochromia	Increased zone of central pallor	Diminished hemoglobin content
Polychromatophilia	Presence of red cells not fully hemoglobinized	Reticulocytosis
Poikilocytosis	Variability of cell shape	Sickle cell disease Microangiopathic hemolysis Leukemias Extramedullary hematopoiesis Marrow stress of any cause
Anisocytosis	Variability of cell size	Reticulocytosis Transfusing normal blood into microcytic or macrocytic cell population
Leptocytosis	Hypochromic cells with small central zone of hemoglobin ("target cells")	Thalassemias Obstructive jaundice
Spherocytosis	Cells with no central pallor, loss of biconcave shape MCHC high	Loss of membrane relative to cell volume Hereditary spherocytosis Accelerated red blood cell destruction by reticuloendothelial system
Schistocytosis	Presence of cell fragments in circulation	Increased intravascular mechanical trauma Microangiopathic hemolysis
Acanthocytosis	Irregularly spiculated surface	Irreversibly abnormal membrane lipid content Liver disease Abetalipoproteinemia
Echinocytosis	Regularly spiculated cell surface	Reversible abnormalities of membrane lipids High plasma-free fatty acids Bile acid abnormalities Effects of barbiturates, salicylates, etc.
Stomatocytosis	Elongated, slit-like zone of central pallor	Hereditary defect in membrane transport of sodium Severe liver disease
Elliptocytosis	Oval cells	Hereditary anomaly, usually harmless

in thalassemias. Heinz bodies may also be seen following splenectomy, since the normal spleen removes all intraerythrocyte inclusions.

Nucleated Red Blood Cells

Normally, maturing red cells lose their nucleus well before they leave the bone marrow. If erythropoietic stress is intense, less mature cells may enter the circulation. In addition to numerous young reticulocytes, nucleated precursors occasionally may be seen. Their presence in the peripheral blood indicates either intense erythropoietic activity in the bone marrow, a damaged bone marrow due to infiltrative disease, or the existence of erythropoiesis in the spleen and other nonmarrow sites where there is less control over erythrocyte release into the blood stream (see Color Plates 38 and 39).

RED CELL METABOLISM

To perform its main function of oxygen transport, the erythrocyte must maintain its biconcave structure for maximal gas exchange, must be deformable to negotiate the small microcirculatory capillaries, and must have a constant internal environment to keep hemoglobin in a reduced form so it can transport the oxygen. Furthermore, the red cell survival must be normal. Its physical and chemical characteristics must be maintained within a narrow spectrum. To do this, erythrocyte metabolism must provide energy and chemical compounds capable of limiting excess oxidation. Abnormalities of these aspects of metabolism produce a shortened red cell survival (hemolysis), and investigation involves categorizing the nature of these metabolic defects. Various diseases producing hemolytic anemia and their laboratory investigation are discussed under Diseases of Red Blood Cells (Chapter 3).

The Red Cell Membrane

The erythrocyte membrane consists of an integral layer of lipids, including phospholipids and cholesterol, which contain an intimate association of proteins. These proteins may be internal or peripheral proteins. The protein–lipid composition is important in maintaining the integrity of the red cell membrane. The membrane also resists an uncontrolled influx of sodium ions, which are present in higher concentration in the plasma, and an efflux of potassium ions, which are present in higher concentration within the red cell. The membrane supports an active transport of sodium ions out of, and potassium ions into, the red cell. The process is critically dependent on an adequate energy source in the form of glucose. The principal external membrane protein is called *glycophorin.* This is a glycosylated protein that contains the majority of the red blood cell antigens. It is probably also responsible for supporting the red blood cell membrane cytoskeleton. The major internal protein is called *spectrin,* which also constitutes the most abundant membrane protein. Spectrin is also an important constituent of normal RBC membrane integrity, and is responsible for strengthening the membrane and resisting sheer stress from the circulatory system. The integrity of spectrin is maintained by providing energy in the form of adenosine triphosphate (ATP). A defective phosphorylation of spectrin is associated with loss of membrane integrity and decreased deformability. It is believed that this is the defect that occurs in hereditary spherocytosis. Loss of the red cell membrane is associated with the production of a *spherocyte* (see Color Plate 10A). An increase in membrane calcium also causes an increase in membrane rigidity. Spherocytes cannot traverse the small pores in the sinusoids of the spleen and are sequestered prematurely or have parts of their membrane removed, which causes their characteristic appearance.

LABORATORY ASSESSMENT OF RED CELL FRAGILITY (MEMBRANE FUNCTION)

Structural abnormalities, as well as some metabolic defects, may make red cells abnormally susceptible to *in vitro hemolysis* as well as *in vivo destruction.* In particular, in the disorder *hereditary spherocytosis,* the spherocytes are particularly fragile when exposed to *osmotic stress.* The test for *osmotic fragility* exposes red cells to increasingly dilute saline solutions in order to determine the point at which the internal flow of water into the erythrocyte causes the red cells to swell and rupture (see Fig. 3–1). Normal disc-shaped cells can imbibe water and swell significantly before membrane capacity is exceeded. Red cells with relatively less surface-area-to-volume ratio (spherocytes) will lyse after much smaller amounts of fluid enter. Spherocytes and other cells that have undergone membrane damage burst when exposed to saline solutions only slightly less concentrated than normal saline. The increased osmotic fragility is enhanced still further by incubating the cells at 37°C for 24 hours before exposing them to hypo-osmolar saline. Osmotic fragility is increased in autoimmune hemolytic anemia, presumably because the cells are more rigid than normal and undergo gradual membrane loss. In *thalassemia, iron deficiency anemia,* and *sickle cell disease,* red cells have excess membrane and are more than normally resistant to osmotic damage.

AUTOHEMOLYSIS

Normal red cells readily survive 48 hours of incubation at 37°C without any exogenous energy source. Red cells with defective ion transport or energy generation tend to hemolyze after 48 hours in their own defibrinated plasma with no added nutrients. The *autohemolysis test* can be used as a screening test for hereditary spherocytosis, since there is markedly increased autohemolysis that is virtually abolished by incubating the cells with an energy source (glucose or ATP). In the enzyme defect *glucose-6-phosphate dehydrogenase (G-6-PD) deficiency,* autohemolysis is modestly increased and neither ATP nor glucose has any effect. Cells with the enzyme deficiency *pyruvate kinase (PK) deficiency* show marked autohemolysis that is partially alleviated by ATP, but not by glucose. For *G-6-PD deficiency* and *PK deficiency,* however, better screening tests are readily available, as will be discussed below.

Erythrocyte Metabolic Pathways

EMBDEN-MEYERHOF PATHWAY

The majority of the energy needed by RBCs is provided by the *Embden-Meyerhof glycolytic pathway.* Through this pathway, each molecule of glucose is metabolized to produce 2 molecules of ATP (Fig. 2–9). This pathway functions anaerobically, and therefore glucose is not fully metabolized to yield the maximum number of ATP molecules. The red cell requires energy for several metabolic functions, which include:

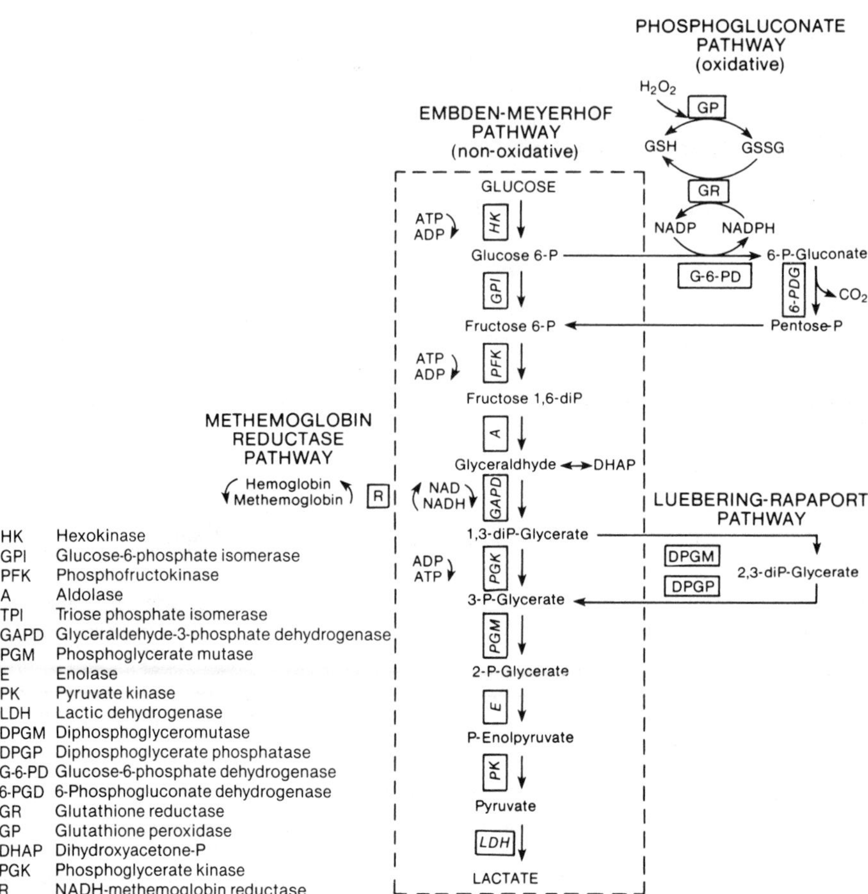

Figure 2–9. Red cell metabolic pathways. The anucleate red cell depends almost exclusively on the breakdown of glucose for energy requirements. The Embden-Meyerhof pathway (nonoxidative or anaerobic pathway) is responsible for most of the glucose utilization and generation of ATP. In addition, this pathway plays an essential role in maintaining pyridine nucleotides in a reduced state to support methemoglobin reduction (the methemoglobin reductase pathway) and 2,3-diphosphoglycerate synthesis (the Luebering-Rapaport pathway). The phosphogluconate pathway couples oxidative metabolism with pyridine nucleotide and glutathione reduction. It serves to protect red cells from environmental oxidants. (From Hillman and Finch,[4] p 14, with permission.)

- maintenance of hemoglobin as a respiratory pigment,
- maintenance of the electrolyte gradients between plasma and the erythrocyte cytoplasm,
- maintenance of the oxidation-reduction metabolic pathways, and
- the synthesis of lipids and nucleotides.

The defective production of energy can affect any or all of these pathways, which may then lead to shortened red cell survival.

Pentose Phosphate Pathway

As already mentioned, the Embden-Meyerhof pathway provides a net of 2 molecules of ATP and is probably the major energy source of the erythrocyte. Another major erythrocytic metabolic pathway is the *pentose phosphate pathway,* in which glucose is converted into *6-phosphogluconate* in the presence of the enzyme *glucose-6-phosphate dehydrogenase.* A pyridine nucleotide cofactor, nicotinamide adenine dinucleotide phosphate (NADP), is converted in this process to a reduced NADPH + H^+ form. This reduced cofactor provides reducing potential in the form of hydrogen ions for a compound called *glutathione,* which is the major reservoir of reducing potential in the erythrocyte. A series of intermediary steps are involved in this process, which is a self-rejuvenating process in the presence of several enzymes (see Fig. 2–9). The deficient production of reduced glutathione and NADP, which may occur in G-6-PD deficiency, is associated with increased oxidative stress on the erythrocyte membrane and many internal proteins. In particular, the globin chains of hemoglobin may become oxidized and lose the ability to keep ferrous iron (Fe^{2+}) in the reduced state. This allows the development of oxidized ferric (Fe^{3+}) iron and an unstable hemoglobin, which then cannot function as a respiratory pigment. The net result is shortened red cell survival and hemolysis. Approximately 5–10% of glucose is metabolized by the pentose phosphate pathway. An inability to neutralize oxidant stress produced by drugs or genetic deficiencies of the various enzymes can cause the accumulation of hydrogen peroxide and other oxidants. This can be visualized on supravital stains as the appearance of denatured globin aggregates *(Heinz bodies)* (see Color Plate 16B).

The commonest disorder associated with defective oxidative neutralization is deficiency of the enzyme *glucose-6-phosphate dehydrogenase.* This enzyme is pivotal to the generation of NADPH, is remarkably polymorphic, and is inherited through the X-chromosome. More than 50 structural variants are known in addition to the normal variants called type A and type B. Type A migrates faster than type B on electrophoresis, and it is found predominantly in blacks. Type B is found more commonly in whites. Many other structural variants have been found that may have normal or near normal activity; however, other variants may be dysfunctional or deficient. Since inheritance is X-linked, abnormalities are more commonly seen in men. Glucose-6-phosphate dehydrogenase deficiency is discussed in the section dealing with hemolytic anemias (Chapter 3).

Methemoglobin Reductase Pathway

Other pathways that are important in red cell metabolism are the *methemoglobin reductase pathways* (NAD^+ and $NADP^+$ methemoglobin reductase, respectively). These systems are responsible for the maintenance of hemoglobin in a reduced or ferrous state. The ferrous hemoglobin is an oxygen transporter by virtue of the maintenance of heme iron in the reduced, or ferrous, state (Fe^{2+}). The two pathways are responsible for the reduction of NAD^+ and $NADP^+$, and require the specific methemoglobin reductase enzymes. In the absence of these enzymes, there is accumulation of methemoglobin, which is the oxidized form of heme (ferric heme, Fe^{3+}). This form of hemoglobin is called *methemoglobin,* and has lost its ability to combine with respiratory oxygen.

The Formation of 2,3-Diphosphoglycerate (2,3-DPG)

Another integral pathway crucial to normal hemoglobin function is the Luebering-Rapaport Shunt, which is responsible for the production of *2,3-DPG* (see Fig. 2–9). This organic phosphate compound is important because it enhances oxygen displacement from hemoglobin and thus facilitates the delivery of oxygen to tissues where there is a low oxygen tension. This compound is present in the red cell in higher concentrations than in any other cell. It has an especially high affinity for Hemoglobin A and does not combine with some other hemoglobins, particular fetal hemoglobin (Hemoglobin F). This compound is thus responsible for shifting the hemoglobin dissociation curve to the right (see Hemoglobin: Oxygen Dissociation—Fig. 10–1), and is important when considering the age of stored blood for transfusion.

Tests to Evaluate the Pentose Phosphate Pathway

Clinically apparent dysfunction occurs only when the G-6-PD enzyme activity is less than 25% of normal. Defective function is uncovered by exposing red cells to an oxidizing stress. Nucleated erythrocytes and reticulocytes may still have the capacity to generate enough G-6-PD to resist oxidant stress in some forms of G-6-PD deficiency. In type A G-6-PD deficiency, only the mature erythrocyte is deficient in the enzyme.

The Ascorbate-Cyanide Test

This test challenges hemoglobin with hydrogen peroxide generated from sodium cyanide and sodium ascorbate. After incubation for one or two hours, brown methemoglobin is seen with *G-6-PD deficiency, PK deficiency, paroxysmal nocturnal hemoglobinuria,* and *unstable hemoglobins,* whereas normal blood remains bright red. The ascorbate-cyanide test is sensitive enough to detect the minimally reduced activity that occurs in G-6-PD heterozygotes and in homozygotes with temporarily increased activity levels; it is not, however, specific for G-6-PD deficiency.

The NADPH Fluorescent Test

This test is specific for *G-6-PD deficiency* and its effect on NADP. If G-6-PD is present, reducing activity is generated, converting NADP to fluorescent NADPH, which appears as a readily visible spot under ultraviolet light. Blood samples up to several weeks old are suitable for use, and the results are moderately sensitive.

The Methylene Blue-Methemoglobin Test

Muddy brown *methemoglobin* evolves from the transparent red hemoglobin solution if G-6-PD is severely deficient. This test can detect homozygote-deficient women or deficient hemizygotes, but is not sensitive enough to detect female heterozygotes.

Specific enzyme assays and electrophoretic characterization permit the definitive diagnosis of G-6-PD deficiency. Except in rare cases or for characterizing unusual genetic variants, the above screening tests provide all the information needed for clinical diagnosis. The oldest procedure, now rarely used, is to induce *Heinz bodies* by incubating the blood with the oxidant drug *acetylphenylhydrazine.* The screening tests mentioned above are, however, better screening procedures and use chemical endpoints to demonstrate whether or not there is sufficient G-6-PD to generate protective reducing activity.

Young cells have higher G-6-PD levels than older ones, regardless of the genetic variant that is present. If the enzyme is defective, older cells are preferentially destroyed during a mild to moderate hemolytic event. *Reticulocytes* generated to replace lost cells have higher activity levels. False negative test results often occur if blood is examined just after a hemolytic episode, because the reticulocytes and nonhemolyzed remaining cells are, by definition, those with adequate levels. Newly generated reticulocytes have still higher levels, and this can affect the results for 3–10 days after a hemolytic episode. The ascorbate-cyanide test is usually sensitive enough to detect reduced activity under these circumstances, but the test should be repeated after red cell production is stabilized.

Erythrocyte Senescence and Hemoglobin Catabolism

During its lifespan of 120 days, the erythrocyte travels approximately 200–300 miles. In the process of aging, there is a slow metabolic down-grading of the red cells. Many enzymes show reduced function and the cells become more sensitive to osmotic lysis. Approximately 1% of the red cells are removed from circulation daily by the reticuloendothelial system. These cells are replaced by reticulocytes from the bone marrow. In addition to the metabolic changes, the loss of the red cell membrane leads to less deformability. As these senescent red cells are removed in the extravascular reticuloendothelial system, the hemoglobin molecule is broken down into its component parts. Approximately 5–7 g of hemoglobin are catabolized daily. The iron is salvaged, as was mentioned in the section Iron Metabolism. The globin portion of the hemoglobin molecule is broken down into amino acids that are recirculated to the amino acid pool. The porphyrin component of the heme molecule is broken down by a series of catabolic steps into a compound called *bilirubin,* which is a brownish-yellow pigment. Bilirubin is bound to albumin and transported to the liver. In the liver it is conjugated by the addition of glucuronides to form a *diglucuronide compound,* which is water-soluble and excreted in the bile (see Liver Function Tests—Chapter 12). A small proportion of this compound is reabsorbed and re-excreted (Fig. 2–10). By bacterial action in the bowel, the bilirubin conjugate is further broken down into *urobilinogen* and *stercobilinogen* and excreted in the stool. A small amount of these compounds are reabsorbed through the enterohepatic circulation and excreted in the urine.

MEASUREMENT OF RED CELL SURVIVAL

Red cell lifespan can be measured by several techniques. The most commonly used technique is the *random method,* where a radioactive label (either ^{51}Cr or ^{111}In) is attached randomly to red cells of all ages after removal of an aliquot of blood from the patient. The rate at which the label disappears corresponds to the progressive destruction of an unselected cell population. The usual endpoint is the half-disappearance time, which under normal conditions is 28–35 days (with ^{51}Cr). With accelerated destruction, the endpoint may be less than a week or even hours. Radioactive chromate is an effective red cell label because it binds specifically to hemoglobin. Its biologic half-life is not excessively long; it emits an easily counted high-energy gamma ray and it does not affect the survival of the cell that incorporates it. Chromium labeling can be used to measure the survival time of the patient's own cells, or that of transfused, homologous cells in the patient. After introduction of the labeled cells, the baseline radioactivity level indicates the proportion of the total circulating cells that bear the label. This figure is necessary for later comparisons and, with suitable calculation of dilution, it demonstrates the patient's *red cell volume* (see Erythrocytosis, p. 120).

Survival is measured by observing blood samples at intervals in order to deter-

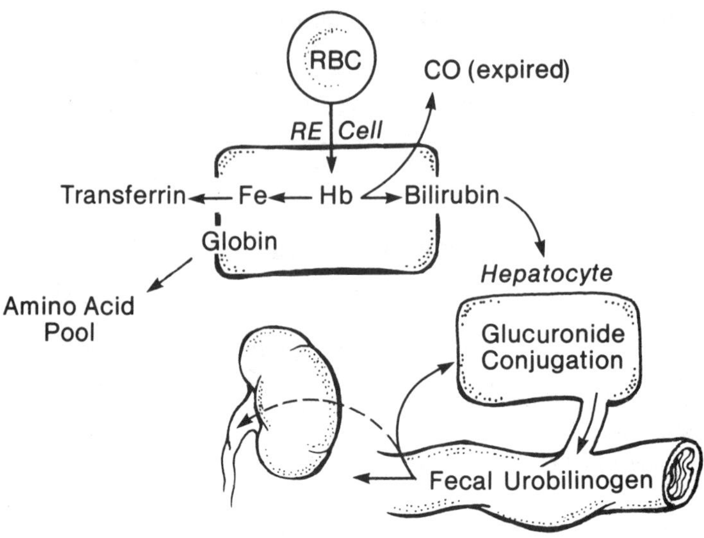

Figure 2–10. Red cell destruction by the reticuloendothelial system. Normally, senescent red cells are phagocytized by reticuloendothelial cells and the hemoglobin is broken down into its essential components. The iron recovered is returned to transferrin for new red cell production and the amino acids from the globin portion of the molecule are returned to the general amino acid pool. The protoporphyrin ring of heme is broken at the alpha methene bridge and its alpha carbon exhaled as carbon monoxide. The remaining tetrapyrrole leaves the reticuloendothelial cell as indirect bilirubin and travels to the liver where it is conjugated for excretion in the bile. In the gut, the bilirubin glucuronide is converted to urobilinogen for excretion in stool and urine. (From Hillman and Finch,[4] p 19, with permission.)

mine the amount of radioactivity remaining in the circulation. Normally, half of the initial dose will have disappeared in 28–35 days. This figure is often used inaccurately as the half-life of red cells. The half-life of normal red cells is 60 days. ^{51}Cr half disappearance time is less because 1% or more of the radioactive label elutes from the red cells every day and is lost to counting. A ^{51}Cr half-time ($T_{1/2}$) of less than 25 days indicates accelerated destruction. This can be as low as 3–5 days in severe intrinsic hemolytic conditions, or can be measured in minutes or hours if there is antibody-mediated destruction.

With markedly accelerated destruction, the ^{51}Cr label from hemolyzed cells accumulates at the site of cell damage. It has been shown that the spleen is responsible for most hemolysis in some intrinsic hemolytic conditions, and is responsible for the removal of damaged cells in other conditions. The accumulation of radioactivity in the liver or spleen can give an insight into the different pathogenetic mechanisms. Intravascular hemolysis occurs with strong complement binding antibodies such as anti-A and anti-B, or with toxic, chemical, or physical damage to the cells.

Hemoglobin Release and Degradation

Free Hemoglobin. Only 5–10% of normal red cell destruction occurs in the vascular system through the process of intravascular hemolysis. When red cells are destroyed within the bloodstream, hemoglobin enters the plasma. Here it dissociates into alpha and beta dimers and complexes with *haptoglobin,* an alpha$_2$ globulin normally present in concentrations of 30–200 mg/dl. This quantity is sufficient to dispose of up to 100 mg of free hemoglobin per 100 ml of plasma. This complex is transported to the liver cell for further catabolism, promoting conservation of the iron in heme and preventing renal losses. Haptoglobin levels, therefore, fall, and the reduction of measurable haptoglobin is one important laboratory sign of *intravascular hemolysis.* Haptoglobin may also drop when the reticuloendothelial system is the site of hemolysis (extravascular hemolysis), since haptoglobin may leak from the spleen or other sinusoids into the bloodstream. As little as 1–2 ml of RBC hemolysis in the intravascular compartment can totally deplete plasma haptoglobin. Another plasma protein, *hemopexin,* also augments the capacity of the plasma to conserve hemoglobin, binding preferentially to *heme.* Low or absent haptoglobins are often found in any chronic hemolytic process, and typically return to normal a week after the cessation of hemolysis.

Haptoglobin. Haptoglobin levels are measured either chemically or, more easily, by immunologic techniques, in particular radial-immunodiffusion or electrophoresis.

Once the binding capacity of haptoglobin has been exceeded, free hemoglobin appears in the plasma. Since free hemoglobin is a small molecule, it can be excreted in the urine. *Hemoglobinemia* and *hemoglobinuria* occur when the haptoglobin capacity for binding hemoglobin dimers is saturated.

Other Tests of Intravascular Hemolysis

Urinary Hemosiderin. With chronic intravascular hemolysis and hemoglobinuria, pigment is reabsorbed by the renal tubules and may ultimately appear as iron granules within renal cells. Some renal tubular cells are desquamated as a normal process. A sample of urine can be collected, centrifuged, and stained for iron. The presence of intracellular iron granules within the desquamated renal tubular cells is indicative of chronic intravascular hemolysis with iron loss in the urine.

Methemalbumin. With intravascular hemolysis and the release of pigment into the plasma, the plasma color may change depending on the type of hemoglobin present. *Oxyhemoglobin* is bright red and *methemoglobin* is dark brown. Similarly, the color of the serum or urine depends on the nature of the pigment released into the plasma. Methemoglobin is the oxidized version of hemoglobin with iron converted into the ferric state (Fe^{3+}). Free metheme may be bound to the other transport conservation protein, *hemopexin* (mentioned above), and transported to the liver for further catabolism. Hemopexin has the capacity to bind 50–100 mg/dl of heme. Once this capacity is exceeded, metheme binds to albumin. The various hemoglobin compounds may be detected by spectroscopic analysis of the plasma, and show specific absorption spectra. Methemalbumin has a typical absorption peak at 630 nm, and forms a characteristic hemochromogen color at 558 nm after the addition of ammonium sulfide as performed in the *Schumm's test.* Both the presence of methemalbumin and a positive Schumm's test are indicative of intravascular hemolysis. Methemalbumin remains stable in the plasma until more hemopexin is synthesized to activate transport molecules. Therefore, methemalbumin is more indicative of a chronic intravascular hemolysis (Fig. 2–11).

The catabolism of iron following disassembly in senescent red cells has been discussed under the section of iron metabolism earlier in this chapter. A more complete discussion of the clinical disorders responsible for shortened red cell survival and hemolysis is presented in the section on diseases of red cells (see Chapter 3).

Lactic Dehydrogenase (LDH). With rupture (hemolysis) of the erythrocyte, its internal enzymes are released and may be measured in the bloodstream. Lactic

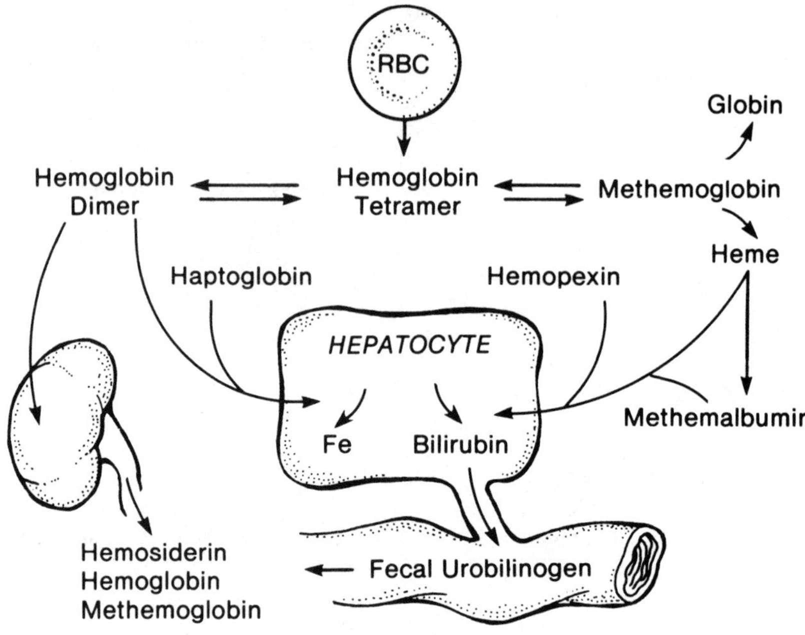

Figure 2–11. Intravascular red cell hemolysis. Red cells can also undergo intravascular hemolysis with the release of hemoglobin into circulation. The free hemoglobin tetramer is unstable and rapidly dissociates into alpha beta dimers, which bind to haptoglobin and are removed by the liver. Hemoglobin may also be oxidized to methemoglobin and dissociate into its globin and heme moieties. To a limited extent, free heme can be bound by hemopexin and/or albumin for subsequent clearance by hepatocytes. Both pathways help recover heme iron for the support of hematopoiesis. Once haptoglobin is depleted, unbound hemoglobin dimers are excreted by the kidney as free hemoglobin, methemoglobin, or hemosiderin. (From Hillman and Finch,[4] p 20, with permission.)

dehydrogenase is one such enzyme, and it is usually elevated in clinically significant hemolysis (see Chapters 3 and 12).

Indirect Bilirubin. Bilirubin, the breakdown product of heme catabolism, also usually accumulates in significant hemolysis, especially the unconjugated or indirect fraction, prior to its delivery to the liver for conjugation and excretion (see Chapters 3 and 12).

PERIPHERAL BLOOD: WHITE CELLS

Circulating blood contains approximately 4,000–11,000 white cells per microliter. The normal peripheral blood white cells comprise, morphologically and functionally, distinct populations of three main types: granulocytes, lymphocytes, and monocytes. These cells constitute the normal leukocyte population, but a small number of circulating white cells may be in the penultimate stage of maturation. The morphologic characteristics of the nucleus and cytoplasm of these cells defines the specific categories and level of maturation, and the relative percentage of these cells may provide information on different disease states. The absolute numbers of the different types of cells may also provide clues as to whether a primary marrow disorder is present, or whether abnormalities are reactive to a secondary disease process.

White Blood Cell Count

White cells are distinguished from circulating red cells by the presence of a nucleus (see Color Plates 4 and 6). Automated counting procedures enumerate all nucleated cells as white cells. If large numbers of nucleated red cells are present, they too are counted and the white cell count may have to be suitably corrected. In spite of this, the total white count is usually determined without difficulty. The *differential white count* gives the proportions of the different cell types that constitute the total number of white cells. Differential counts are sometimes omitted if the total count is normal and there is no clinical or laboratory evidence of hematologic abnormality. However, many neoplastic, inflammatory, and immunologic conditions alter cellular proportions despite a normal level for total white cells.

Like red cell counts, white counts use a small sample of diluted blood and are subject to sampling and dilutional errors. Because blood contains far fewer white than red cells, the dilution is less, and a larger volume of blood is examined than in red cell counting. Most laboratories use automated methods for white cell counting, either by electronic particle counting or by light-scattering principles. Manual dilution and visual examination of hemocytometer counts remain reliable when carefully performed. Manual methods are usually performed to corroborate exceedingly high or low electronic white cell counts.

Visual examination of stained blood films remains the mainstay of differential white cell counting, but automated procedures are gaining acceptance. Two different automated approaches are in use. In one of these, a sophisticated computer program for pattern recognition is linked with a lens that scans the stained blood film. This is fundamentally the same approach as that of the human eye and brain. The count is usually done on 100, 200, or 500 cells. A completely different technology separates the various kinds of white cells by manipulating the chemical properties of the medium in a continuous flow system, and then enumerates the individual populations by light-scattering and absorbance techniques. Much larger numbers of white cells are sampled in the automated approach (10,000 cells).

Granulocytes

In adults, half or more of circulating white cells are granulocytes, the cytoplasm of which contains readily visible granules of various chemical and enzymatic compositions. As previously discussed, there are three main types of granulocytes, termed *neutrophils, eosinophils,* and *basophils* (see Color Plates 4 and 6). The staining characteristics of the granules define the cell type: specifically, neutral staining characterizes neutrophils, reddish (eosinophilic) staining granules characterize eosinophils, and bluish granules define basophils. The *myeloblast* is the earliest cell recognizably committed to granulocytic identity (see Fig. 2–2 and Color Plates 2 and 33), and typically contains no granules. Specific granules are first seen in the *promyelocytes,* the next developmental phase after differentiation from a myeloblast. In health, maturation occurs only within the bone marrow. Granulocytes normally develop and mature at no other site, and once released from the marrow cannot reproduce. With intense stimulation to increase circulating granulocytes, immature cells of this series may appear in the blood. Immature or abnormal granulocytes sometimes enter the circulation if bone marrow control mechanisms are deranged by malignant processes, or when hematopoietic activity occurs outside of the marrow, as may happen in neoplastic myeloproliferative diseases.

NEUTROPHILS

The cytoplasmic granules of neutrophils react with both basic and acidic stains, producing "neutral" or light purple granules on the most commonly used Wright-Giemsa stain preparations. In the mature cell, nucleochromatin is condensed into discrete lumps or lobes connected by thin strands of material. These cells are called *polymorphonuclear leukocytes* because there are so many (poly-) possible forms (morph-) that these flexibly linked nuclear lumps can assume. Acceptable shortened terms for this polysyllabic description are *PMNs* and *"polys."* Less mature neutrophils have larger nuclei that are not separated into lobes. The state that precedes maturity is called a *band cell* because its nucleus is shaped like a curved band.

Neutrophils are actively motile, and large numbers can congregate at sites of tissue injury within a short time. They are attracted to sites of injury and inflammation by a process called *chemotaxis.* Microbial products, the products of cellular injury, and many plasma proteins can exert a chemotactic effect on neutrophils. Neutrophils constitute the body's first line of defense when tissue is damaged or foreign material gains entry into the body. Their function is closely aligned to other defense systems of the body, including antibody production *(immunoglobulins)* and activation of the *complement system* (see Chapter 7). The interaction of these systems with neutrophils enhances their ability to *phagocytize* and degrade particles of many sorts. They are capable of releasing enzymes into their own cytoplasm, destroying ingested or phagocytized material, and they also can release enzymes into the surrounding medium. One way to identify abnormal or ambiguous immature cells as members of the neutrophil series is to elicit these enzyme reactions with cytochemical techniques (see section on Cytochemical Staining). The neutrophil granules may be divided into *primary granules,* which appear at the *promyelocyte stage,* and *secondary granules,* which appear at the *myelocyte stage* and predominate in the mature granulocytes. The *primary* granules contain *myeloperoxidase* and *acid phosphatase* as well as other acid hydrolytic enzymes, whereas the *secondary* granules contain *alkaline phosphatase* and the enzyme *lysozyme.*

The principle function of neutrophils is the phagocytosis and removal of debris, particulate material, and bacteria, as well as the killing of microbial organisms. Their only proven useful role is preventing invasion by pathogenic microorganisms, and localizing and killing them following successful invasion. The circulating neutrophils released from the bone marrow may align themselves closely to the blood vessel and are called *marginating neutrophils,* or may remain within the circulating bloodstream (see Fig. 2–3). It is probably the marginal neutrophils that are released to tissue sites when needed. Normally the rate at which new cells enter the blood from the bone marrow is equal to the rate at which cells egress to the tissues. Egress from the circulation by neutrophils is random, and a mature neutrophil remains in the bloodstream for approximately 7–10 hours before it exits to the tissues and body cavities. There is no evidence that neutrophils ever return to the bone marrow from the blood, and therefore this functional pathway may be considered to proceed in one direction only. The abnormalities in production and distribution within the bloodstream will be considered in Diseases of White Blood Cells.

Eosinophils

Eosinophils are granulocytes with a two-lobed nucleus and moderately large, refractile granules that stain deep red with the acidic dye eosin (see Color Plate 6A). Although capable of phagocytosis, eosinophils are not bactericidal. The eosinophil contains several enzymes that inactivate mediators of acute inflammation and, like the neutrophil, it contains *histaminase.* The biologic role of eosinophils seems to be the modulation of cellular and chemical activities in immunologically mediated inflammation. Although during development these cells resemble developing neutrophils, they have distinct terminal stem cells as well as differing chemistries, kinetics, and functions. The normal range for eosinophils is 0–700 cells per microliter. Unlike the neutrophil, the eosinophil probably returns from tissues to blood and from blood to marrow under normal circumstances. It may also respond to the same chemotactic stimuli as neutrophils. The eosinophil is more sluggish and inefficient in phagocytosis and the killing of bacteria. In inflammation much of their function is unknown. Eosinophils also have a unique ability to damage larvae of certain helminth parasites.

Basophils

Basophils constitute less than 1% of normal circulating leukocytes. Their large, coarse cytoplasmic granules stain deeply with blue basic dye and are brilliantly stained by metachromatic dyes (see Color Plate 6B). The granules contain acid-mucopolysaccharides, hyaluronic acid, and large amounts of histamine. Basophils in the circulation serve no known function. Cells very similar to blood basophils are plentiful in skin, in the mucosa of the respiratory tract, and in connective tissue. These cells, called *mast cells,* contain histamine and other materials in their granules responsible for causing allergic tissue reactions. Tissue basophils, but not blood basophils, have immunoglobulin E (IgE) receptors adherent to the cell membrane; these receptors react with allergens and IgE to induce the release of vasoactive mediators, which have many different effects. The massive release of granule contents may evoke sudden death (anaphylactic shock). Many of the mediators cause smooth muscle contraction and increase vascular permeability. Basophils also release chemotactic factors and other chemical mediators of inflammation.

Abnormal Granulocyte Morphology

It is abnormal for more than 8–10% of the circulating neutrophils to be band forms, or for there to be any earlier precursors at all in the peripheral blood. Certain morphologic abnormalities may be seen in mature granulocytes that may be indicative of an acquired or hereditary abnormality.

Acquired Abnormalities

Toxic Granulation. In the cytoplasm of neutrophils from severely ill or infected patients or from those in whom tissue destruction or inflammation has occurred, more prominent, coarsely staining cytoplasmic granules can be seen (see Color Plate 19). These are thought to be abnormally activated, enzyme-containing granules rather than inclusion bodies or phagocytized material. Frequently, the cytoplasm of these stimulated cells is vacuolated or takes a more basic stain than normal. Cytoplasmic vacuolization is another abnormal finding that, together with toxic granulation, is often seen accompanying bacterial sepsis.

Döhle Bodies. Neutrophils may sometimes contain large, round, pale blue masses in the periphery of the cytoplasm called Döhle bodies (see Color Plate 20). These may occur with severe infections, burns, malignancies, or extensive cell lysis, but may also be found in normal pregnancy. The masses seem to be aggregated, rough endoplasmic reticulum. Their presence reflects the same metabolic alterations that stimulate rapid neutrophil degranulation and toxic granulation.

Azurophilic Granules. As granulocytes and other leukocytes develop, they may have numerous small, smoothly rounded, red cytoplasmic granules that contain a variety of lysosomal enzymes. As specific granules develop, these azurophilic granules decline sharply, but a few may persist in the cytoplasm of mature lymphocytes, monocytes, or granulocytes. They may have no pathologic significance.

Hypersegmentation and Macropolycytes. Disorders of folic acid or vitamin B_{12} metabolism produce many morphologic abnormalities, of which megaloblastic red cell development is the most conspicuous. Other rapidly proliferating cells also manifest abnormal developmental changes. Granulocytic cells tend to be abnormally large, especially metamyelocytes in the marrow (Giant metamyelocytes) and neutrophils in the peripheral blood. These neutrophils have nuclei with seven or eight lobes instead of the normal three–five lobes, and an abundant but morphologically normal cytoplasm (see Color Plate 25).

Hereditary Abnormalities

Alder-Reilly Anomaly. In this disorder, the neutrophils contain giant, dark-staining granules filled with polysaccharides. Patients with this disorder have systemic abnormalities of mucopolysaccharide metabolism leading to gargoylism in Hunter's syndrome, Hurler's syndrome, and other mucopolysaccharidoses.

May-Hegglin Anomaly. These neutrophils contain large blue or pinkish bodies, resembling Döhle bodies, that distort the cytoplasm of myeloid and monocytic cells. Moderate thrombocytopenia and abnormal platelet morphology often accompany leukopenia in this condition, but the patients generally remain in good health.

Pelger-Huet Phenomenon. Two forms of this morphologic anomaly may occur, the acquired and the inherited variety. The inherited disorder represents a purely morphologic aberration in which the neutrophils have a bilobed or monolobed nucleus and coarse chromatin, but are functionally normal. In the acquired disorder, a similar morphology may be seen in persons with myeloproliferative diseases. These mature neutrophils are often mistaken for immature or band forms.

Chediak-Higashi Anomaly. Chediak-Higashi syndrome is a rare autosomal recessive disorder of lysosomal function and structure, leading to the accumulation of giant lysosomes containing various hydrolases and other enzymes. This change is most conspicuous in neutrophils, but it also affects many epithelial cells, nerve cells, and the pigment-containing melanocytes in the skin, hair, and eyes. Anemia, thrombocytopenia, decreased leukocyte counts, and increased susceptibility to infection characterize a frequently downhill clinical course. Aleutian mink, prized for the color of their fur, suffer from a similar form of partial cutaneous albinism and severe susceptibility to infection. The function of these unusual leukocytes is abnormal, which contributes to the susceptibility to infections.

Lymphocytes

Lymphocytes constitute the second most numerous leukocyte in the peripheral blood. These cells are essential components of the immune defense system; their primary function is to interact with antigens and mount an immune response. The latter may be 1) *humoral,* in the form of antibody production; 2) cell mediated, with elaboration of *lymphokines* by lymphocytes; or 3) cytotoxic, with the production of *cytotoxic killer lymphocytes.* Not only are the absolute quantities of these cells important, but so are the relative proportions of their different subclasses. This is well demonstrated in the devastating disease acquired immunodeficiency syndrome (AIDS), in which the infecting virus selectively attacks one lymphocyte subtype. The role of the lymphocyte in immune function is discussed in the section devoted to Immunology (Chapter 7).

Circulating blood lymphocytes constitute a tiny fraction (<5%) of the total lymphocyte pool. Dense concentrations are found in the lymph nodes, the spleen, and the mucosa of the alimentary and respiratory tracts, while diffuse numbers exist in the bone marrow, liver, skin, and chronically inflamed tissue. There is a continuous circulation of lymphocytes from one compartment to another, which is normally maintained in equilibrium. There are two primary subtypes, T-lymphocytes and B-lymphocytes, each performing unique immunologic functions (see Fig. 2–2). In healthy adults, about 75–80% of the circulating lymphocytes are T cells and 10–15% are B cells, while the remainder exhibit neither characteristic and are termed "null" cells. *T-lymphocytes* are responsible for *cell-mediated immunity* and modulating *immune responsiveness. B-lymphocytes* are largely responsible for *humoral immunity* and *antibody production.* T-lymphocytes appear to recirculate much more widely than do their B-lymphocyte counterparts, and have a longer life span (months or years compared with weeks or months). Most lymphocytes in the blood and lymphatic tissues are small cells less than 10 μm in diameter. They have deep-staining nuclei that are round or slightly indented, and coarse, ill-defined aggregates of chromatin (see Color Plates 4, 21–23). Nucleoli are usually not present. The cytoplasm often stains intensely blue, and in most cases is seen as a scanty rim around the nucleus. Larger lymphoid cells occur less frequently, constituting approximately 10% of the circulating lymphocytes. These cells are between 12–16 μm in diameter with an abundant cytoplasm, often containing azurophilic granules. They may represent *natural killer-cytotoxic lymphocytes* (see Color Plate 21), and probably represent active, antigenically stimulated cells.

LYMPHOCYTE SUBPOPULATIONS

The process of T- and B-lymphocyte development may be studied in the laboratory by quantitating secretory products (lymphokines or antibodies), or by using specific reagents to identify the cell surface characteristics (phenotypic or immunologic). The use of monoclonal antibodies specifically directed against single cell membrane receptors has enabled the characterization of several lymphocyte subpopulations whose functional diversity is only now becoming appreciated. The goals of these cells in *immune function* and their *laboratory detection* are discussed in the section on Immunology (Chapter 7).

ATYPICAL LYMPHOCYTES

Most immune activities occur outside of the bloodstream, but altered immune responsiveness sometimes produces characteristic changes in circulating lymphocytes. The *"atypical lymphocyte,"* or Downey cell, is a T-lymphocyte in a state of immune activation, and is classically associated with *infectious mononucleosis.* In infectious mononucleosis, the inciting agent is the Epstein-Barr virus (EBV), but other viral stimuli such as the cytomegalovirus (CMV) may also stimulate immune responsive (atypical) lymphocytes (see Color Plate 22).

Monocytes

Monocytes constitute 5–8% of circulating blood leukocytes. Only small numbers of monocytes circulate at any one time. These cells share a stem cell with neutrophils, but their maturation pathways subsequently diverge (see Fig. 2–2). Their precursor cells *(monoblasts)* are well demonstrated by staining with *esterase stains.* The mature monocyte circulates only briefly in the peripheral blood, and then enters the tissues to become a *macrophage.* Known by many names, it appears that "fixed" and "wandering" macrophages, histiocytes, the Kupffer cells of the liver, sinusoidal macrophages in the spleen and lymph nodes, peritoneal macrophages, and the macrophages that line the pulmonary air spaces all originate from the same primordial cell population. Their placement within the tissues seems to influence subsequent maturation and function. For example, the enzymatic compositions of pulmonary and peritoneal macrophages are quite different. Within the tissues, these macrophages may fuse into one another and become multinucleated giant cells that are especially prominent in *granulomatous inflammation.* Inflammation may stimulate monocytes to migrate from the blood into the tissues, but at a slower rate than neutrophils. They are particularly evident in subacute and chronic inflammation. These cells play a vital role in many host defense mechanisms. They are particularly active in the phagocytosis and killing of microorganisms, as well as many complex interactions with immunogens and with the cellular and protein constituents of the immune system. They may initiate and regulate the magnitude of the immune response. They are also responsible for antigen recognition and processing. By processing and presenting antigens to responsive T- and B-lymphocytes, monocytes initiate both cell-mediated and humoral immune responses. They also secrete various soluble, biologically active substances called *monokines,* among them interleukin-1 (see Fig. 2–2). This factor promotes the proliferative response and expression of T cell membrane receptors. Their interaction with lymphocytes, in particular T-lymphocytes, is highly integrated and complex and is further discussed in Chapter 7.

Blood monocytes characteristically are large (16–20 μm), with delicate nuclear chromatin. They have elongated, indented, or folded (kidney-shaped) nuclei and abundant, greyish-blue, translucent-looking cytoplasm (see Color Plate 6C). More immature forms, which circulate under conditions of monocytic stress or abnormal marrow proliferation, have a larger nucleus, sometimes a nucleolus, and more basophilic cytoplasm with more azurophilic granules than the mature forms. It is not clear how conditions such as tuberculosis or other inflammatory or immunologic events influence monocyte production, but bone marrow response can clearly be demonstrated.

Abnormal Differential White Cell Counts

Since the differential white count is reported in percentages, the total white count must be known in order to understand the pathophysiologic significance of the differential. Proportions change, either because there is a true increase in the numbers of preponderant cells *(absolute increase)* or because of a decline in the numbers of one cell type, which makes the remaining cells appear increased *(relative increase).*

Circulating white cell counts are remarkably volatile. Absolute and relative values can change within minutes or hours of stimulation. The most dramatic variations in the differential count occur following the release of *corticosteroid* hormones. Steroids cause lymphocytes and eosinophils to disappear from the circulation within 4–8 hours. Circulating granulocytes increase somewhat later, probably because of reduced egress from the bloodstream. *Epinephrine,* the hormone of the adrenal medulla, causes *granulocytosis* within minutes, probably by mobilizing mature neutrophils from "storage" or noncirculating locations. Most of the physiologic stimuli that induce neutrophil leukocytosis (e.g., exercise, emotional stress, exposure to extreme temperatures) appear to act by stimulating epinephrine output. Still unexplained is how a localized, acute, inflammatory stimulus induces the bone marrow toward sustained increases of neutrophil production and release. Tables 2-6, 2-7, and 4-4 list conditions that affect neutrophil numbers.

Lymphocyte proportions often reflect relative changes caused by absolute alterations in granulocyte levels. Conditions that increase absolute lymphocyte numbers are shown in Table 2-8. Relative lymphocytosis is common in acute viral syndromes and other infectious conditions that cause neutropenia. In some acute leukemias, a relative preponderance of lymphocytes may be noted in the peripheral blood

Table 2-6. CONDITIONS CAUSING NEUTROPHILIA (>8000 PMNs/μl)

Physiologic response to stress:
- Physical exercise
- Exposure to extreme heat or cold
- Following acute hemorrhage or hemolysis
- Acute emotional stress
- Childbirth

Infectious diseases:
- Systemic or severe local bacterial infections
- Some viruses (smallpox, chicken pox, herpes zoster, polio)
- Some rickettsial diseases (especially Rocky Mountain spotted fever)
- Some fungi, especially if there is acute tissue necrosis

Inflammatory diseases:
- Acute rheumatic fever
- Rheumatoid arthritis
- Acute gout
- Vasculitis and myositis of many types
- Hypersensitivity reactions to drugs

Tissue necrosis:
- Ischemic damage to heart, abdominal viscera, extremities
- Burns
- Many carcinomas and sarcomas

Metabolic disorders:
- Uremia
- Diabetic ketoacidosis
- Eclampsia
- Thyroid storm

Drugs:
- Epinephrine
- Lithium
- Histamine
- Heparin
- Digitalis
- Many toxins, venoms, and heavy metals

Table 2–7. CONDITIONS CAUSING NEUTROPENIA (<1500 PMNs/μl)

Infectious diseases:
- Some bacteria (typhoid, tularemia, brucellosis)
- Some viruses (hepatitis, influenza, measles, mumps, rubella, infectious mononucleosis)
- Protozoa (especially malaria)
- Overwhelming infection of any kind

Chemical and physical agents:
- Dose-related, universal marrow depressants (radiation, cytotoxic drugs, benzene)
- Idiosyncratic drug reactions (numerous)

Hypersplenism:
- Liver disease
- Storage diseases

Other disorders:
- Some collagen-vascular diseases, especially lupus erythematosus
- Severe folic acid or vitamin B_{12} deficiency

Table 2–8. CONDITIONS AFFECTING LYMPHOCYTE COUNTS

Lymphocytosis (>4000 lymphocytes/μl in adults; >7200/μl in children):
- Infectious diseases:
  - Bacterial (whooping cough, brucellosis, sometimes tuberculosis, secondary syphilis)
  - Viral (hepatitis, infectious mononucleosis, mumps, many exanthems, cytomegalovirus)
  - Other (infectious lymphocytosis, toxoplasmosis)
- Metabolic conditions:
  - Hypoadrenalism
  - Hyperthyroidism (sometimes)
- Chronic inflammatory conditions:
  - Ulcerative colitis
  - Immune diseases (serum sickness, idiopathic thrombocytopenic purpura)

Lymphocytopenia (<1000 lymphocytes/μl in adults; <2500/μl in children):
- Immunodeficiency syndromes:
  - Congenital defects of cell-mediated immunity
  - Immunosuppressive medication
- Adrenal corticosteroid exposure:
  - Adrenal gland hyperactivity
  - ACTH-producing pituitary gland tumors
  - Therapeutic administration of steroids
- Severe, debilitating illness of any kind:
  - Congestive heart failure
  - Renal failure
  - Far-advanced tuberculosis
- Defects of lymphatic circulation:
  - Intestinal lymphangiectasia
  - Disorders of intestinal mucosa
  - Thoracic duct drainage

when the neutrophil count is decreased because of disease or chemotherapy. Conditions affecting other circulating white cells are shown in Table 2–9.

The Shift to the Left

When immature granulocytes become prominent in the differential white count, the condition is sometimes called a *"shift to the left."* The term derives from early studies that used tabular headings to report the number of each cell type. The cell types were listed across the top of the page, starting with blasts on the left and placing mature neutrophils on the right side. Large numbers of immature cells provoked entries in the left hand columns, normally empty except for a few bands. Numbers thus shifted to the left-hand columns when immature cells were numerous. The causes and significance of altered white cell levels can be are shown in Tables 2–6 through 2–9.

ERYTHROCYTE SEDIMENTATION RATE

This test determines the rate at which erythrocytes fall to the bottom of a vertical tube of anticoagulated blood within a specified period. Measurement of the distance from the top of the column of sedimented erythrocytes to the top of the fluid level in a given period determines the erythrocyte sedimentation rate (ESR). Anticoagulated blood placed in a vertical, small-bore tube exhibits settling (sedimenting) of the red

Table 2–9. CONDITIONS AFFECTING OTHER CIRCULATING WHITE CELLS

Monocytosis (>800 monocytes/µl in adults):
- Infections (tuberculosis, subacute bacterial endocarditis, hepatitis, rickettsial diseases, syphilis)
- Granulomatous diseases (sarcoid, ulcerative colitis, regional enteritis)
- Collagen-vascular diseases (lupus, rheumatoid arthritis, polyarteritis)
- Many cancers, lymphomas, and myeloproliferative disorders

Eosinophilia (>450 eosinophils/µl):
- Allergic diseases (asthma, hay fever, drug reactions, allergic vasculitis, serum sickness)
- Parasitic infections (trichinosis, echinococcus, hookworm, schistosomiasis, amebiasis)
- Skin disorders (some psoriasis, some eczema, pemphigus, dermatitis herpetiformis)
- "Hypereosinophilic" syndromes (systemic eosinophilia associated with pulmonary infiltration and sometimes cardiovascular disturbances)
- Neoplastic diseases (Hodgkin's disease, extensive metastases or necrosis of solid tumors)
- Miscellaneous (collagen-vascular diseases, adrenal cortical hypofunction, ulcerative colitis, L-tryptophan eosinophilic myalgia syndrome (TEM))

Basophilia (>50 basophils/µl):
- Chronic hypersensitivity states in the absence of the specific allergen (exposure to the allergen triggers cell lysis and rapid drop in basophil count)
- Systemic mast cell disease
- Myeloproliferative disorders

Table 2–10. FACTORS INFLUENCING ERYTHROCYTE SEDIMENTATION RATE

1. Plasma factors (factors that reduce the zeta potential)
   a. Fibrinogen concentration
   b. Globulin concentration, particularly gamma globulins
   c. Serum cholesterol
2. Red cell factors
   a. Increased ESR
      - Anemia (particularly hematocrit range 0.3–0.4)
      - Red cell surface area: microcytes sediment more slowly than macrocytes
      - Rouleaux: decreased surface area
      - Sickle cells fail to form into rouleaux and therefore have a low ESR
   b. Conditions causing increased ESR
      - Pregnancy
      - Hyperglobulinemia
      - Hyperfibrinogenemia

cells at a rate determined largely by the relative density of the red cells with respect to the plasma. The actual rate of fall is greatly influenced by the ability of the erythrocytes to form into *rouleaux.* Rouleaux are clumps of red cells joined not by antibodies or covalent bonds, but merely by surface attraction *(zeta potential).* This represents the ability of red cells to aggregate together. If the proportion of globulin to albumin increases, or if *fibrinogen* levels are especially high, rouleaux formation is enhanced and the sedimentation rate increases. A high concentration of asymmetric macromolecules in the plasma also reduces the mutually repellent forces that separate suspended red cells and enhance the formation of rouleaux. Other factors that affect the sedimentation rate include the ratio of red cells to plasma and the plasma viscosity. Table 2–10 is a list of the plasma factors and red cell factors that influence the ESR.

In normal blood, relatively little settling occurs because the gravitational pull of individual red cells is almost balanced by the upward current generated by the displacement of plasma. If the plasma is extremely viscous or cholesterol levels are very high, the upward trend may virtually neutralize the downward pull of individual or clumped red cells.

Measurement of ESR

In the *Wintrobe method* for ESR, undiluted anticoagulated blood is allowed to stand for one hour in a tube 100 mm tall and 2.8 mm in diameter. Normal values are up to 8 mm/hour for men and 15 mm/hour for women. The *Westergren technique* uses a 200-mm column in which the anticoagulated blood, diluted 20% with saline or sodium citrate solution, is allowed to settle for one hour. *Normal values are up to 15 mm/hour for men and 20 mm/hour for women,* rising somewhat in both sexes after the age of 50. The Westergren method is generally recommended as the standard method because of its simplicity and reproducibility.

Interpretation

Nonspecific increases in globulins and increased fibrinogen levels occur when the body responds to injury, inflammation, or pregnancy. A rise in ESR accompanies most inflammatory diseases, whether localized or systemic, and occurs when smoldering chronic inflammatory processes flare up.

The observed rate of settling varies as the concentration of red cells in plasma changes. Controversy exists over reporting ESR results in a "corrected" form that takes hematocrit level into account. Hematocrit has a much greater potential effect on the Wintrobe method. The Westergren technique is somewhat less affected by hematocrit because, in this method, the blood is substantially diluted.

Erythrocyte sedimentation rate really has three main uses: 1) as an aid in detecting inflammatory process, 2) as a monitor of disease course or activity, and 3) as a screen for occult inflammatory or neoplastic conditions. The test, however, is relatively nonsensitive and nonspecific since it is influenced by many technical factors. Nevertheless, it remains a useful test and is widely employed. It must be emphasized that a normal ESR cannot be used to exclude organic disease; however, most acute and chronic inflammatory and neoplastic conditions are associated with an increase in sedimentation rate. The elevated ESR with pregnancy returns to normal by the third or the fourth week postpartum. Sedimentation rates of greater than 100 mm/hour are seen in plasma cell dyscrasias such as multiple myeloma, where high immunoglobulin concentrations cause increased RBC rouleaux. This can also be seen in collagen-vascular diseases, malignant diseases, and tuberculosis.

SPECIAL LEUKOCYTE STUDIES

White cells on a freshly made blood film retain enzyme activity and can alter added substrates. This is most useful when cells are morphologically so abnormal that it becomes difficult to detect their cell line of origin. Enzyme studies are also useful in assessing cellular maturation and in evaluating departures from normal differentiation. The development of monoclonal antibody technology has also facilitated the identification of cell origin, particularly that of immature hematopoietic cell precursors. These are also useful when categorizing immature or undifferentiated cells in acute leukemia.

Leukocyte Alkaline Phosphatase

Among the enzymes in neutrophilic granules is a phosphatase capable of hydrolyzing phosphate-containing substrates into a product that binds to highly colored dyes. Leukocyte alkaline phosphatase (LAP) can be roughly quantitated by scoring the size and intensity of the stained granules. Normal levels fall between 10–130 out of a maximum of 400. Generally, 100 cells are counted, and the intensity of the staining is graduated from zero (no staining) to four (heavy and intense staining). Leukocyte alkaline phosphatase increases in polycythemia vera and myelofibrosis, and decreases in chronic granulocytic leukemia and paroxysmal nocturnal hemoglobinuria (PNH). It is normal or elevated in leukemoid reactions to infections. Since all of these conditions have increased the numbers of immature circulating neutrophils, LAP scores can be helpful in distinguishing among them. Leukocyte alkaline phosphatase is unrelated to serum alkaline phosphatase (see also Color Plate 27).

Leukocyte Peroxidase

Myeloid and monocytic cells have cytoplasmic granules that contain enzymes with peroxidase activity capable of transferring hydrogen from a donor compound to hydrogen peroxide. Lymphoid and erythroid cells lack these enzymes. There is little clinical use in testing mature cells for myeloperoxidase content, but stains to demonstrate cytoplasmic peroxidase are extremely useful in distinguishing immature myeloid cells from immature lymphoid cells. In acute myelocytic leukemia (especially M1, see Chapter 4), greater than 75% of the blasts will be peroxidase-positive; whereas in acute lymphocytic leukemia, a similar disease morphologically (L2, see page 154), very few (if any) of the blasts have peroxidase activity.

Sudan Black B

Sudan Black stains neutral fats and other lipids that, in circulating leukocytes, tend to be most conspicuous in the same cytoplasmic structures that have peroxidase activity. In the acute leukemias, intense Sudan Black staining, either generalized or clumped, is characteristic of acute myelocytic leukemia. The monocytic and monoblastic cells of M4 and M5 leukemias usually have fine, scattered granules, and in the lymphoblastic leukemias very few, if any, cells take the Sudan Black stain.

Leukocyte Esterases

Myeloid and monocytic cells contain numerous enzymes that hydrolyze ester bonds. By selecting appropriate substrates and reaction conditions, hematologists can distinguish monocytic cells from myeloid cells. This is most useful in classifying the acute leukemias, in which abnormal maturation and morphology reduce the usefulness of the usual differentiating criteria. Chloroacetate esterase is normally present only in promyelocytes, but is sometimes present in leukemic myeloblasts and is characteristically present in Auer rods. Monocytic and lymphoid cells lack this esterase; for these cells the substrate used is naphthol AS-D chloroacetate. Chloroacetate esterase activity is not affected by prior fluoride treatment.

Nonspecific Esterase

Nonspecific esterase is most abundant in monocytic cells, but may be weakly present in granulocytes, lymphocytes, or even normoblasts. The discriminating feature, besides the intensity and distribution of the reaction, is that sodium fluoride inhibits the strong esterase activity of monocytes, but does not reduce the stain reactivity of granulocytes or other cells. The usual substrate used in testing is alpha-naphthyl acetate.

Periodic Acid-Schiff

In the periodic acid-Schiff (PAS) stain, compounds that can be oxidized to aldehydes are localized by brilliant fuchsia staining. Many elements in multiple tissues are PAS positive, but in blood cells, the PAS-positive material of diagnostic importance is cytoplasmic glycogen. Early granulocyte precursors and normal erythroid precursors are PAS negative. Mature red cells remain PAS negative, but granulocytes acquire increasing PAS positivity only with maturation. Monocytes and lymphocytes may have scattered granules and give a positive test.

In acute granulocytic leukemia, myeloblasts and monoblasts are either negative or weakly positive in a finely granular pattern. Leukemic lymphoblasts, especially in childhood acute lymphoblastic leukemia, often have coarse clumps or masses of PAS-positive material in a block granular fashion within their scant cytoplasm. The staining pattern is usually heterogeneous, with some cells containing PAS-positive chunks and others virtually unstained (see Color Plate 28).

Erythroid precursors contain PAS-positive material in erythroleukemia (M6, see page 142) and in scattered cases of thalassemia and anemias. Conspicuous PAS staining in the erythroid line, however, creates a strong likelihood of erythroleukemia.

Terminal Deoxynucleotidyl Transferase (TdT)

Terminal deoxynucleotidyl transferase is an enzyme marker for immature lymphoid cells. This enzyme is a DNA polymerase that is found in immature lymphoid precursors and also in the majority of patients with acute lymphoblastic leukemia. The test is performed on fixed cell preparation smears by using a labeled antibody to TdT, labeled either with an enzyme or a fluorescent marker. The enzyme is normally present in the nucleus of the immature cells, which would show either positive fluorescence or cytochemical staining if present.

Chromosome Studies

The normal human chromosomal karyotype consists of 22 pairs of autosomes and one pair of sex chromosomes. Chromosome studies can be performed on cells that are capable of division by inducing mitosis. If the cell division is arrested at a phase in mitosis and the nuclei of the cells are lysed by osmotic swelling, preparations of these paired chromosomes can be made and photographed. The cut out photographs of the individual chromosomes can then be arranged in order of decreasing size and compared with one another and with standard morphologic nomenclature (Fig. 2–12). In addition, these chromosomes can also be stained by various methods, producing several bands. Depending on the location of the band and the intensity of the staining, the bands are subclassified. Breakpoints, exchanges of genetic material between chromosomes, and other abnormalities can then be analyzed. Excess chromosomal material can also be seen. Specific abnormalities of chromosomal material can be used diagnostically (for example the Philadelphia chromosome in chronic myelogenous leukemia) or prognostically (4;11 translocations in acute lymphoblastic leukemia have a worse prognostic feature), or to follow therapy and diagnose relapse in leukemia. Chromosomal markers have become an integral part of the investigation of many malignant hematologic disorders. Chromosomal studies can also be used to assess bone marrow engraftment following bone marrow transplantation. The usefulness of chromosomal methods in hematologic diseases is discussed more fully in the section on white cell disorders. The expansion of chromosomal analyses by using molecular and genetic probes has characterized breakpoints on specific chromosomes that may be important in understanding the development

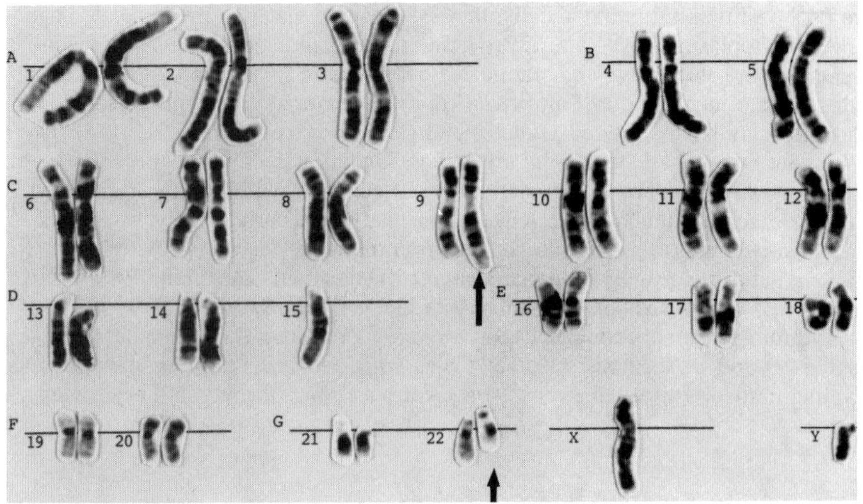

Figure 2–12. Human chromosomal preparation showing Philadelphia chromosome. (*Arrows* denote t 22:9.) (Courtesy of Dr. E. Himoe, Division of Genetics, Georgetown University, Washington, DC.)

of disease, specifically cancer (oncogenes). Recent studies have shown that oncogenes can be relocated and activated as a result of chromosomal translocations. In addition, several chromosomes contain fragile sites that may be important breakpoints in permitting unregulated cell growth. In the future, analysis of the chromosomal constitution of affected cells in many disorders may provide clues to diagnostic, prognostic, and etiologic aspects of malignant disorders. The banding techniques have clearly outlined subchromosomal structure and permitted more refined chromosomal mapping. Molecular probe analysis has remarkably expanded the application of chromosomal studies in disease, primarily in the area of leukemia diagnosis and prognosis. Newer leukemia classifications will presumably be based not only on morphology, but also on cytogenetic and immunologic characterizations. In this way, subcategories of leukemia with more refined and precise prognostic and therapeutic implications will be outlined.

REFERENCES

1. Burns, HF and Forget, BG: Human Hemoglobin: Molecular, Genetic and Clinical Aspects. WB Saunders, Philadelphia, 1986.
2. Dacie, JV and Lewis, SM: Practical Hematology, ed 6. Churchill Livingstone, Edinburgh, 1985.
3. Henry JB: Todd, Sanford, and Davidson's Clinical Diagnosis and Management by Laboratory Methods, ed 17. WB Saunders, Philadelphia, 1984.
4. Hillman, RS and Finch, CA: Red Cell Manual, Ed 5. FA Davis, Philadelphia, 1985.
5. Metcalf, D: The Hemopoietic Colony Stimulating Factors. Elsevier, Amsterdam, 1985.
6. Pittiglio, DH and Sacher, RA: Fundamentals of Hematology and Hemostasis. FA Davis, Philadelphia, 1987.
7. Williams, JW, et al: Hematology. McGraw-Hill, New York, 1983.

CHAPTER

3

Diseases of Red Blood Cells

OUTLINE

TESTS

CHAPTER

3

DISEASES OF RED BLOOD CELLS

ANEMIA: DEFINITION AND CLASSIFICATION

The main function of the erythropoietic marrow is production of erythrocytes capable of transporting the respiratory pigment hemoglobin to the tissues for oxygen delivery. Adequate numbers of erythrocytes must be produced and their hemoglobin must be quantitatively normal and maintained in a functional state for oxygen delivery. The red cell concentration must be kept within normal limits; therefore, the red cell destruction must be balanced by the red cell production. Furthermore, the red cell membrane must be deformable by passage through the microcirculation. Internal red cell metabolism has been developed to maintain hemoglobin in a state capable of transporting oxygen. Other metabolic activities of the cells are directed at maintaining the cell's deformability and survival in the peripheral blood. Abnormalities of these functions may be associated with disorders of erythrocyte development or distribution, and may produce accelerated erythrocyte destruction. *Anemia* is often the end result of these abnormalities, and is defined as a *decrease in the concentration of hemoglobin.*

Anemia may also be thought of as a reduction in the red cell mass, producing decreased oxygen-carrying capacity to meet the tissue demands. This reduction in red cell mass may occur if the production of red cells is defective, or if their destruction or loss exceeds the capabilities of the bone marrow to replace them. Anemias may be classified on the basis of the degree of *hemoglobinization* of the red cells, i.e., *hypochromic,* or *normochromic;* or the *size of the red cells,* i.e., *microcytic, normocytic,* or *macrocytic;* or they may be classified according to the category of disorder that is responsible for the anemia.

There are three main categories:

1. Disorders of Red Cell Formation
   a. Deficiency diseases
   b. Hypoproliferative anemias—reduced or absent functional marrow
   c. Ineffective erythropoiesis—refractory anemia

2. Excessive Loss of Red Cells
   a. Hemorrhage
   b. Hemolysis
3. Abnormal Distribution

Characterization of the type and severity of anemia is achieved by the performance of the *hemoglobin concentration,* or *hematocrit,* and the *red cell indices* mentioned in Chapter 2. Effective red cell production is determined by the *reticulocyte count,* which assesses the number of functional erythrocytes made by the marrow. One of the most important laboratory tests in evaluating any patient with anemia is the examination of the *peripheral blood smear.* This gives many clues as to the etiology of the anemias. However, in many instances a *bone marrow specimen* also must be examined to enable categorization of the type of anemia. Specialized tests help define the exact etiology. The laboratory tests that will be ordered are dependent on the classification of the anemia and its possible cause, as will become apparent in this chapter.

DISORDERS OF RED CELL FORMATION

Anemias Due to Deficiency States

IRON DEFICIENCY AND THE HYPOCHROMIC ANEMIAS

Deficiencies of the essential minerals and nutrients required for erythropoiesis commonly produce anemias. The most prevalent worldwide cause of anemia is iron deficiency. Iron metabolism is discussed in Chapter 2. Iron deficiency anemia commonly produces *hypochromic, microcytic* erythrocytes. The mean cell hemoglobin is usually below 27 pg/liter, and the mean cell volume is below 80 fl. The reason the cells are microcytic is because continued synthesis of erythrocytes occurs. There is little incorporation of iron into protoporphyrin, and the rate-limiting enzyme heme synthetase (ferrochelatase) requires iron to switch off heme synthesis (see Fig. 2–4). If iron is deficient, cell division will continue for several additional cycles, producing smaller cells. Since inadequate amounts of iron are present, less hemoglobin is also present per individual red cell, producing the hypochromia. There are four main conditions associated with hypochromic, microcytic anemia. These are:

- iron deficiency anemia,
- thalassemia syndromes,
- anemia of chronic disease, and
- sideroblastic anemia.

Iron Deficiency Anemia

Iron deficiency is by far the commonest cause of anemia. The most common causes of iron deficiency are 1) blood loss (all ages, especially menstruating women), 2) nutritional deficiency (infants), and 3) increased iron demand (pregnancy, lactation, adolescence) (Table 3–1). Iron metabolism is delicately balanced in the body to prevent excessive iron absorption, since iron is an abundant element in nature (Chapter 2). Consequently, iron deficiency generally ensues because the body can only moderately adapt to iron deficiency due to *blood loss* (particularly continuing blood loss). As was mentioned in Chapter 2, the normal diet contains 10–15 mg of iron per day. Normally the body can absorb 10% of this iron, and this

Table 3–1. MAJOR CAUSES OF IRON DEFICIENCY

Major causes
Dietary inadequacy
Malabsorption
Gastrectomy
Achlorhydria
Steatorrhea
Celiac disease
Pica
Increased iron loss
Menstruation
Gastrointestinal bleeding
Hemoptysis
Hematuria
Hemodialysis
Increased iron requirements
Infancy
Adolescence
Pregnancy
Lactation

balances the amount of iron lost through desquamation of cells, particularly from the gastrointestinal tract and skin. In order to maintain this steady state, 1 mg of iron needs to be absorbed per day. In situations of excess bleeding or, for that matter, associated with normal bleeding in menstruation, iron loss from hemorrhage needs to be replaced. Since the average menstrual cycle is associated with 60 ml of blood loss per month, this translates to 30 mg of iron and, consequently, women require an extra milligram of iron per day to be absorbed to also maintain the steady state. Maximal iron absorption is up to 25% of the dietary iron and can occur in situations of depletion. Women can absorb up to this amount to maintain the steady state. However, young menstruating women, particularly those with heavy blood losses, are commonly iron depleted. A normal pregnancy also depletes the body of 600–700 mg of iron. Since body stores contain 500–1500 mg of iron, one pregnancy can deplete the body's stores, especially if iron supplements are not given.

Iron deficiency anemia is especially common during times when iron demands are greatest, as occurs in infancy, during the adolescent growth spurt, and in pregnancy. Chronic blood loss can occur at any age, but is particularly prevalent in older adults, especially from gastrointestinal and genitourinary sources. Malignancies of the gastrointestinal tract especially are associated with iron deficiency anemia.

When negative iron balance occurs, iron deficiency anemia develops only after depletion of the body stores. Following depletion of body stores, serum iron falls and plasma iron binding capacity increases. Following this, hemoglobin synthesis is reduced and defective hemoglobinization of the developing red cells occurs. Red cells are produced that are *pale (hypochromic)* and *small (microcytic)* (see Color Plate 30). The red cell indices of hemoglobin concentration, namely the mean cell hemoglobin and mean cell hemoglobin concentration, are reduced. When iron deficiency anemia is severe, tissue iron depletion also occurs and is associated with changes in various tissues, particularly the nails (koilonychia) and tongue (glossitis) and produces marked fatigue due to depletion of the muscle enzymes and myoglobin, the muscle respiratory pigment (Table 3–2).

TABLE 3–2. SEQUENTIAL CHANGES IN THE DEVELOPMENT OF IRON DEFICIENCY

	Normal	Iron Depletion	Iron Deficient Erythropoiesis	Iron Deficiency Anemia
Iron Stores / Erythron Iron				
RE Marrow Fe	2-3+	0-1+	0	0
Transferrin IBC (μg/100 mL)	330±30	360	390	410
Plasma ferritin (μg/mL)	100±60	20	10	<10
Iron absorption (%)	5-10	10-15	10-20	10-20
Plasma iron (μg/100 mL)	115±50	115	<60	<40
Transferrin saturation (%)	35±15	30	<15	<10
Sideroblasts (%)	40-60	40-60	<10	<10
RBC Protoporphyrin	30	30	100	200
Erythrocytes	Normal	Normal	Normal	Microcytic/ Hypochromic

From Hillman and Finch,[16] p 60, with permission.

Dietary depletion of iron is an uncommon cause of deficiency in adults; however, in infants it is more common. The newborn infant begins life with 350–500 mg of iron: all further increments come from the diet. Iron requirements are greatest in the first year of life when expanding red cell production requires daily intake of 1 mg/kg to keep pace with growth. Adolescence, pregnancy, and lactation also impose severe stress on iron balance. The commonest victims of inadequate dietary intake are small children whose diet consists largely of milk. In the United States, fortified food products and generally varied diet make poor intake alone a rare cause of iron deficiency in older children and adults. A borderline iron balance may, however, occur under conditions of increased requirement such as rapid growth spurts, onset of menstruation, or repeated pregnancies. Adult men and postmenopausal women almost never become iron deficient from diet alone, no matter how poor their diets, unless other problems coexist. In less developed countries, the combination of poor diet, frequent parasitic infestations, and repeated pregnancies make iron deficiency anemia a widespread and severe health problem.

Chronic bleeding, often unnoticed, may occur from the gastrointestinal tract. Peptic ulcer, gastritis, hiatal hernia, diverticulitis, and neoplasms are the usual causes. In many cases the patient is asymptomatic or, at the very least, unaware of blood loss. Heavy use of alcohol or aspirin may cause painful gastritis, but the patient may not notice the small, continuous blood loss.

Excessive menstrual loss is a common cause of iron deficiency in women. In adolescent girls, with their frequently erratic diets and often irregular, heavy menstrual periods, the pubertal growth spurt may tip iron balance into a deficiency state. Consecutive pregnancies exert a cumulative effect by depleting iron stores.

The *urinary tract* is another avenue of loss. Tumors, stones, or inflammatory disease affecting kidneys, ureters, or bladder may cause blood loss in the urine. A rare cause of urinary-related iron deficiency is excretion of large amounts of hemosiderin in patients with chronic hemolytic states.

A person may have reduced body iron without being anemic (see Table 3–2, which shows the sequential changes in development of iron deficiency). Many individuals with normal hemoglobin levels are chronically iron-depleted but do not develop iron deficiency anemia until some stress—for example increased demand, repeated blood donation, or acute and chronic hemorrhage—accentuates the negative iron balance. In a largely white population of middle to lower income status, 20% of menstruating women were found to be iron deficient, but less than half of these women had iron deficiency anemia. Of the anemias found in the entire study population, half were due to iron deficiency alone. Table 3–3 lists the laboratory findings in iron deficiency. Iron deficiency may easily be differentiated from the other 3 conditions by the markedly *reduced serum iron* and markedly *elevated total iron-binding capacity* (Table 3–4). The *saturation of transferrin* is usually below 5% in iron deficiency anemia, and the *serum ferritin,* a test reflecting iron stores, is less than 5 ng/ml, indicating markedly reduced or absent iron stores. The *free erythrocyte protoporphyrin,* which represents the substrate for iron incorporation into heme, is markedly increased since heme synthesis is reduced, and therefore the precursor product accumulates. Tests of tissue iron such as *bone marrow iron* show absent iron stores in iron deficiency anemia. Table 3–4 lists laboratory findings characteristic of iron deficiency anemia compared with the other causes of hypochromic, microcytic anemias, namely thalassemia, anemia of chronic disease, and sideroblastic anemia.

Table 3–3. LABORATORY FINDINGS IN IRON DEFICIENCY

Blood Count
- Microcytic, hypochromic red cells if Hgb < 12 g/dl (men), < 10 g/dl (women)
- Leukopenia may occur
- Platelets high with active bleeding
- Reticulocytes lower than expected for degree of anemia

Bone Marrow
- Erythroid hyperplasia
- Stainable iron very low or absent

Other
- Serum iron very low, iron-binding capacity high, percent of saturation very low
- Serum ferritin < 10 ng/dl
- Free erythrocyte protoporphyrin high
- RBC survival time slightly low
- RDW high

Hgb = hemoglobin; RBC = red blood cells; RDW = red cell distribution width.

Table 3–4. DIFFERENTIAL DIAGNOSIS OF MICROCYTIC HYPOCHROMIC ANEMIA

	Serum Iron	TIBC	Serum Ferritin	FEP	HbA_2	HbF	RDW
Iron deficiency	Low	High	Low	High	nl	nl–low	High
Alpha-thalassemia	High	nl	High	nl	nl	low	
Beta-thalassemia	High	nl	High	nl	High	High (varies)	High
Anemia of chronic disease	Low	Low	High	High	nl	nl	nl
Sideroblastic anemia	High	nl	High	Low	nl	nl	High

TIBC = total iron-binding capacity; FEP = free erythrocyte protoporphyrin; nl = normal; HbA_2 = Hemoglobin A_2; HbF = Hemoglobin F; RDW = red cell distribution width.

Iron deficiency anemia is a symptom, not a primary disease entity. The cause of the iron deficiency anemia always needs to be established and specific treatment directed to this cause. However, correction of the iron-deficient patient requires replacement of therapeutic doses of iron continuous enough to replenish the body's stores. This may require iron replacement therapy for 3–6 months. The iron-deficient patient who receives therapeutic iron develops reticulocytosis within 2–3 days, which often spuriously increases the mean cell volume. The reticulocytosis is visible as a polychromatophilia on examination of a peripheral blood smear (see Color Plate 30B).

Anemia of Chronic Disease

Since chronic disorders may present with a hypochromic, microcytic anemia, it is important that these conditions be distinguished from iron deficiency anemia. Chronic infections, inflammatory processes, and malignant neoplasms can present with hypochromic, microcytic anemias. The basic defect is in the iron utilization for erythropoiesis. There appears to be a block in delivery of iron from the reticuloendothelial iron stores to the developing red cell. Consequently, the red cells are deficient in iron, whereas the body stores have abundant iron. Usually the peripheral blood smear shows a normochromic, normocytic picture, but with advanced states the cells may be hypochromic and microcytic. Microcytosis is usually not as severe as with iron deficiency anemia, and mean cell volume values of less than 70–75 fl are rare. Anemias are usually of moderate severity, with hemoglobins in the 7–11 g/dl range.

Table 3–4 shows the profile of iron studies in the anemia of chronic disease. Typically, the serum iron values are low, as is the total iron-binding capacity. This latter point differentiates this form of hypochromic anemia from that of iron deficiency anemia. The percentage saturation of transferrin is usually higher than that seen with iron deficiency anemia, and is in the 7–15% range. A major discriminating feature, of course, is the fact that the serum ferritin value is increased with values of 50–2,000 ng/ml. This point can be used to discriminate between chronic disease and iron deficiency anemia, since serum ferritin values are less than 10 ng/ml in iron deficiency states.

Sideroblastic Anemias

The sideroblastic anemias are a group of disorders characterized by abnormalities of heme metabolism. The diagnostic feature of these disorders is the presence of nucleated red cells with iron granules ("ringed sideroblasts") in the marrow, and the appearance of a *dimorphic peripheral blood picture,* found particularly in the primary types (Table 3–5 and Color Plate 15A). In the sideroblastic anemias, the body has adequate, even abundant, iron, but is unable to incorporate it into hemoglobin. The iron enters the developing red cell, but accumulates in the perinuclear mitochondria of normoblasts in primary sideroblastic anemia. The dimorphic pattern in the peripheral blood shows two apparent populations of erythrocytes, with one population of fairly normal cells and another population of hypochromic, irregularly shaped, generally small erythrocytes. The bone marrow shows an increased erythropoietic activity and is therefore hypercellular, but circulating reticulocyte counts are generally not increased. As previously mentioned, this reflects ineffective erythropoiesis.

There are several conditions that can produce this apparent abnormality where iron is trapped in the mitochondria and cannot be fully utilized in hemoglobin synthesis. These are listed in Table 3–5, Classification of Sideroblastic Anemias. In general, the sideroblastic anemias are associated with more than 15% ringed sideroblasts and may be classified as having congenital and acquired causes. Once the secondary disorders listed in the table are excluded, the condition is termed idiopathic or primary. This disorder represents a clonal disturbance of erythropoiesis and is discussed in the disorders classified as the myelodysplastic syndromes (see Chapter 4, Disorders of White Blood Cells). Specifically, however, primary or idiopathic sideroblastic anemia is characterized by abnormal erythropoietic maturation (dys-erythropoiesis) and abormal iron utilization with the typical ringed sideroblasts. Ringed sideroblasts may be less prominent in the secondary disorders.

The laboratory data are reflective of impaired iron utilization with normal or increased iron stores. The red cell indices may vary, depending on which population of cells predominates. Consequently, the MCV may be low, normal, or even increased. The MCH and MCHC are often low but may be normal. White cell abnormalities may also be seen. With defects in the synthesis of porphyrin or the ring insertion of iron, regulation of iron absorption is disturbed and systemic accumula-

Table 3–5. CLASSIFICATION OF SIDEROBLASTIC ANEMIAS

Inherited
- Rare sex-linked

Acquired
- Primary (idiopathic) (see myelodysplasias)
- Secondary
  1. Associated with other myeloproliferative syndromes (leukemias, polycythemia vera)
  2. Pyridoxine-deficient or responsive anemias
     a. Vitamin B_6 deficiency
     b. Drugs: isoniazid, cycloserine
     c. Alcoholism
  3. Disorders of hemoglobin synthesis
     a. Folate deficiency, B_{12} deficiency
     b. Lead poisoning
     c. Erythropoietic porphyria

From Pittiglio, DH and Sacher, RA: Clinical Hematology and Fundamentals of Hemostasis. FA Davis, Philadelphia, 1987, p 51, with permission.

tion of iron may develop. The serum iron is usually greater than normal, with a high percentage saturation of transferrin. Serum ferritin values are also markedly elevated. Serum B_{12} and folic acid levels are normal. Other laboratory tests are also reflective of ineffective erythropoiesis, with an elevated lactate dehydrogenase.

Treatment is usually aimed at correcting a secondary cause; however, in the primary disorders, patients are usually unresponsive to the various vitamin supplements, in particular pyridoxine.

Thalassemia Syndromes

These will be discussed in the section on Hemolytic Anemias.

Lead Poisoning

Anemia and disordered heme synthesis accompany lead poisoning, and provide the major diagnostic clues for this common, preventable disorder. In adults, lead exposure is usually occupational. In children, the most common cause is pica, a tendency to consume inedible materials. Lead-containing paint formerly was a cause of this problem, but has largely been eliminated. Children are also sensitive to the lead levels in polluted atmospheres.

Lead depresses enzyme activity at the beginning, the middle and the end of heme synthesis. Defective delta-amino-levulinic dehydratase activity causes *delta-amino-levulinic acid* (ALA) to accumulate. Urine ALA levels have long been used as a rough screening test for lead toxicity. Coproporphyrin metabolism is depressed, and the insertion of ferrous iron into protoporphyrin is inhibited, because lead also inhibits heme synthetase (see Fig. 2–4). Depression of heme synthetase causes red cells to accumulate excessive protoporphyrin; *elevated red cell protoporphyrin* levels constitute the best laboratory test for quantifying lead toxicity. Table 3–6 lists the laboratory findings in lead poisoning.

Table 3–6. LABORATORY FINDINGS IN LEAD POISONING

Anemia
Hemoglobin 9–11 g/dl
MCHC moderately low
Reticulocytosis 2–7%
RBC changes
Ratio of protoporphyrin to hemoglobin >5.5 μg/g (>17 in severe cases)
Basophilic stippling
Moderate anisocytosis and poikilocytosis
Diminished osmotic fragility
Blood lead usually >40 μg/ml
Bone marrow
Erythroid hyperplasia
Ringed sideroblasts
Urine
ALA excretion >20 mg/liter
Coproporphyrin III >0.5 mg/liter
Porphobilinogen normal

MCHC = mean corpuscular hemoglobin concentration; ALA = delta-amino levulinic acid.

VITAMIN B₁₂ AND FOLIC ACID DEFICIENCY

Although vitamin B_{12} and folic acid deficiency are the commonest causes of *megaloblastic anemia,* diagnosis and therapy of this condition requires an understanding of the differential diagnosis and laboratory evaluation of other causes of anemia with macrocytic red cells.

As was mentioned in Chapter 2, *macrocytosis* occurs when the mean cell volume (MCV) is greater than 100 fl. Erythrocytic macrocytosis can easily be determined with the aid of an automated electronic particle counter, which gives an accurate and reproducible value for the MCV. The finding of macrocytic indices does not imply megaloblastic anemia, since other conditions can give a macrocytosis (Table 3–7). An elevated MCV, however, is an abnormal finding and may precede, by months or years, the onset of a megaloblastic anemia. Megaloblastic anemia may be masked in the presence of complicating infections, inflammatory disease, or iron deficiency.

Spurious macrocytosis can occur with automated measurements, and the finding of an elevated MCV must always be corroborated by examination of the peripheral blood smear. The earliest sign of megaloblastic anemia reflected in the peripheral blood is hypersegmentation of the polymorphonuclear leukocytes. Red cell morphology can also help distinguish the other causes of macrocytosis from megaloblastic anemia. In liver disease, the macrocytosis is usually associated with the presence of *round macrocytes.* B_{12} or folate deficiency (megaloblastic anemia), with *oval macrocytes,* reticulocytosis with *basophilic round macrocytes* and altered red cell morphology can also help distinguish the macrocytosis of other myeloproliferative disorders (see Color Plate 12). In general, a bone marrow examination is essential to establish whether megaloblastic anemia is present, although examination of the bone marrow cannot distinguish vitamin B_{12} deficiency from folic acid deficiency. Clinical features are, however, often helpful in differentiating pernicious anemia from folic acid deficiency (Table 3–8). Table 3–9 outlines the laboratory findings in megaloblastic anemias.

Table 3–7. DIFFERENTIAL DIAGNOSIS OF MACROCYTOSIS (MCV > 100 FL)

Actual
- Megaloblastic anemias
- Liver disease
- Reticulocytosis
- Myeloproliferative diseases (leukemia, myelofibrosis)
- Multiple myeloma
- Hypothyroidism
- Aplastic anemia
- Drugs (post-chemotherapy, alcohol)

Spurious
- Auto-agglutination/cold agglutination disease

From Sacher, RA: Pernicious Anemia and Other Megaloblastic Anemias. In Rakel, R (ed): Conn's Current Therapy. WB Saunders, Philadelphia, 1988, with permission.

Table 3–8. SEVEN CLINICAL "P"S OF PERNICIOUS ANEMIA

1. Pancytopenia
2. Peripheral neuropathy
3. Posterior spinal column neuropathy
4. Pyramidal tract signs
5. Papillary (tongue) atrophy
6. pH elevation (gastric fluid)
7. Psychosis (megaloblastic madness)

Adapted from Sacher, RA: Pernicious Anemia and Other Megaloblastic Anemias. In Rakel, R (ed): Conn's Current Therapy. WB Saunders, Philadelphia, 1988.

Causes of Megaloblastosis

The two most common problems leading to megaloblastic anemia are vitamin B_{12} (cobalamin) deficiency and a deficiency of folic acid (see Chapter 2). As was discussed in Chapter 2, cobalamin deficiency is almost always due to vitamin B_{12} malabsorption. Pernicious anemia is the commonest cause and is due to lack of *intrinsic factor,* the essential cofactor needed for vitamin B_{12} absorption in the terminal ileum. Intrinsic factor is normally produced by the parietal cells of the gastric mucosa, and is deficient in any condition that decreases its production such as atrophic gastritis and gastrectomy. Occasionally, dietary deficiency (veganism) and altered metabolic states or bacterial overgrowth with organisms requiring intestinal B_{12} for their metabolism may produce B_{12} deficiency by competition for available B_{12} with the host. These conditions may be differentiated, as was discussed in Chapter 2, by testing vitamin B_{12} absorption using the *Schilling Test.*

Megaloblastic anemia due to folic acid deficiency may have many different causes (Table 3–10). In general, a deficiency of folic acid is nearly always due to a dietary cause. Stores of folic acid are only sufficient for 3 months. These can rapidly be depleted in conditions of excess folic acid demand such as pregnancy, rapid growth in adolescence and infancy, rapid cell turnover that may occur with hemolytic anemias, poor folate intake, and alcoholism. Folic acid deficiency may also occur with malabsorption syndromes, and its absorption may be competitively inhibited by means of concommitant drugs such as birth control pills and some anticonvulsants. Sprue and other enteropathies often depress absorption of both vitamin B_{12} and folic acid. Many drugs cause megaloblastosis by interfering with DNA synthesis, some as antagonists of folic acid or as inhibitors of purine or pyrimidine synthesis, and others, especially alcohol, through less clearly defined pathways. Several rare, genetically determined enzyme defects (e.g., Lesch-Nyhan syndrome, orotic aciduria) cause megaloblastosis in addition to other signs and symptoms.

Pernicious Anemia

Classic or *"Addisonian"* pernicious anemia is a chronic disease with an apparent familial predisposition. The disease complex includes atrophy of the gastric mucosa, megaloblastic blood cell changes caused by vitamin B_{12} deficiency, a high incidence of autoimmune phenomena, and neurologic manifestations. Clinical features are often most helpful in differentiating pernicious anemia from folic acid deficiency. Table 3–8 lists the *seven clinical "P"s of pernicious anemia* helpful with this distinction. Dysplastic changes of the oral mucous membranes and tongue are also common. The atrophic gastric mucosa secretes neither intrinsic factor nor

Table 3–9. LABORATORY FINDINGS IN MEGALOBLASTIC ANEMIA

Blood count
- Severe anemia (Hgb to 3 g/dl)
- Macrocytosis (MCV 100–140 μm^3), with anisocytosis
- Ovalocytes and macro-ovalocytes numerous
- WBCs, platelets often low
- Hypersegmented neutrophils >5%
- Reticulocytes disproportionately low for anemia

Bone marrow
- Marked erythroid hyperplasia
- Megaloblastic nuclear appearance in all 3 cell lines
- Storage iron normal or high

Blood chemistry
- Bilirubin high (indirect)
- Serum iron high
- LDH very high
- Serum gastrin high (pernicious anemia)

Other studies
- Schilling test abnormal (pernicious anemia)
- Antibodies to gastric cells, intrinsic factor (pernicious anemia)
- Serum, RBC levels of vitamin B_{12} low (vitamin B_{12} deficiency)
- Urine methylmalonate high (vitamin B_{12} deficiency)
- Serum, RBC levels of Folate low (Folic acid deficiency)
- Histamine—fast achlorhydria (pernicious anemia)

MCV = mean corpuscular volume; LDH = lactate dehydrogenase; WBC = white blood cells; RBC = red blood cells.

hydrochloric acid; therefore the gastric secretions of individuals with pernicious anemia are associated with a lack of acidity and a higher pH. Neither the red cell morphology of the peripheral blood nor the bone marrow examination will distinguish between the megaloblastic anemia of B_{12} deficiency and folic acid deficiency. This distinction is initially made by performing a serum B_{12} or folic acid level; however, the Schilling Test is the foundation for the laboratory diagnosis of pernicious anemia once megaloblastic anemia has been established.

Pernicious anemia becomes apparent in middle adulthood or later. The incidence is highest in persons of northern European origin. No clear pattern of genetic transmission exists, but blood relatives of an affected patient are at a higher risk for part or all of the disease complex. Patients with pernicious anemia as well as their hematologically normal relatives frequently have autoantibodies against stomach parietal cells and intrinsic factor and related thyroid autoantibodies.

Therapy for pernicious anemia is simple and effective. Vitamin B_{12} is given by injection, bypassing the absorption defect and permitting the resumption of normal hematopoiesis. Injected vitamin B_{12} corrects the neurologic symptoms, but affects neither the patient's stomach acidity nor the increased liability (about three times

Table 3–10. CAUSES OF FOLATE DEFICIENCY

Dietary
Infancy
Pregnancy and lactation
Malnutrition
Alcoholism
Intestinal malabsorption
Malabsorption syndromes
Drug interaction: phenytoin, oral contraceptives
Increased demand
Infancy and adolescence
Pregnancy and lactation
Increased cellular turnover
Chronic hemolytic anemias
Psoriasis/exfoliative dermatitis
Excess loss
Hemodialysis
Peritoneal dialysis
Defective synthesis
Liver disease
Antifolate drugs
Alcoholism

normal) to develop gastric carcinoma. Thyroid and adrenal hypofunction are more prevalent in these patients than in the general population.

Other Causes of Impaired Absorption of Vitamin B_{12}

Gastrectomy, either total or partial, causes intrinsic factor deficiency and may lead, in months or years, to vitamin B_{12} deficiency. Prolonged deficiency of intrinsic factor (IF) can cause such severe atrophy of the ileal absorption site that therapeutic administration of IF takes some time to promote adequate vitamin B_{12} absorption. *Resection of the ileum,* or ileal diseases such as *celiac disease* and *regional enteritis,* are associated with inflammatory damage to the site of absorption. Organisms within the intestine occasionally affect luminal vitamin B_{12} stores for their own use. This can occur with bacterial overgrowth owing to altered intestinal flow patterns *("blind loop" syndrome)* or with manifestations of the *fish tapeworm, Diphyllobothrium latum.* The tapeworm problem is largely confined to northern Scandinavia where incompletely cooked fish is consumed by a population with a high genetic disposition to pernicious anemia.

Folic Acid Deficiency

The specifics of folic acid metabolism were discussed in Chapter 2. In general, however, as was mentioned, folic acid deficiency usually occurs as a result of dietary deficiency or drug-induced antagonism. Dietary deficiency is particularly noticeable at times of increased demand, as has previously been mentioned. Table 3–10 outlines causes of folic acid deficiency.

The Effects of Drugs

Alcohol is undoubtedly the commonest pharmacologic cause of folic acid deficiency, but the mechanisms are complex and poorly understood. Alcohol seems to impair absorption and also to interfere with folate-dependent enzymatic reactions. In addition, chronic alcoholics often have defective diets, multiple vitamin deficiencies, reduced hepatic function, and poor or absent tissue stores of folic acid. Since alcohol also influences iron absorption and pyridoxine pathways, it is not surprising that alcoholics so often have complex and severe hematologic problems.

Folic acid antagonists are pharmacologic agents given precisely because they interfere with folate-dependent steps in cell multiplication. Methotrexate is a cytotoxic agent widely used for treating leukemias and other malignancies (lymphomas). Their depressive effects on the marrow can sometimes be prevented by simultaneously administering *leucovorin (folinic acid)*. Folinic acid is a reduced form of folic acid that bypasses the antifolate activity of the chemotherapeutic agent methotrexate. It is usually administered parenterally to "rescue" systemic antifolate effects of the drug, enabling a higher antimitotic dose to be given.

Oral contraceptives, phenytoin, and related *anticonvulsants,* and the *antituberculosis* drug *cycloserine* seem to reduce folic acid absorption. Patients taking these drugs should be observed for the development of megaloblastic anemia. Principles of treatment of folic acid deficiency involve reversal of the initial effects of the deficiency by supplementation, replenishment of folate stores, and subsequent maintenance of sufficient dietary intake to ensure adequate folate nutrition.

Hypoproliferative Anemias and Syndromes of Bone Marrow Failure

Anemia resulting from the quantitative reduction of functional bone marrow may occur because of a decrease in the absolute number of stem cells, or due to qualitatively abnormal stem cells. The result is a deficiency in the number of committed cell precursors oriented towards erythroid development. Obviously abnormalities of stem cells may affect other cell lines as well, producing leukopenia and thrombocytopenia. Decreased proliferation (hypoproliferation) may support production of some marrow cells, and the severity of the specific cytopenia is reflective of the amount of functional bone marrow. When platelets, white cells, and red cells are all decreased in the peripheral blood, the condition is called *pancytopenia.* Aplastic anemia represents the most severe disease of the spectrum of the hypoproliferative anemias, and is characterized by a peripheral blood pancytopenia in association with a reduction or depletion of the hemopoietic stem cells in the marrow. Cellular marrow is replaced by fat, producing marked marrow *hypocellularity* (see Color Plate 8A). Occasionally, the disorder may start with an isolated anemia, leukopenia, or thrombocytopenia, and mild to moderate forms of the disease do occur. The severe form, however, is characterized by a hematocrit of less than 20% with marked reticulocytopenia, a granulocyte count of less than 500/μl and a platelet count of less than 20,000/μl. Table 3–11 lists a differential diagnosis of pancytopenia.

Aplastic Anemia

Aplastic anemia is a serious, but fortunately rare, disorder with an incidence of approximately 1 case per hundred thousand population. In some cases an association has been seen with *drug exposure (chloramphenicol* and *phenenylbutazone),* and a long list of drugs has been incriminated in association with aplastic anemia. In other cases, the condition may have been preceded by some infection, in particular *viral infections* including *hepatitis, cytomegalovirus,* and *Epstein-Barr virus.* Expo-

Table 3–11. CAUSES OF PANCYTOPENIA

Marrow failure syndrome

- Quantitative reduction of hematopoietic tissue (bone marrow deficiency)
  1. Hypoproliferative and aplastic anemias
     - Fanconi's anemia
     - Idiopathic anemia
       - Viral infections
         - Hepatitis B virus
         - Epstein-Barr virus
         - Cytomegalovirus
         - Parvovirus
     - Bacterial (tuberculosis)
     - Neoplasms
       - Clonal hematopoietic diseases
       - Secondary (metastatic) malignancies
         - Carcinomas
         - Lymphomas
       - Myelodysplastic syndromes
     - Toxic
       - Drugs
         - Chloramphenicol
         - Phenylbutazone
         - Chemotherapy
         - Others (idiosyncratic)
       - Irradiation
     - Autoimmune disease
       - SLE
       - Rheumatoid arthritis
       - Autoimmune pancytopenia
  2. Bone marrow replacement
     - Myelofibrosis
       - Idiopathic
       - Secondary (metastatic malignancy, TB)
       - Lymphomas
       - Granulomatous disease

Ineffective hematopoiesis

- Megaloblastic anemias
- Myelodysplastic syndromes

Hemodilution

Hypersplenism/splenomegaly

Immune destruction (autoimmune diseases)

sure to other *toxins* such as chemical solvents, *benzene, irradiation,* or *cytotoxic drugs* is also associated with aplastic anemia. *Irradiation* tends to produce rapid aplasia, and exposure to the *cytotoxic drugs* in cancer treatment may produce variable aplasia with variable recovery, depending on the drug used. These agents are expected to produce marrow hypoplasia, which is usually dose-dependent and self-limiting. Aplastic anemia associated with drugs not ordinarily expected to produce hypoproliferative anemia is thought to be an *idiosyncratic reaction.*

Other conditions known to be associated with hypoproliferative anemias include *autoimmune diseases* such as *lupus erythematosus.* Antibodies against stem cells or T cell inhibition of stem cells are suspected as immune mediators of injury. Some patients have a truly inherited disposition to aplasia, as occurs with *Fanconi's anemia.* Children with this disorder appear to have a deficiency in cellular DNA repair. This condition is associated with other constitutional abnormalities including abnormal kidneys and abnormal facial characteristics and digits. Aplasia or hypoplasia of the thumb is a common association. Other skeletal malformations occur in approximately two thirds of patients. Aplastic-hypoplastic anemia also occurs in association with other clonal hematologic neoplasms. It may herald the onset of an acute leukemia by months or even years, and may also be associated with *paroxysmal nocturnal hemoglobinuria* (PNH).

Laboratory Findings

Patients with aplastic anemia usually have pancytopenia with reticulocytopenia; however, a deficiency of a specific cell line can predominate (e.g., anemia, or leukopenia, or thrombocytopenia). A bone marrow must always be performed and shows *hypocellularity* of all elements, with a relative predominance of supporting marrow cells (plasma cells, lymphocytes, and reticulum cells) (see Color Plate 8A). If immature cells are seen, a myelodysplastic process should be suspected (preleukemia). If many lymphocytes predominate, a collagen-vascular disorder may be suspected as a co-association. Chromosomal studies are important to exclude Fanconi's anemia, in particular when this disease occurs in children. The acidified serum test and leukocyte alkaline phosphatase (LAP) test should be performed to exclude the condition paroxysmal nocturnal hemoglobinuria. In PNH, the LAP score is low (see Chapters 2 and 4).

Severe aplastic anemia is a fatal disease in the majority of patients. Patients classified as having severe aplasia have three out of the four following criteria:

1. neutrophil count of less than 500/μl
2. platelet count of less than 20,000/μl
3. reticulocyte count of less than 10,000/μl and
4. a markedly hypocellular marrow with less than 20% hematopoietic cells remaining for longer than three weeks.

The disease was associated with a 50% six-month mortality; however, many patients now survive longer because of improvement in clinical support measures. If the patient is less than 40 years of age and has an HLA-matched sibling bone marrow donor, the prognosis is very much better, with a high likelihood of cure following bone marrow transplantation. The prognosis is especially better for children and young adults. Patients who have been multiply transfused appear to have a worse prognosis, although the overall results of bone marrow transplantation in aplastic anemia show a 70–80% recovery.

Bone Marrow Replacement

Pancytopenia may also occur when the bone marrow is replaced by nonhematopoietic cells, as occurs in *secondary or metastatic malignancy,* or when there is an abnormal growth of hematopoietic cells replacing the normal bone marrow (e.g., leukemia, multiple myeloma) (see Chapter 4). When neoplastic cells infiltrate the hematopoietic marrow, pancytopenia develops if the process is extensive, but red cell production is depressed before other cell lines are affected. Leukemias, multiple myeloma, lymphoma, and carcinomas of the prostate, lung, and breast are the commonest tumors involved. Diagnosis rests on demonstrating the presence of malignant cells, but the presence of bizarre or randomly immature blood cells in the circulation tends to raise suspicion, especially if there are suggestive roentgenogram changes.

Myelofibrosis is replacement of hematopoietic marrow by fibrous connective tissue elements. Myelofibrosis is discussed in more detail under The Myeloproliferative Syndromes in Chapter 4. In this situation, either because of a primary clonal hematologic disease or due to secondary malignancy, the bone marrow is replaced by fibrous tissue. Hematopoietic development is usually taken over by other reticuloendothelial organs, particularly the spleen and the liver. Since those organs are less discriminating in preventing abnormal cells from being released into the blood stream, numerous misshapen and bizarre erythroid elements are seen in the peripheral blood in these conditions.

Hypoproliferative Anemia Associated with Other Diseases

Chronic infections, noninfectious inflammatory diseases such as rheumatoid arthritis and lupus erythematosus, slowly progressive neoplasms, and longstanding renal failure all depress bone marrow function by mechanisms not clearly understood. The laboratory findings are of a normochromic, normocytic anemia, usually of moderate degree (7–11 g/dl hemoglobin) with normal or near normal red cell survival, reduced serum iron and transferrin levels, and normal or increased storage iron in the marrow (see Anemia of Chronic Diseases, p 80). The bone marrow may be somewhat less cellular than normal, but those cells that are present have a normal appearance and are in normal proportions. Treatment is aimed at correction of the underlying disease, which if achieved is associated with improvement in the hematologic parameters.

Bone marrow aplasia sometimes follows viral hepatitis; other viral infections have also been implicated in sporadic cases. Tuberculosis may depress bone marrow function, but its other possible hematologic effects include pancytopenia caused by splenomegaly, or leukocytosis so severe as to resemble leukemia. Hypothyroidism may also be associated with a macrocytic anemia. Because metabolic activity is low, the low hemoglobin level does not cause tissue hypoxia; thus, erythropoietin is not stimulated and the bone marrow adjusts to lowered equilibrium.

Pure Red Cell Aplasia

In this disorder, there is hypoplasia of the erythrocyte precursors only, producing a severe anemia with reticulocytopenia. A bone marrow aspirate shows absence of erythroid precursors with normal myeloid and platelet elements. Peripheral blood indices usually show normochromic, normocytic red cells; however, occasionally macrocytosis may be seen. This disorder may occur transiently in association with other hemolytic anemias (e.g., sickle cell disease or spherocytosis) and may be caused by an infection from a parvovirus. This type of crisis has been termed *"aplastic crisis,"* and may be associated with an acute drop in hemoglobin or hematocrit. Patients may require blood transfusions if recovery does not occur within a short period. *Red cell aplasia* has also been seen in association with certain drugs, and may also occur with vitamin deficiency (particularly pyridoxine and riboflavin). In addition, a more common association of pure red cell aplasia with a tumor of the thymus gland (thymoma) is recognized. The condition is often corrected with removal of the thymus, or may respond to corticosteroid treatment. A congenital form of red cell aplasia presents with severe anemia in infancy, but is not associated with suppression of the white cell or platelet counts or skeletal abnormalities, as is seen in Fanconi's anemia. A condition termed *transient erythroblastopenia of childhood* (TEC) occurs as an acquired self-limited condition in early infancy. The origin is also thought to be a parvovirus infection, but may be immune-mediated. It is usually self-limiting in several weeks, but may require transfusion therapy or corticosteroid.

Refractory Anemia and Ineffective Erythropoiesis

Refractory Anemia

The refractory anemias constitute a group of disorders that are characterized by abnormal red cell production, generally unresponsive to any treatment. These disorders are often considered *preleukemic syndromes,* a term that is inaccurate because the majority of these disorders do not evolve into acute leukemia. However, the more unstable the bone marrow growth and the more abundant immature cells, particularly blasts, are in the bone marrow, the greater the likelihood for leukemic transformation. These conditions are more appropriately classified as *myelodysplastic syndromes,* and include the following conditions in which refractory anemia is often a major feature:

- refractory anemia with ring sideroblasts,
- refractory anemia with excess blasts,
- paroxysmal nocturnal hemoglobinuria,
- refractory anemia with excess blasts in transformation. (see Myelodysplasias and Preleukemic syndromes, Chapter 4)

The hallmark of these conditions is ineffective erythropoiesis in which the marrow is usually markedly hypercellular and shows an abundance of abnormal erythroid precursors. In many instances, the red cell precursors show megaloblastic features. In PNH, the marrow is more usually hypocellular and all marrow elements are decreased. These conditions are clonal abnormalities of marrow precursor cells, and consequently leukopenia and thrombocytopenia may coexist. In addition, cytogenetic abnormalities occur in almost half the patients with myelodysplastic syndromes involving, most commonly, chromosomes 5, 7, or 8 (see Chapter 4).

Paroxysmal Nocturnal Hemoglobinuria

Paroxysmal nocturnal hemoglobinuria (PNH) is a rare, acquired disorder characterized by the proliferation of an abnormal clone of hemopoietic cells in the bone marrow, erythrocytes with increased sensitivity to complement fixation and intravascular hemolysis. Despite the name, the majority of patients manifest with chronic intravascular hemolysis characterized by the presence of hemosiderin in the urine and not frank hemoglobinuria. Half of the cases of PNH develop between the ages of 20 and 40. In some cases, a similar PNH-like defect may occur in association with other hematologic malignancies such as leukemia, myelofibrosis, and aplastic anemia. Despite the descriptive name, episodic urinary excretion of hemoglobin after a night's sleep occurs in only 25% of cases.

Cellular Defects

The pathognomonic feature of PNH is strikingly increased susceptibility to complement mediated red cell lysis. Not every circulating cell is equally affected. Blood from PNH patients contains cells with three different degrees of complement sensitivity: 25–30 × normal, 3–5 × normal, and normal. The relative proportions of these populations determines how severely the patient is affected. Severity differs markedly from patient to patient, but tends to follow an episodic, gradually worsening course in the majority of affected individuals.

The membrane of PNH cells has both morphologic and chemical abnormalities. Scanning electron microscopy reveals strange pits and protuberances on the red cell surface. Chemical analysis reveals deficient acetylcholinesterase activity and the presence of abnormally constituted glycoproteins. It is probable that both acetylcholinesterase deficiency and complement sensitivity are manifestations of some underlying, still undefined causal phenomenon rather than having a cause and effect relationship.

Laboratory Findings

Paroxysmal nocturnal hemoglobinuria is diagnosed by demonstrating that red cells experience excessive hemolysis when exposed to low ionic strength solutions (sugar or sucrose lysis test). This test is often used as a screening test; however, the definitive test of PNH is the demonstration of excessive hemolysis when exposed to complement-containing serum at low pH (Ham's acid hemolysis test). The acid hemolysis test is less sensitive but more specific than the sugar water test; therefore, the latter is usually performed as a screening test. Patients with PNH usually have chronic, compensated hemolysis; however, unlike most patients with ongoing hemolysis, they have low iron stores and may be frankly iron deficient. Iron depletion occurs because hemoglobin and hemosiderin are excreted in the urine after complement-mediated intravascular hemolysis releases hemoglobin into the plasma (see Chapter 2).

Bone marrow aplasia is a common presenting symptom in PNH, causing leukopenia and thrombocytopenia along with depressed red cell production. Fifteen percent of patients with aplastic anemia may have PNH-like red cells. Thrombotic and infectious manifestations are other common presenting events and like aplastic crises, they may occur episodically throughout the disease. Reticulocytosis remains disproportionately low for the degree of hemolysis, even between frankly aplastic episodes. Hemolysis may be exacerbated during sleep, or by drug or dietary exposure; however, no clear pattern of inciting substances can be described. Transfusion of blood products containing even small amounts of plasma precipitates hemolysis reliably. If red cell transfusions are necessary, washed or deglycerolized frozen cells should be used to eliminate all the complement-containing plasma.

ANEMIAS CAUSED BY EXCESSIVE RED CELL LOSS

Hemorrhagic Anemia

A sudden drop in hemoglobin or hematocrit is associated either with acute blood loss or acute destruction of erythrocytes. This distinction is quite easy when bleeding is clinically apparent. The identification of hemolysis is also evident when laboratory criteria for hemolysis are present (see Hematologic Methods, Chapter 2). Internal bleeding may be more difficult to detect and may be associated with laboratory features compatible with extravascular hemolysis, since extravasated blood is also removed by the reticuloendothelial system (see Chapter 2). Laboratory data usually found in hemolytic anemia, including elevated bilirubin, elevated LDH, and decreased haptoglobin, are more usually associated with hemolysis than bleeding. Reticulocytosis, however, is commonly seen in hemorrhage and hemolysis.

Excessive Loss of Red Cells

Hemorrhage

Acute, massive blood loss does not cause immediate anemia. Rapid hemorrhage acutely decreases the intravascular blood volume and stresses the compensatory circulatory adjustments. Enough hemoglobin may remain to sustain life, but if circulatory mechanisms fail, hemoglobin cannot get to the tissues and oxygenation is impaired. After acute blood loss, the body adjusts by maintaining circulation through the most vital vascular beds by speeding up heart rates and expanding circulatory volume at the expense of the extravascular fluid. It is this volume adjustment that causes anemia. As extravascular fluid enters the bloodstream, it dilutes the remaining cells and the hematocrit drops over the next 48–72 hours.

Hematologic Response to Acute Blood Loss

Acute blood loss stimulates the bone marrow immediately. The platelet count and the number of circulating granulocytes increase before the hematocrit falls. Thrombocytosis between 600,000 and 800,000 per microliter and leukocytosis between 10,000 and 30,000 per microliter may occur within a few hours, accompanied in extreme cases by an outpouring of immature platelets and neutrophils. Since there is no storage reservoir of erythrocytes in the bone marrow, it may take up to several days or weeks to replenish the erythrocytes lost during hemorrhage. Erythropoietin levels rise within six hours, and reticulocytosis becomes apparent within 24 hours, reaching a peak in seven to ten days. If the hemorrhage is severe enough, "shift reticulocytes" and the presence of later stage normoblasts may be seen in the bloodstream.

If iron stores are normal, the rate of red cell production increases twofold–threefold. Iron-deficient patients cannot increase hematopoiesis appropriately when the hematocrit falls. Patients who receive therapeutic iron to supplement an erratic, inadequate, or borderline supply may show fourfold–sevenfold rises in erythropoietic activity. Reticulocytosis ceases when lost red cells are restored, usually within 30 days if no further bleeding occurs. Persistently elevated reticulocyte counts suggest continuing blood loss or red cell destruction.

If blood is shed into the body cavities, the lumen of the alimentary tract, or the soft tissues, nonviable red cells and hemoglobin accumulate and must be degraded. These changes may cause elevation of blood urea and bilirubin levels. Blood loss to the exterior does not, of course, have this effect. Chronic blood loss, due to continuous low-level bleeding, does not disrupt the blood volume since fluid adjustments occur automatically. However, as red cells are lost, also lost is the iron in their hemoglobin, and chronic blood loss commonly induces a state of iron deficiency anemia.

Hemolytic Anemias

Hemolytic anemia is a disorder that is associated with a *shortened red cell survival.* Usually there is either an *intracorpuscular* or *extracorpuscular* abnormality that limits the erythrocyte lifespan. The extent and severity of the anemia is dependent on the rate of destruction and removal of red cells, and balanced by the compensatory increase in bone marrow erythrocyte production. The normal bone marrow is capable of increasing its work activity by six to eightfold, so that an anemia may not be apparent until the red cell lifespan is shortened to approximately 20 days. Hemolytic anemias may be classified into disorders associated with an *intrinsic defect (intracorpuscular)* or those associated with an *extrinsic abnormality (extracorpuscular).* Table 3–12 lists conditions characterized by hemolysis.

Table 3–12. CLASSIFICATION OF HEMOLYTIC ANEMIAS

Intrinsic defects
- Hereditary defects
  - Abnormalities of the red cell membrane
    - Hereditary spherocytosis
    - Hereditary elliptocytosis
    - Hereditary pyropoikilocytosis
    - Hereditary stomatocytosis and xerocytosis
  - Inherited erythrocyte enzyme disorders
    - Glucose-6-phosphate dehydrogenase deficiency
    - Other enzyme deficiencies
      - Pyruvate kinase deficiency
      - Pyrimidine-5′-nucleotidase deficiency
  - Disorders of hemoglobin production
    - Hemoglobinopathies
    - Sickle cell syndromes
      - Sickle cell disease
      - Sickle cell trait
      - HbS beta-thalassemia syndrome
      - Hemoblogin C disease
      - Hemoglobin SC disease
    - Methemoglobins/hemoglobin M
    - Unstable hemoglobin
    - Thalassemia syndromes
      - Alpha-thalassemia
      - Homozygous beta-thalassemia
      - Heterozygous beta-thalassemia
      - Thalassemia heterozygotes with other hemoglobinopathies
  - Acquired defects
    - Paroxysmal nocturnal hemoglobinuria

Extrinsic defects
- Non-immune destruction
  - Microangiopathic and macroangiopathic hemolytic anemia
  - Chemical and toxic agents
  - Infections causing hemolysis
  - Hypersplenism
  - Systemic disorders
- Immune hemolytic anemias
  - Primary
  - Secondary (associated with chronic lymphocytic leukemia, lymphomas and carcinomas)
  - Drug-induced
  - Infections

INTRINSIC DEFECTS

Hereditary Defects

Abnormalities of the Red Cell Membrane

An appreciation of the pathophysiology of hemolysis due to abnormalities of the erythrocyte membranes requires a basic understanding of the structure of the red cell membrane (see Chapter 2). The membrane has a skeletal component that consists of a protein chain adjacent to the cell membrane. The structural integrity of the erythrocyte is dependent on its ability to withstand shear forces during its passage through the microcirculation. It is the membrane's skeletal proteins that enable the erythrocyte to withstand such forces, and disorders of these proteins are associated with shortened red cell survival, i.e., hemolysis. The erythrocyte should be deformable and have an appropriate cell surface-area-to-volume ratio in order to withstand shear forces and osmotic stress. The chemical composition of the membrane is one of a lipid bilayer consisting of cholesterol and phospholipids, forming approximately 50% of the chemical structure, that are arranged in close aposition with the membrane proteins. Some membrane proteins traverse the lipid layer, whereas others are internally distributed and some are distributed only on the periphery of the membrane lipids. The *integral proteins* traverse the lipid membrane, whereas the *peripheral proteins* are situated on the internal aspect of the cell membrane. The skeletal proteins of the membrane comprise several proteins called *spectrin, actin,* and some other proteins (see Chapter 2). The cytoskeleton is anchored to the plasma cell membrane via a protein called *ankyrin.* These proteins may be separated by electrophoretic methods and are classified according to their molecular weight and migration on electrophoretic gels. Although classification will probably be more refined and will be categorized on the basis of the molecular defect, current classifications are morphologic and include *five main disorders:* 1) *hereditary spherocytosis,* 2) *hereditary elliptocytosis,* 3) *hereditary pyropoikilocytosis,* 4) *hereditary stomatocytosis,* and 5) *hereditary xerocytosis.* Table 3–12 outlines the hereditary defects of the red cell membrane.

Hereditary Spherocytosis. Hereditary spherocytosis (HS) is a fairly common hemolytic condition that is usually transmitted as an autosomal dominant trait in Caucasian people. In 25% of cases, no inheritance pattern is identified and these persons are thought to have developed this disorder due to a spontaneous mutation. Recently, molecular abnormalities of the skeletal proteins have been identified in some cases of HS (e.g., deficient synthesis of spectrin). In many cases, however, the molecular defect has not been identified. In the United States, HS affects approximately 2.2 per 10,000 whites, but the anemia is relatively mild and sometimes goes undiagnosed until late adulthood. Patients with HS, like those with other chronic hemolytic anemias, have marked susceptibility to formation of bilirubin stones in the gallbladder. Often it is the gallbladder, not the blood problem, that causes patients to seek medical attention.

Cellular Changes. The basic defect in the erythrocyte is loss of membrane, resulting in decreased surface area. This produces a cell with the lowest surface-area-to-volume ratio, namely the *spherocyte* (see Color Plate 10A). As previously described, the reduced surface-area-to-volume ratio makes these cells more susceptible to osmotic lysis, and consequently increases osmotic fragility (see Chapter 2, p 51). These cells are also less deformable and cannot easily negotiate the microcirculation. The reason for the loss of membrane is still unexplained; however, it is thought to occur in passage through the splenic sinusoids. The primary defect, however, is probably an abnormality in the skeletal protein producing a defect of deformability. As the cells negotiate the splenic sinusoids, with each circulatory passage more and more membrane is removed (microspherocytes formed) until the cell is ultimately sequestered. A formerly held belief that cells in HS were metabolically depleted because of extra ATP consumption and problems with sodium and calcium influx, is presently in doubt. However, it is possible that calcium may interact adversely with spectrin to produce defective deformability.

As mentioned in Chapter 2, a spherocyte is the structure that has the lowest surface area compared with volume, and is consequently extremely sensitive to any increase in intracellular fluid (osmotic fragility). Further understanding of the molecular structure of the red cell membrane will enable a more precise classification to be developed, and it is apparent that deficiencies of membrane proteins may lead to spherocytic, elliptocytic, or other morphologic abnormalities in red cell shape, characterized in most cases by shortened red cell survival, i.e., hemolysis. Hereditary spherocytosis is the commonest of these disorders.

Clinical Features. The condition may present a clinical spectrum characterized particularly by varying degrees of *anemia, jaundice, and splenomegaly,* and the presence of *spherocytosis* and *stomatocytosis* in the peripheral blood. Since spherocytes are sequestered and destroyed in their passage through the spleen, the majority of cases benefit substantially by removal of the spleen (splenectomy). Patients may have a mild hemolytic state and be relatively compensated; however, with physical and infectious stress they may manifest an exaggerated anemia *(hemolytic crisis).* Some patients may have a severe hemolytic anemia requiring red cell transfusions. In addition, in response to fever, infections, and stress, patients may experience a sudden decrease in marrow production and manifest with an exaggerated anemia *(aplastic crisis).* Other clinical manifestations of hereditary spherocytosis include skeletal abnormalities due to a continuous marrow hyperproliferation, and chronic leg ulcers and gallstones, which may occur in other hemolytic conditions as well (notably sickle cell disease). A small percentage of patients also have a history of neonatal jaundice.

Laboratory Findings—Red Cell Morphology: The laboratory findings in hereditary spherocytosis are listed in Table 3–13. The characteristic cells seen in the peripheral smear are the *spherocyte* (see Color Plate 10A), which are uniformly

Table 3–13. LABORATORY FINDINGS IN HEREDITARY SPHEROCYTOSIS

Blood count
Mild anemia (Hgb 9–12 g/dl)
MCV normal or slightly low, MCHC high
Spherocytes in peripheral blood
Platelets slightly low if spleen present
Reticulocytes 5–7%
Red cell studies
Osmotic fragility very high
Autohemolysis after 48 hr at 37°C
10–50% (normal <4%)
Glucose or ATP abolishes high autohemolysis
Chemistry
Bilirubin slightly high (indirect)
Urine urobilinogen high
Haptoglobin low

round cells with more intensely staining hemoglobin and the absence of the central pale area usually seen in a normal red cell. In addition, there is an increased, diffuse *polychromatophilia,* which represents the marrow erythropoietic (reticulocyte) response and is often proportional to the degree of anemia. Since the spherocyte has a normal hemoglobin content but smaller surface area, the mean cell hemoglobin concentration (MCHC) is increased. Other features of a hemolytic process are also present, including an elevated indirect serum bilirubin, an elevated lactate dehydrogenase (LDH), and a decreased serum haptoglobin.

Definitive diagnosis of hereditary spherocytosis is confirmed by demonstrating an abnormal *osmotic fragility test* (Fig. 3–1) which, as was mentioned in Chapter 2, assesses red cell membrane function.

Autohemolysis is often markedly increased, and especially after incubation at 37°C for 24–48 hours. This may be corrected by the addition of glucose (see Chapter 2, p. 51).

Treatment. In symptomatic patients, splenectomy is the treatment of choice because it removes the major source of red cell sequestration and destruction. Patients should be maintained on folic acid as a prophylaxis against aplastic crises. Splenectomy does not cure the defect, but removes the site of sequestration.

Hereditary Elliptocytosis. This condition is also an inherited disorder associated with a defective membrane protein skeleton structure. The condition is associated with a morphologic abnormality in the peripheral blood smear, and the pres-

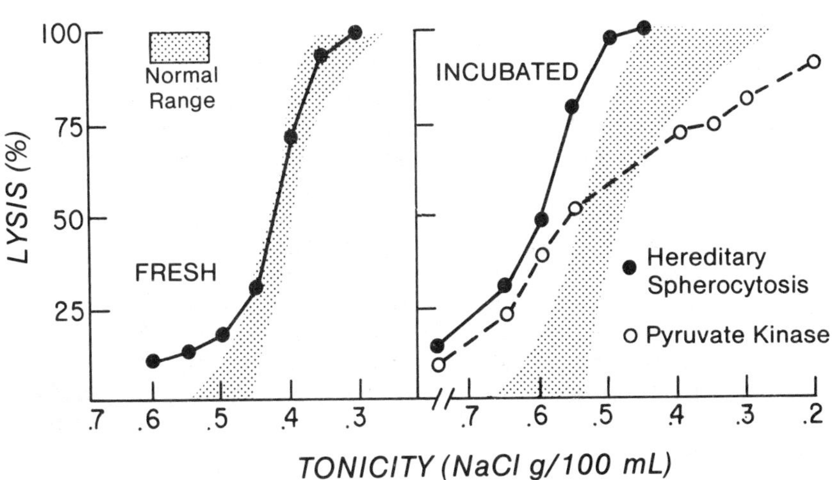

Figure 3–1. Osmotic fragility test. This test may be used to identify patients with defects in red cell membrane (hereditary spherocytosis) or intracellular metabolism (pyruvate kinase deficiency). The osmotic fragility test involves subjecting the red cells to stress of increasingly hypotonic salt solutions. When performed on a fresh blood sample, there is displacement of the hereditary spherocytic curve to the left, representing increased susceptibility to hemolysis. Often this is limited to a small tail of cells that are unusually susceptible to lysis. After incubation, the defect is magnified. In contrast, pyruvate kinase-deficient blood shows a mix of sensitive cells and cells resistant to osmotic lysis. (From Hillman and Finch,[16] p 96, with permission.)

ence of elongated, *elliptical cells* (see Color Plate 18). It is inherited as an autosomal dominant trait in most cases. A variant of this condition is another disorder called *hereditary pyropoikilocytosis.* The erythrocytes show marked variation in shape (poikilocytosis) with many teardrop forms, spherocytes, and microspherocytes, as well as fragmented cells. There is also a heat instability. When heparinized patient blood is subjected to a temperature of 45°C, the morphologic changes are exaggerated. There are several variants that are categorized by the degree of hemolysis and the type of morphologic abnormality. These conditions are often clinically insignificant and often represent a "cosmetic" abnormality on the peripheral blood smear. Patients with mild *hereditary elliptocytosis* usually have normal osmotic fragility and autohemolysis. These tests may be abnormal in the more severe cases.

Hereditary Stomatocytosis and Hereditary Xerocytosis. Two other rare disorders of red cell membrane permeability are *hereditary stomatocytosis* and *hereditary xerocytosis.* These conditions are characterized by red cell morphologic abnormalities, namely increased numbers of *stomatocytes* and an elevated mean cell volume in hereditary stomatocytosis, and an increased number of target cells in *hereditary xerocytosis.* Occasionally patients may present with hemolytic anemias that show a good response to splenectomy. These diseases reflect abnormalities in the red cell membrane cytoskeleton, causing alteration in ionic fluxes and accumulation of abnormal intracellular electrolytes.

Inherited Erythrocyte Enzyme Disorders

Deficiency of erythrocyte enzymes *(enzymopathies)* may be associated with abnormal metabolic functions that may decrease erythrocyte survival. The spectrum of hemolysis produced is dependent on the nature of the enzyme deficiency and its importance in erythrocyte function. Erythrocyte metabolic pathways are discussed in Chapter 2. Although many enzymes are important for normal erythrocyte function, except for glucose-6-phosphate dehydrogenase deficiency, other enzyme deficiencies are extremely uncommon.

Glucose-6-Phosphate Dehydrogenase Deficiency. Glucose-6-phosphate dehydrogenase (G-6-PD) is the initial enzyme involved in the *pentose phosphate pathway* of erythrocyte metabolism. It catalyzes the removal of hydrogen from *glucose-6-phosphate* to produce *6-phosphogluconate* (6-PG) and requires cofactors *nicotine-adenine-dinucleotide phosphate* (NADP), which is reduced to NADPH (see Chapter 2, Fig. 2–9). This is an important reaction because NADPH is a source of reducing potential for the erythrocyte to resist oxidant stress. Deficiency of this enzyme is associated with an inability to neutralize oxidation stress, which produces instability of the hemoglobin molecule and consequent hemolysis. This is especially provoked by oxidant drugs. NADPH is an electron donor that is active in many biologic systems. Its reducing capacity is important for the red cell's *glutathione system,* which is the main reservoir of protection of hemoglobin against oxidative stress and irreversible denaturation.

A gene on the X-chromosome determines the structure of G-6-PD, which exhibits remarkable polymorphism in human populations. A mutant expression of the X-chromosome is fully expressed in the male *(hemizygote)* who inherits this mutant gene. Female heterozygotes are usually normal; however, homozygous females with two mutant X-chromosomes can exhibit G-6-PD deficiency and clinical disease. A heterozygote female may exhibit partial expression of the disorder, depending on which X-chromosome is inactivated. Since only a single X-chromosome is operative in any single cell, random inactivation of the second X-chromosome occurs in females *(Lyon hypothesis).* Depending on the degree of inactivation of a normal X-chromosome, a mutant X-chromosome may be expressed in heterozygous females. Normal G-6-PD is termed the *B variant,* and is present in 99% of the Caucasians in the United States. A variant G-6-PD that differs from the B variant by a single amino acid is found in approximately 16% of American black males and is called *A variant.* A common defective *variant of A* is called A^-, which occurs in 9–13% of American blacks. The designation A^- is because there is generally a decreased functional expression of G-6-PD. The amino acid difference between A and B variants creates differing electrophoretic mobilities, which can be demonstrated in the laboratory. Approximately 20% of black females are heterozygous for the G-6-PD A variant. Nearly all heterozygotes have functionally adequate red cells. There is a relationship between the possession of G-6-PD, type A and resistance to malaria for reasons similar to those discussed under Sickle Cell Disease. Most persons with the A^- variant do have comfortably adequate activity levels, except when subjected to oxidant drug stress. The function of G-6-PD is assessed clinically by subjecting red cells to oxidative stress (see Chapter 2). Specific variants can be characterized by their *electrophoretic mobility, thermal stability,* and other enzyme *kinetic studies. Isoenzymes* are enzymes with the same biologic function but differing physical or chemical properties, including electrophoretic mobility. There are many isoenzymes of G-6-PD that have been described. The A and B variants are the most common.

Clinical Patterns. Glucose-6-phosphate dehydrogenase deficiency may have a varied clinical presentation. The commonest clinical patterns are 1) neonatal jaundice, 2) congenital hemolytic anemia, 3) drug-induced hemolysis, and 4) favism.

Patients with the A^- enzyme experience no difficulty under normal conditions. Most remain unaware that hematologic abnormality exists, except that the A^- enzyme has about 15% of normal activity—enough for most purposes. Red cell number, function, and survival are normal unless and until some acute oxidative stress occurs. Activity of G-6-PD declines as the red cell ages, no matter what variant is present. When the enzyme is defective, the effects of this decline become more noticeable. Aging red cells are especially susceptible to oxidative challenge by drugs, systemic infection, metabolic acidosis, and other stresses. Oxidative stress induces rapid intravascular destruction of susceptible cells, leading to hemoglobinemia, hemoglobinuria, and a sudden drop in hematocrit. The hemolytic crisis is self-limited because eventually the only cells left are those younger cells with sufficient enzyme levels to withstand the stress. Prompt erythropoietic response results in reticulocytosis and the introduction of still more young cells that are well supplied with active enzyme. Thus, drug-induced hemolysis is the commonest clinical manifestation of G-6-PD deficiency and is usually self-limiting.

Drugs that hemolyze G-6-PD deficient cells are those that either act as direct oxidants themselves or produce peroxide activity. *Primaquine,* an antimalarial drug, is notable in this respect; an older term for the red cell defect G-6-PD deficiency is *Primaquine Sensitivity.* Primaquine is a drug that was used for malarial prophylaxis in the Korean War. Since many black patients were treated with the drug, the association was quickly made between acute hemolysis and the antimalarial oxidant drug primaquine. Hence the term Primaquine Sensitivity and the association with black patients. The severity of the hemolysis depends on the nature of the G-6-PD variant and the degree of deficiency. The signs of intravascular hemolysis occur approximately three days after taking the drug, when the patient presents with anemia, jaundice, and hemoglobinuria. Many sulfa drugs, quinine derivatives, nitrofurans, and antipyretic-analgesic drugs can induce hemolysis in G-6-PD-deficient patients. Susceptibility seems to vary among different individuals. The presence of coexistent fever, metabolic disease or hepatic or renal failure increases the likelihood that symptoms will occur.

Another G-6-PD variant is the *Mediterranean enzyme variant.* This occurs in whites, especially those of Greek, Italian, and some Jewish populations. The *Mediterranean variant* has severely reduced activity, so that even very young cells have little capacity to generate NADPH. Hemolytic episodes are more severe, are triggered by a greater variety of stimuli, and are less likely to be self-limited than in patients with the A$^-$ variant. Infants with the deficiency may present with severe *neonatal jaundice. Favism,* a susceptibility to massive hemolysis after exposure to the fava bean, occurs especially in persons with the Mediterranean type G-6-PD deficiency. Serum factors and immune mechanisms are involved in this type of hemolysis, although the exact pathogenesis is not clearly understood. Patients with this variant and other more unusual severe variants may have a *chronic hemolytic anemia* associated with chronic intravascular hemolysis. Laboratory findings in this case include a chronic intravascular hemolytic anemia with decreased haptoglobin, increased LDH and bilirubin, an elevated reticulocyte count, and the presence of hemosiderin in the urine, which is indicative of a chronic intravascular hemolysis. See Chapter 2 for assessment of the phosphate pentose pathway and G-6-PD.

Typically, following drug exposure, there is an acute drop in hemoglobin and hematocrit. This is associated with a brisk reticulocyte count elevation. Reticulocyte counts may go as high as 50% or more. *Screening tests* during the acute intravascular hemolytic phase may be normal with the A$^-$ deficiency because of the presence of the high reticulocyte count. During the asymptomatic phase, however, they will be abnormal and will indicate deficiency. The nature of the G-6-PD can be confirmed by *gel electrophoresis. Enzyme studies* can then identify the specific abnormality and will facilitate quantitation of the deficiency.

During the acute intravascular hemolytic event, the peripheral blood may show *fragmented red cells* and, more typically, the *"blister cell."* Because of oxidative denaturation of hemoglobin, the hemoglobin appears to separate from the superficial erythrocyte membrane, which appears as a clear *"blister."* Since hemoglobin has become denatured and oxidized, Heinz bodies will also be detected (see Color Plate 16). Other laboratory findings indicative of acute intravascular hemolysis, as outlined in Chapter 2, can also be seen during acute crisis, particularly in the Mediterranean type.

Other Enzyme Deficiencies. *Pyruvate Kinase Deficiency.* Although numerous, rare enzyme abnormalities have been detected, the next most common defect, representing approximately 95% of the remaining enzyme abnormalities other than G-6-PD, is *pyruvate kinase deficiency.* The rest of the defects are metabolic curiosities involving the entire range of available enzymes. *Pyruvate kinase* is the enzyme that catalyzes the conversion of 2-phospho-enol-pyruvate into pyruvate, and represents an energy-producing final step of the glycolytic pathway (see Fig. 2–9). The effect of pyruvate kinase deficiency would also be considered to be more profound in older red cells that lack the oxidative phosphorylation metabolic capability. This step, therefore, represents the major source of energy production for nonreticulocyte red blood cells. It is associated with the generation of two molecules of adenosine triphosphate (ATP). Pyruvate kinase-deficient cells are also more preferentially removed in the spleen, and patients have a chronic hemolytic anemia. The clinical features, however, may vary considerably. Failure to generate sufficient ATP results in defective control of ions, so that excessive sodium and calcium enter the cell and membrane phospholipids may sustain damage.

Defective PK and other glycolytic enzymes may induce hemolytic anemia, which is characterized by *increased autohemolysis* after incubation at 37°C, and increased indirect bilirubin. The major clinical features are anemia, jaundice, and splenomegaly. The anemia is a nonspherocytic hemolytic anemia, since spherocytes are not seen. Pyruvate kinase deficiency is inherited as an autosomal recessive trait; therefore, both sexes are affected equally.

Pyrimidine-5'-Nucleotidase Deficiency. This condition, which is associated with deficiency of the enzyme responsible for metabolism of pyrimidine residues in the developing red cell, is associated with a chronic, congenital hemolytic anemia whose striking feature is the presence of marked basophilic stippling (see Color Plate 16C). These patients may also present with anemia, jaundice, and splenomegaly, which may be quite prominent. Patients may benefit from the removal of the spleen. This is a rare disorder, and diagnosis is made by special enzyme assays, usually performed by a reference laboratory.

Disorders of Hemoglobin Production

Disorders of Globin Synthesis (Hemoglobinopathies). *Normal Maturational Changes.* In the earliest embryonic stages, unique hemoglobins are produced by the yolk sac derivatives. By six weeks, fetal cells begin producing hemoglobin F, which dominates the oxygen-carrying mechanism until birth. Beta chain production can be detected by the sixth month of intrauterine life. At birth, up to 30% of the hemoglobin in each red cell is hemoglobin A, and the change from fetal to adult hemoglobin progresses rapidly. At six months of age, 80–90% of the hemoglobin present is hemoglobin A and from one year onwards, hemoglobin F constitutes less than 2% of the total. Delta chain production is insignificant before birth. Adult red cells contain 1–2% hemoglobin A_2, a level achieved at about one year. Each red cell in a given individual contains the same proportions of the same hemoglobins. Figure 3–4, later in the chapter, shows the sequence of hemoglobin chain development.

Hemoglobin Variants. The most common abnormal hemoglobin is *hemoglobin S* or *sickle hemoglobin,* in which the normal *glutamic acid* at the sixth position in the beta chain is replaced by the neutral amino acid *valine.* Hemoglobin S is by far the commonest hemoglobinopathy. Amino acid #6 occurs at the outer surface of the richly intertwining globin chain configuration, at the area where alpha and beta chains shift position during oxygenation and deoxygenation. Other substitutions can and do occur within the folded globin chain at contact points between the other globin chains, or near the heme insertion. Each substitution produces a different hemoglobin, of which several hundred have been discovered.

Substitutions within the globin chains may cause altered solubility, altered ability to withstand oxidation, instability, increased propensity for methemoglobin production, or increased or decreased oxygen affinity. Some substitutions produce very little in the way of clinical abnormalities.

Genes determining globin chain structures are codominant; this means that the gene product is detectable no matter which allele is on the opposite chromosome. Heterozygotes with two different genes for globin structure will have two kinds of hemoglobin. Heterozygous subjects with hemoglobinopathies, then, will usually have hemoglobin A and the other abnormal substituted variant. People who have two different abnormal alleles have red cells that contain two different abnormal hemoglobins (double heterozygotes) and no normal hemoglobin A at all (e.g., sickle cell [SC] disease). If the same abnormal allele is present on both chromosomes, the individual is homozygous for the hemoglobinopathy and all the hemoglobin is the same type expressing the same abnormality.

The existence of a hemoglobinopathy is demonstrated by *hemoglobin electrophoresis.* For the common hemoglobin abnormalities, no further diagnostic proof is needed. More detailed study becomes necessary with rare abnormal hemoglobins, and may include hemoglobin synthesis, protein characterization, and physical properties. Only two hemoglobinopathies are sufficiently common to warrant detailed consideration here.

Sickle Cell Syndromes. Sickle cell syndromes include all the conditions in which sickle hemoglobin (HbS) is present: *heterozygous AS, homozygous SS,* the presence of *S with other beta chain abnormalities* such as *SC disease,* and the presence of *hemoglobin S in association with defective expression of globin chains,* e.g., *S thalassemia.*

Sickle Cell Disease: Sickle cell disease is a disorder in which the patient lacks a normal hemoglobin A and hemoglobin S is present. Therefore, an individual with sickle cell disease has a homozygous expression of S hemoglobin. The sickle cell gene frequency is high among American blacks, and is reminiscent of their equatorial African heritage. The gene frequency in equatorial Africa ranges between 5–20%. The frequency of the carrier state in the United States is approximately 8%, with the incidence of the homozygous state at birth being 0.16%. Possession of the sickle gene is believed to confer some advantage against (falciparum) malaria infection.

Pathophysiology: When hemoglobin A releases its oxygen, one alpha and one beta chain change their relative positions. They resume their previous positions when reoxygenation occurs. Hemoglobin S has the hydrophobic amino acid valine in place of the hydrophilic amino acid glutamic acid at the sixth position on the beta chain. In the deoxygenated configuration, this substitution assumes critical importance. The valine residue represents a key-like surface structure that just fits into a complementary site on an adjacent, deoxygenated molecule. As one molecule locks into the next, the deoxygenated hemoglobin forms filaments that intertwine into elongated, cable-like, polymeric masses that are insoluble at high concentrations. The initial shape change is reversible. If oxygen is restored, the adjacent sites unlock, the beta chain returns to the oxygenated configuration, and solubility resumes.

Deoxygenated hemoglobin S can link with adjacent molecules of hemoglobin A or of other abnormal hemoglobins, but the association is not long-lasting. Whether or not insoluble aggregates will form depends on the proportion of hemoglobin S to other hemoglobins, on the absolute concentration of hemoglobin S, and on the degree of deoxygenation. The presence of hemoglobin A guards, to a modest extent, against polymerization; *hemoglobin F exerts a very strong protective effect.* Persons heterozygous for hemoglobin S and hemoglobin A have only 30–40% hemoglobin S in each cell. The high concentration of hemoglobin A is a deterrent to sickling. Except in nonphysiologic conditions of extreme deoxygenation (in laboratory testing), the cells do not sickle, even though individual molecules may undergo the shape change. High intracellular levels of hemoglobin F can protect even homozygous hemoglobin S from sickling.

It is likely that erythrocytes of patients with sickle cell disease undergo intravascular sickling and unsickling many times as they circulate. Initially sickling may be a reversible effect, but with repeated episodes of sickling, the cells become so-called *"irreversibly sickled cells."* These cells are less flexible and less deformable to the physical demands of the circulation. Some cells gradually lose their mechanical and osmotic resistance and undergo intravascular dissolution, whereas others withstand individual stresses but are destroyed at an above-normal rate by the reticuloendothelial system. Red cells in hemoglobin S disease experience a chronically shortened lifespan.

The likelihood of *sickling* increases with *low oxygen tensions* (hypoxia), *lowered pH* (acidosis), and *increased body temperature* (fever). In those parts of the circulation where blood flow is slow, tissue oxygen levels are low, or metabolic waste products accumulate, sickling is a danger. Sickle cells pass poorly through tiny vessels. This causes blood viscosity to rise and blood flow to become more stagnant, which in turn aggravates the problems of poor tissue perfusion, increased acidity, and decreased oxygenation.

Clinical considerations: Persons homozygous for hemoglobin S (SS) suffer from *sickle cell anemia,* a lifelong, variably severe, hemolytic anemia punctuated by superimposed episodes of exaggerated hemolysis *(hemolytic crisis),* bone marrow aplasia *(aplastic crisis),* and *painful* vaso-occlusive episodes. Continuous hemolysis causes erythropoietic hyperplasia of such magnitude that the bones may be deformed by the mass of proliferating erythroid marrow. Sickle cell anemia rarely becomes clinically apparent before 6 months of age because protective amounts of hemoglobin F remain in each cell. Intrauterine development is usually normal because hemoglobin F is not affected by abnormalities of beta chain production.

The most common clinical manifestation of sickle cell anemia is the vaso-occlusive crisis, which probably occurs as a result of impairment of blood flow from the irreversibly sickled cells, and is perpetuated by deoxygenation and devitalization of the tissues affected. Consequently, depending on which vessels are affected, clinical features may vary tremendously, but the most common manifestations are bone pain and tenderness from micro-infarcts in the bones. Ischemia and infarction can occur in many other sites involving parenchymal organs such as the lungs, liver, spleen, and kidney, and the central nervous system and eyes. In childhood the spleen may be enlarged; however, because of recurrent vaso-occlusive crisis involving this organ, the spleen gradually becomes fibrosed and atrophied. Consequently, persons with sickle cell anemia have functional asplenia and are prone to infections from capsulated organisms, particularly *pneumococcus* and *H. influenzae.* In children, infarctive crises affecting the developing bones are common as well as skeletal abnormalities from hyperproliferation of the bone marrow in response to the chronic hemolytic state. With successive episodes of infarction involving parenchymal tissues, there is loss of tissue reserve and symptomatic disease of that organ may occur. In adults, pulmonary involvement is very common and patients often present with infections and pneumonia.

Inexplicable episodes of marrow aplasia occur, some secondary to parvovirus infection, during which hemolysis continues and erythropoiesis ceases. There is a remarkable drop in the hematocrit and reticulocyte count, which leads to a dangerous level of anemia. The *aplastic crises* can occur from folic acid deficiency, and patients must be maintained on continuous folic acid for life.

The exaggerated *hemolytic crises* are difficult to differentiate from the chronic hemolytic state, especially since an increase in jaundice may be secondary to gallstones. Gallstones are very common in patients with any chronic hemolytic anemia, and the clinical features may be very similar to acute intravascular hemolytic crises. In acute intravascular sickling, the hematocrit drops but the reticulocyte count rises, as do the other laboratory parameters of intravascular hemolysis (Table 3–14 shows the characteristic laboratory findings in sickle cell anemia).

Sickle Cell Trait: Heterozygotes, with one hemoglobin S gene and one hemoglobin A gene, have sickle cell trait but usually have no clinical disease. The heterozygous hemoglobin SA state appears to offer significant protection against malarial infection with *Plasmodium falciparum.* This apparently beneficial effect may explain why this otherwise deleterious gene has persisted with such high incidence in areas where malaria is endemic. Patients also have generally no hematologic symptoms and a normal life expectancy with normal patterns of morbidity and mortality. The presence of the gene, however, has potential implications with regard to anesthesia and air travel in unpressurized aircraft. Reduction of oxygen tension can cause the development of sickling. Oxygen tension needs to be sustained at greater than 100 mmHg during anesthesia.

Table 3–14. LABORATORY FINDINGS IN SICKLE CELL ANEMIA (HEMOGLOBIN S DISEASE)

Blood count
- Hgb low (usually 6–10 g/dl)
- Marked poikilocytosis, inclusion bodies
- Irreversibly sickled cells 6–18% of RBCs on smear
- WBCs 10–20 × $10^3/\mu l$
- Platelets high
- Reticulocytes 10–20% (except in aplastic crises)

Bone marrow
- Marked erythroid hyperplasia
- Storage iron high

Blood chemistry
- Bilirubin high (especially indirect)
- Serum iron high, iron-binding capacity normal, % saturation high

Other tests
- Sickle prep (solubility test) positive (Note: if anemia is severe, it may be necessary to remove some plasma)
- Hgb electrophoresis shows Hgb S
- Red cell survival low
- Erythrocyte sedimentation rate abnormally low

Hgb = hemoglobin; RBC = red blood cells; WBC = white blood cells.

Persons with sickle cell trait usually have normal hematologic values with a normal peripheral blood smear. A sickle solubility test is positive, and hemoglobin electrophoresis reveals 55–60% hemoglobin A and 35–45% hemoglobin S.

Hemoglobin S/Beta-Thalassemia Syndrome: This condition occurs as a result of the inheritance of one sickle gene and one beta thalassemia gene. The severity of the clinical disease will depend on the amount of normal beta chain synthesized. These individuals manufacture normal amounts of alpha chains but, depending on the degree of impairment of the beta chains and which beta chain is affected, may express varying proportions of hemoglobin A or hemoglobin S. Consequently, patients may have a mild disorder or may express a clinical severity similar to sickle cell anemia (see also Thalassemia Syndromes).

Hemoglobin C Disease: Hemoglobin C resembles hemoglobin S with an amino acid substitution at the sixth position on the beta chain. In this case, *glutamic acid* is replaced by *lysine.* Hemoglobin C is less soluble than hemoglobin A because the positive charge on the lysine interacts with adjacent negatively charged groups. It is not clear whether *in vivo* crystallization occurs, but red cells with hemoglobin C as a dominant molecule are more rigid and more liable to fragmentation than normal red cells. About 2–3% of American blacks carry the hemoglobin C gene. The heterozygous state (HbC trait) does not cause anemia or shortened red cell lifespan. Although target cells may be seen in the blood smears, there is no anemia and no shortening of red cell survival.

One in 6,000 American blacks is homozygous for hemoglobin C (CC). This causes a mild, hemolytic anemia with striking red cell morphologic abnormalities (see Color Plate 13). There are numerous target cells, microspherocytes, and intracellular crystals (tactoids), but hemoglobin levels remain in the range of 8–12 g/dl. The biochemical findings of hemolysis exist to a modest extent. Since the disease has few intrinsic complications and does not interact adversely with other diseases, patients often remain unaware of their condition until it is detected during hemoglobin screening programs or during medical care for some other condition.

Hemoglobin SC Disease: This condition is a chronic hemolytic anemia associated with the inheritance of one abnormal gene carrying the C trait and another gene carrying the S trait. Consequently, individuals with SC disease are double heterozygotes. This condition occurs with a gene frequency of up to 0.25% of the population in Western Africa, and occurs in the United States in approximately 1 in 833 blacks. Clinical features can be very similar to those of patients with SS disease; however, they generally tend to be milder. Curiously, patients with SC disease tend to develop more aseptic necrosis of the femoral head, which is a common arthritic complaint of this disorder.

The hematologic features of SC disease generally show a mild anemia with reticulocytosis and numerous target cells in the peripheral smear. Occasional sickle cells may also be seen.

Hereditary Persistence of Fetal Hemoglobin: This condition is generally a benign disorder, which manifests a persistence of fetal hemoglobin synthesis into adult life. The regulation of beta-gamma switching is unknown; however, different degrees of persistence of the gamma globin gene activity occur. The homozygous condition is associated with 100% of fetal hemoglobin and usually manifests with erythrocytosis (see Polycythemias). Occasionally the presence of this gene may coexist with other hemoglobin abnormalities such as hemoglobin S and hemoglobin C. In the case of the persistence of fetal hemoglobin in the presence of hemoglobin S, the clinical expression of S-hemoglobin is attenuated and may exhibit a mild clinical disease.

The presence of fetal hemoglobin is easily detected in the laboratory by the fact that it is *resistant to acid and alkali denaturation,* whereas adult hemoglobin (hemoglobin A) is not. Consequently, a smear that is made and placed in an acid or alkaline medium will lyse the hemoglobin A-containing cells, whereas the hemoglobin F-containing cells will be intact. Staining will identify hemoglobin F inside the intact red cells (see Color Plate 50). In hereditary persistence of fetal hemoglobin, there is *homogeneous distribution* of HbF (present uniformly in all cells). In other conditions where fetal hemoglobin is increased, such as thalassemia, there is a heterogeneous distribution (see Fig. 3–4 later in this chapter).

Other Hemoglobinopathies: Genetic disorders causing substitution of internal nonpolar amino acids of the globin chains can produce significant alterations of structure or function of the hemoglobin molecule. These variants may alter the affinity of the hemoglobin molecule for oxygen, or may allow oxidation of the iron from the ferrous to the ferric state, or may produce hemoglobin molecules that are unstable and precipitate to form Heinz bodies. In general, these diseases are found in the heterozygous state, since homozygosity is usually incompatible with life.

Methemoglobins/Hemoglobin M: As was mentioned in Chapter 2, *methemoglobinemia* occurs when hemoglobin is oxidized to the ferric form of iron (Fe^{3+}). Since this molecule is unable to transport oxygen, the patient presents with cyanosis and hypoxemia. In general, these patients do not have a hemolytic anemia. They do, however, have an abnormal hemoglobin that can be detectable on hemoglobin electrophoresis.

Unstable Hemoglobin: Inheritance of a gene that produces a defect in the structural component of the globin chains can result in instability of hemoglobin. This produces *Heinz bodies,* which are removed in the spleen, producing an inherited

Heinz body hemolytic anemia (see Color Plate 16B). The severity of the disorder is dependent on the nature of the amino acid substitution. The clinical features are those of a hemolytic anemia that is confirmed by laboratory data. Hematologic indices may vary; however, spherocytes are generally not seen in the peripheral blood smear. Laboratory tests for unstable hemoglobins include a *heat stability test* or exposure to certain drugs such as *isopropanol.* In unsplenectomized patients, Heinz bodies are sometimes difficult to detect; however, following splenectomy they may be quite prominent. Oxidant drugs may precipitate episodes of hemolysis in these patients.

Thalassemia Syndromes

The term thalassemia derives from a combination of the Greek words *thalassa* (sea) and *haima* (blood). An early name for the severest form of the disease was Mediterranean anemia because Mediterranean populations were the first ones known to be afflicted. The thalassemia syndromes are characterized by a decreased rate of production of the globin chains. They are classified according to which globin chain is affected; namely: *alpha-thalassemia,* where there is a decreased production of alpha chains, and *beta-thalassemia,* where beta chain production is decreased. These are the commonest thalassemic syndromes and also occur in a geographic distribution very similar to that of malaria. Rarer types of thalassemia do occur affecting some other minor globin chains, namely the delta chain, and occasional hybrid forms may occur (the so-called beta-delta-thalassemia or hemoglobin Lepore syndromes). The difference between the thalassemia syndromes and the disease-producing hemoglobin variants is that, in most cases, all the chains that are synthesized have a normal structure; the amount, however, is decreased.

Molecular Biology of Globin Synthesis

As was mentioned in Chapter 2, the genetic codes for globin synthesis are located on chromosome 11 (gamma, delta, and beta chains) and chromosome 16 (alpha and embryonic chains) (Fig. 3–2). Figure 3–3 shows a diagram of progression from the genetic code to the protein polypeptide. For alpha chain synthesis, each chromosome 16 has two subloci, making a total of four functioning subloci in diploid cells of normal people. The genes that control beta, gamma, and delta chain synthesis form a cluster that has been shown in a well-defined sequence on chromosome 11. The fundamentals of globin synthesis have been discussed in Chapter 2. Thalassemia syndromes may occur as a result of abnormalities in the coding sequence,

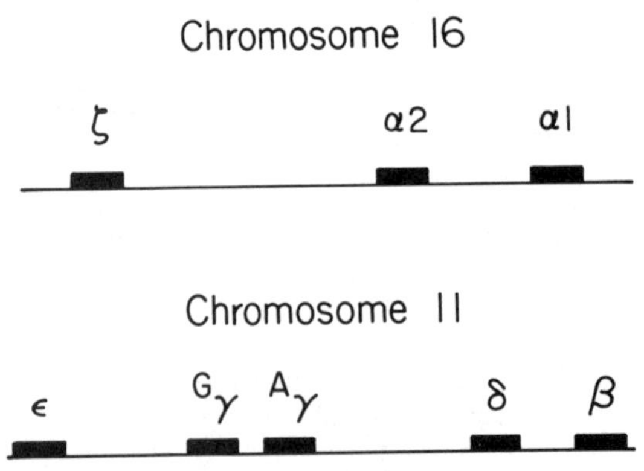

Figure 3–2. Location of the globin genes on chromosomes 16 and 11. (From Pittiglio, DH and Sacher, RA: Clinical Hematology and Fundamentals of Hemostasis. FA Davis, Philadelphia, 1987, p 121, with permission.)

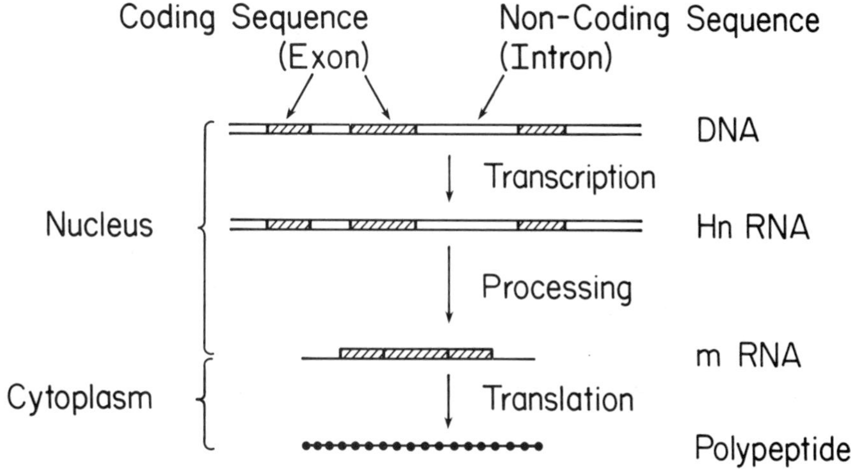

Figure 3–3. Diagram of the progression from gene to peptide. (From Pittliglio, DH and Sacher, RA: Clinical Hematology and Fundamentals of Hemostasis. FA Davis, Philadelphia, 1987, p 122, with permission.)

transcription, processing, or defects in gene translation. The consequence is defective globin chain production. Deletion of all four alpha chain loci causes complete absence of messenger RNA (mRNA) for alpha chain synthesis. Deletion or severe abnormality of two genes causes slightly reduced levels of mRNA, and mild or no reduction in chain synthesis.

Genes for the beta chain are more variable. One form, called beta$^+$ thalassemia, results in markedly deficient but still measurable levels of mRNA, whereas the beta° thalassemia gene produces no mRNA at all. In both these conditions, the DNA present on the chromosome determines the defective activity. A third possibility can occur where chain production involves deletion of the gene itself, with absence of any DNA code for beta chain synthesis. A similar situation can exist for delta chains.

Hemoglobin Products

Defective alpha chain production affects all the hemoglobins except those yolk sac-derived embryonic hemoglobins with unique, separately regulated chains. In red cell precursors with grossly deficient alpha chain supplies, four gamma chains may unite as a gamma tetramer, producing *hemoglobin Barts.* Similarly, four beta chains may unite as a tetramer, producing an abnormal hemoglobin termed *hemoglobin H.* In persons with defective alpha chain production, hemoglobin Barts (γ^4) is conspicuous during fetal existence when gamma is the dominant non-alpha chain. Hemoglobin H (β^4) becomes predominant in postuterine life when beta chain production takes over.

The fetus suffers very little if beta chain genes are defective, since hemoglobin F ($\alpha_2\,\gamma_2$) is perfectly normal. In extrauterine life, inadequate supplies of beta chains cause excess alpha chains to accumulate (Fig. 3–4). Synthesis of gamma or delta chains may rise to compensate for the deficiency of beta chains and produces increased amounts of *hemoglobin A_2* ($\alpha_2\,\delta_2$) and *hemoglobin F* ($\alpha_2\,\gamma_2$). These hemoglobins support oxygen transport to some extent, although they are less efficient at oxygen delivery than hemoglobin A. The level of compensatory hemoglobin F

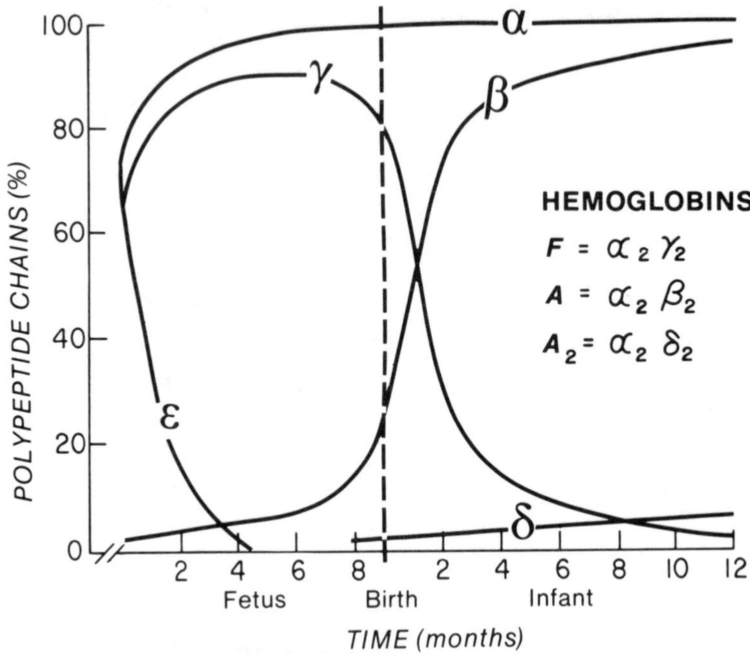

Figure 3–4. Changes in hemoglobin with development. Sequential suppression and activation of individual globin genes in the immediate postnatal period result in a switch from fetal hemoglobin (hemoglobin F: 2-alpha and 2-gamma chains) to adult hemoglobin (hemoglobin A: 2-alpha and 2-beta chains). A small amount of hemoglobin A_2 (2-alpha and 2-delta chains) is also present in the adult. (From Hillman and Finch,[16] p 9, with permission.)

depends on how completely the switch from gamma synthesis to beta chain production occurs. Massive compensatory delta chain production never occurs; therefore, hemoglobin A_2 values are only marginally elevated. Nevertheless, elevation of hemoglobin A_2 is an important laboratory finding in beta-thalassemia, although the values never exceed 7% of the total hemoglobin.

Alpha-Thalassemias

Complete *absence of alpha chain synthesis* causes stillbirth in midpregnancy. The fetus can survive on embryonic hemoglobins only until the second trimester. Once the gamma chain occurs, hemoglobin Barts (γ^4) evolves from all the unpaired gamma chains. This has such high oxygen affinity that although blood reaches the tissues, almost no oxygen is released and the fetus dies from anemia and congestive heart failure *(hydrops fetalis)*.

Persons whose cells have only one (of a possible four) functioning alpha chain loci have *hemoglobin H disease,* which produces a serious, although less severe, hemolytic anemia *(thalassemia intermedia)*. Adult cells have 4–30% hemoglobin H, along with inefficient erythropoiesis and a moderately severe anemia. Cord blood has up to 25% hemoglobin Barts.

Heterozygotes for *alpha-thalassemia* have two or three functioning alpha chain genes and suffer no clinical disability. In certain American black populations, as many as 2% may be heterozygous for alpha-thalassemia. The diagnosis is best made on cord blood, which has up to 5% hemoglobin Barts. Adult blood in alpha-thalassemia heterozygotes does not contain hemoglobin H, and the hematologic findings are mild and nonspecific. The red cells, however, are *hypochromic* and *microcytic,* reflecting the defective hemoglobin synthesis, and the morphology is very similar to that seen in iron deficiency anemia (see Table 3–4). Obviously, since these patients are not iron deficient, they do not respond to iron supplementation and diagnosis can be established on family studies or more sophisticated alpha-beta synthesis tests. Occasionally, *hemoglobin H bodies* may be seen on supravital stain smears (see also Color Plate 32).

Homozygous Beta-Thalassemia

Beta-thalassemia will not manifest itself clinically at birth since the predominant hemoglobin is hemoglobin F ($\alpha_2\ \gamma_2$). When the switch to beta chain production occurs at 3–6 months after birth (see Fig. 3–4), the defective rate of beta synthesis manifests itself as ineffective red cell production with intramedullary hemolysis. The decreased synthesis of beta chains is partially compensated by an increase in gamma chain synthesis, producing an *elevation of hemoglobin F* ($\alpha_2\ \gamma_2$) and an increase in delta chain synthesis, producing an *increase in hemoglobin A_2* ($\alpha_2\ \delta_2$).

When both beta chain genes are defective, patients suffer from a severe, lifelong anemia called *thalassemia major (Cooley's anemia* or *Mediterranean anemia).* Hemoglobin ranges from 2–6 g/dl. Red cells are small, pale, and misshapen with enormous hemolysis and ineffective red cell production. Reticulocytosis runs 15% or more. Nucleated red cells are numerous, and severe splenomegaly and moderate jaundice are present. As alpha chains are produced normally, there is a huge excess of alpha chains that pair with one another and form alpha tetramers. These accumulate and precipitate in the form of intracellular inclusions *(Heinz bodies)* that interfere with intramedullary maturation and induce intrasplenic destruction of those cells that enter the circulation. Splenectomy can permit somewhat enhanced red cell survival, but leads to an increased risk of sudden, overwhelming bacterial infections (see Color Plate 32).

The severe anemia retards growth and causes marrow expansion with skeletal abnormalities due to the widening of productive bone marrow. This is an attempt at compensatory erythroid production. The overwhelming marrow hyperplasia is induced by exaggerated erythropoietin levels. Anemia is not the only stimulus to erythropoietin secretion. Hemoglobins F and A_2, produced to compensate for absent hemoglobin A, yield oxygen to the tissue less readily than does hemoglobin A. This leads to tissue hypoxia greater than would occur if normal hemoglobin were present at the same concentration. Because there is such a brisk erythropoiesis, large quantities of iron are absorbed from the gastrointestinal tract. Iron utilization, however, is poor, and large quantities of storage iron accumulate, first in the reticuloendothelial system and later in parenchymal cells, especially the cells of the heart and liver.

Transfusion therapy ameliorates the anemia and suppresses marrow hyperplasia by diminishing erythropoietic production. However, each unit of red cells adds 250 mg of additional iron to the body's already excessive supply. Careful transfusion therapy can restore patients with thalassemia major to a relatively normal existence, but death usually occurs before age 20 because iron overload induces myocardial failure. Therapy with chelating agents and other drugs to mobilize iron excretion has extended the limited lifespan of these patients well into the third, and occasionally the fourth, decade. Other problems of chronic transfusion therapy also occur (see Chapter 8). In general, the aim is at *hypertransfusion therapy* in order to decrease the skeletal abnormalities, and also to reduce erythroid hyperplasia.

The syndromes caused by $beta^+$ and $beta^\circ$ thalassemia genes are clinically similar, although on electrophoretic analysis they differ in the proportions of hemoglobin A_2 and F. Thalassemia caused by complete deletion of the gene segment controlling both beta and delta chain production is somewhat less disastrous. Absence of the delta-beta segment seems to allow compensatory gamma chain production, and these patients have markedly elevated hemoglobin F values. These patients also have a less severe clinical syndrome of *thalassemia intermedia.*

Heterozygous Beta-Thalassemia

Patients with one normal and one abnormal beta chain gene have relatively few clinical problems. The laboratory findings vary, depending on which abnormal gene is present. Both beta$^+$ and beta$^\circ$ heterozygotes have hemoglobin A_2 levels raised to about 7% of total hemoglobin, and hemoglobin F is variably increased. Heterozygotes for delta-beta thalassemia have normal hemoglobin A_2, but hemoglobin F values that may constitute 5–20% of the total. The hemoglobin F in these syndromes is distributed heterogeneously in erythrocytes. All three types of heterozygotes manifest the syndrome of *thalassemia minor,* characterized by abnormally small, hypochromic red cells with numerous target cells, basophilic stippling, and increased resistance to osmotic lysis. Anemia, however, is mild (hemoglobin levels are usually 10–12 g/dl), and erythropoiesis is only mildly inefficient. If the spleen is removed, Heinz bodies become apparent in circulating red cells. Serum iron and transferrin saturations are normal, but may be elevated (Table 3–15; see also Table 3-4).

The biggest problem with thalassemia minor comes in distinguishing it from iron deficiency anemia (see Table 3–4). Both conditions cause hypochromic, microcytic anemias, often of comparable degree (see also Chapter 3, p 79). Measuring serum iron level or examining the bone marrow for storage of iron allows the distinction to be made. Patients with thalassemia minor can, however, also be iron deficient. When iron levels are low, the characteristic increase in hemoglobin A_2 tends

Table 3–15. LABORATORY FINDINGS IN BETA-THALASSEMIA

	Homozygous	Heterozygous
Hemoglobin	2–5 g/dl	9–11 g/dl
RBC morphology	Pronounced poikilocytosis Basophilic stippling Target cells Nucleated RBCs Heinz bodies	Small hypochromic cells MCH 20–22 pg MCV 50–70 fl
Reticulocytosis	≥15%	Mildly elevated
Platelets, WBCs	Low if splenomegaly present	Normal
Bone marrow	Erythroid hyperplasia so marked that bones are deformed	Mild to moderate erythroid hyperplasia
Hemoglobin A_2	Variable	3.5–7%
Hemoglobin F	10–90% of Hgb present	Slight increase in 50% of patients
Storage iron	Greatly increased, hemosiderosis often fatal	Normal or slightly increased

RBC = red blood cells; WBC = white blood cells; MCH = mean corpuscular hemoglobin; MCV = mean corpuscular volume.

to disappear. This removes the distinctive clue for thalassemia and the patient seems only to be iron deficient. After iron repletion, total hemoglobin fails to achieve normal values, but the abnormal hemoglobin A_2 levels return and more complete diagnosis can be made. Table 3–15 lists major laboratory findings in homozygous and heterozygous beta-thalassemia.

Thalassemia Heterozygotes with Other Hemoglobinopathies

Genes for globin chain structure and for rate of globin synthesis seem to occupy virtually the same genetic locus. It is not clear how functional distinction occurs. The result, however, is that thalassemia genes and hemoglobinopathy genes behave as alleles. The individual with a $beta^{s}$ allele on one chromosome and a beta°-thalassemia allele on the other will have no hemoglobin A, but often has more hemoglobin A_2 and F than that seen in homozygotes for hemoglobin S. Still another allele that causes gamma chain production to continue throughout adult life can be paired with normal, thalassemia, or hemoglobin variant genes. In the latter case, a heterozygous state of sickle hemoglobin and the hereditary persistence of fetal hemoglobin (HPFH) will protect the cells against many hemoglobin S-related problems, so the absence of hemoglobin A causes little difficulty. Furthermore, the finding of coexistent thalassemia genes and sickle genes is not infrequent and not surprising considering the geographic distribution of these two populations.

Acquired Thalassemia Syndromes

Defects in globin chain production, involving particularly the alpha chain locus, can occur in some *myelodysplastic* and *preleukemic* syndromes (see Chapter 4). These defects may be in gene deletion or in transcription, and result in defective amounts of alpha chain being synthesized by the abnormal clone. The clinical features are very similar to hemoglobin H disease, and the patient presents with a hypochromic, microcytic anemia. Bone marrow shows exuberant erythroid response with ineffective erythropoiesis. Hemoglobin electrophoresis confirms the presence of an abnormal hemoglobin, which is fast migrating in the distribution of hemoglobin H (see Fig. 3–5). Hemoglobin H bodies are seen on supravital stains of the erythroid cells. This condition is usually rapidly progressive to acute leukemia. Since it is an acquired form, it can easily be distinguished by previously normal blood counts and presentation at an elderly age.

Laboratory Investigation of the Hemoglobinopathies

While clinical features are obviously extremely important in ascertaining the nature of a chronic hemolytic anemia, laboratory tests ultimately define the disorder and whether an abnormal hemoglobin is present or not.

As with the investigation of any anemia, examination of the peripheral blood smear provides important clues in characterizing a hemoglobinopathy. Red cells are usually normochromic and normocytic, except in the thalassemia syndromes, where they are hypochromic and microcytic. Diffuse polychromatophilia, representing a reticulocytosis, is variably present. Specific morphologic changes are often present in the specific disorders. Irreversibly sickled cells may be seen in sickle cell anemia, and hemoglobin C crystals and clam-shaped cells indicate the presence of hemoglobin C (see Color Plates 13, 16–18, 31, 32). Hemoglobin C disease is also associated with abundant target cell formation (see Color Plate 13). Target cells are also often seen in thalassemias and, in addition, basophilic stippling in this disorder gives a clue about the disordered hemoglobin production (see also Color Plate 16C). Spherocytes are usually not a feature of the hemoglobinopathies, unless splenectomy has been performed (e.g., thalassemia).

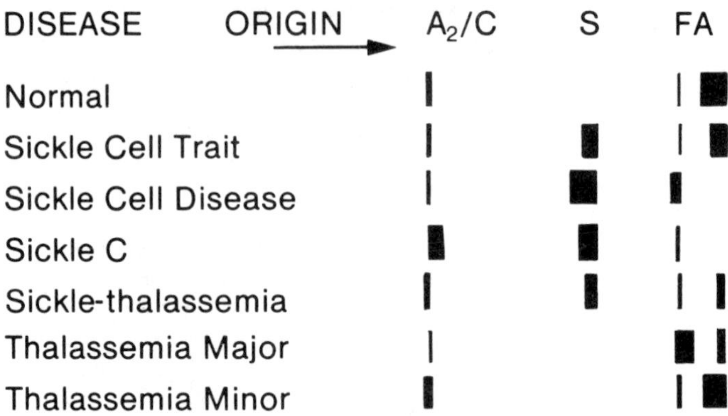

Figure 3–5. Cellulose acetate electrophoretic patterns for common hemoglobinopathies. In the normal individual, 97% of the hemoglobin found in circulating red cells is hemoglobin A. Only small amounts of hemoglobin F and A_2 are detectable. Patients with sickle cell trait and sickle cell disease show increased amounts of hemoglobin S, with a corresponding decrease in hemoglobin A. Sickle cell disease patients may show a variable increase in hemoglobin F. Sickle C patients show an increase in the hemoglobin band in the A_2 position, which in fact is hemoglobin C. Sickle thalassemia patients show increases in the A_2 and S bands and a decrease in the hemoglobin A band, which is more marked than that observed in sickle cell trait patients. Thalassemia major patients show a decrease in hemoglobin A and a marked increase in hemoglobin F. In contrast, the beta thalassemia minor patient shows only a slight increase in hemoglobin F together with an increase in hemoglobin A_2. (From Hillman and Finch,[16] p 93, with permission.)

Initial laboratory tests must include documenting the presence and the degree of the hemolytic anemia, as was outlined in Chapter 2. Although hemoglobin screening tests are performed prior to genetic counseling, laboratory evaluation of hemoglobinopathies should be supported by a strong suspicion of a hemolytic anemia. In general, a bone marrow examination is not necessary. *Hemoglobin electrophoresis* on cellulose acetate, or starch gel electrophoresis at an alkaline pH of 8.6 is the most convenient laboratory test demonstrating the presence of an abnormal hemoglobin (see Fig. 3–5). Hemoglobin separated by this method may be quantified by elution and spectrophotographic analysis or densitometry scanning. Most of the more important hemoglobins are separated by this method. Unfortunately, the method does not discriminate between hemoglobins A and F, and therefore hemoglobin F must be quantitated by another method. Since hemoglobin F is acid and alkali-resistant, whereas hemoglobin A is denatured, particularly at low pHs, this forms the principle of the *acid-resistant hemoglobin assay for hemoglobin F.* Hemoglobin F can therefore be quantitated by treatment with acid, representing the resistant hemoglobin present. This tests forms the basis of the *Kleihauer-Betke test* for the presence of fetal cells in the maternal circulation during pregnancy (see Hemolytic Disease of the Newborn, Chapter 8).

In alpha-thalassemia, since there is decreased synthesis of alpha chains, there is an excess of beta chains. These beta chains may form tetramers, which can easily be demonstrated on supravital staining by the presence of *hemoglobin H crystals.* They produce a "golf ball" morphologic appearance of the red cells, and this is a test for hemoglobin H inclusions. In addition, hemoglobin H migrates differently on hemoglobin electrophoresis and is one of the fast-migrating hemoglobins (see Fig. 3–5).

Clearly the position of a hemoglobin band on hemoglobin electrophoresis can direct the laboratory investigation. The presence of a hemoglobin band in a sickle position can be followed up by performing a *sickle cell screening test,* which is more commonly used prior to hemoglobin electrophoresis. The principle of this test is that a sample of blood placed on a blood smear, covered by a cover slip, and sealed with paraffin or subjected to a reducing agent such as *sodium metabisulfite,* is rendered oxygen-deficient. Since sickle blood is sensitive to oxygen depletion, sickle cells are formed after approximately half an hour of incubation. This is a *screening test for a sickle hemoglobin* and hemoglobin S is subsequently confirmed by hemoglobin electrophoresis.

Unstable hemoglobins can be demonstrated by the presence of *Heinz bodies* (see Color Plate 16B) or by performing an *unstable hemoglobin test.* In most cases, unstable hemoglobins are sensitive to heat and precipitate after exposure to higher temperatures. This forms the basis of the *heat stability test.* The *isopropanol denaturation test* is another method to enable detection of unstable hemoglobins, which precipitate after exposure to this reagent. Test selection clearly must follow a pattern of suspicion, documentation of a hemolytic anemia, and, most often, the demonstration of an abnormal hemoglobin on hemoglobin electrophoresis. In most cases, more refined testing is unnecessary; however, in difficult cases, amino acid analysis and the hemoglobin synthesis ratios of the alpha and non-alpha chains to one another may be needed. Hemoglobin synthesis ratios are valuable in a research setting to confirm milder cases of thalassemia where the relative synthesis of the two chains are compared. Molecular biologic techniques are currently performed in the research setting to define DNA abnormalities or alterations of messenger RNA expression. In the future, these tools may be available in antenatal testing, or perhaps even in routine laboratory testing.

Acquired Defects

Paroxysmal Nocturnal Hemoglobinuria

This condition was already discussed under Refractory Anemia and Ineffective Erythropoiesis. The condition is a clonal hematologic disorder that is characterized by abnormal marrow growth and membrane sensitivity to complement-mediated lysis.

Extrinsic Hemolytic Anemia

Hemolysis from extracellular causes may be broadly categorized into those that are *immune-mediated* (mediated through an immune antibody) and the *nonimmune hemolytic anemias.* The immune hemolytic anemias are also discussed in the section dealing with immunohematology in Chapter 8.

Nonimmune Destruction

Erythrocytes may have a shortened intravascular survival if subjected to the harmful effects of abnormal or unusual physical or chemical stress, and forces within the circulation that may cause erythrocyte damage. The cell membrane may be damaged by heat, radiation, chemicals, enzymes, and toxins. Internal forces form within the red cells, or parasitic infestations in the erythrocyte may cause the cell to rupture. These processes are acquired hemolytic anemias that do not require the presence of or cooperation with the humoral antibody system or complement activation. The mechanisms of red cell damage are listed in Table 3–16.

Table 3–16. EXTRACORPUSCULAR DEFECTS—NONIMMUNE HEMOLYTIC ANEMIA MECHANISMS FOR RED CELL DAMAGE

Mechanism	Pathogenesis
Mechanical pressure	
In heart and great vessels	Artificial valves
In microcirculation	Hemolytic uremic syndrome (HUS) Thrombotic thrombocytopenic purpura (TTP) Disseminated intravascular coagulation (DIC)
Membrane disorders	
Loss of membrane	Hypersplenism
Lipid peroxidation	Oxidant drugs
Lipid dissolution	*Clostridium perfringens* (Welchii)
Thermal damage	Burns
Intracellular pressure	
Parasites	Malaria
Water (osmotic)	Drowning
Altered energy production	Lead poisoning

Physical Trauma (Angiopathic Hemolytic Anemia)

Red cells that encounter physical obstacles within the vascular bed lose small parts of their membranes and undergo continuous reduction in their surface areas, causing a change in the surface-to-volume ratio. Cracks or other defects in *prosthetic heart valves* induce a chronic hemolytic process because of damage to passing red cells *(macroangiopathic hemolytic anemia).* Patients whose capillaries are partially occluded by tiny fibrin strands and clots may experience an acute hemolytic process termed *microangiopathic hemolytic anemia (MAHA),* in which red cells show morphologic evidence of fragmentation. These *schistocytes* are fragments of red cells produced by the mechanical injury as cells pass through and are "chopped" and destroyed (see Color Plate 14). Microangiopathic hemolytic anemia occurs particularly in conditions associated with the syndrome of *disseminated intravascular coagulation (DIC)* where there is a diffuse, intravascular clotting process with deposition of fibrin strands (see Chapter 6). Microangiopathic hemolytic anemia also occurs in the rare disorder *thrombotic thrombocytopenic purpura (TTP),* which is also discussed in Chapter 6. Hemolysis is an integral part of this syndrome, and occurs as a result of mechanical fragmentation within the microcirculation. Typically, in the syndromes of MAHA, the platelet count is often decreased; whereas in fragmentation associated with prosthetic valves, the platelet count is normal. Thrombocytopenia and MAHA also occur in another condition, characterized by renal insufficiency, called *hemolytic uremic syndrome.* Microangiopathic hemolytic anemia may also occur in association with some epithelial malignancies, particularly gastric carcinoma, and following drug therapy with the agent mitomycin-C.

A mild mechanical hemolytic state may occur in long distance runners and following repetitive traumatic stress exerted upon the vascular channels of the foot with strenuous marching. This condition is termed *march hemoglobinuria,* and can occur with karate exercises and bongo drumming. In most of these conditions, plasma haptoglobin declines and plasma-free hemoglobin accumulates. The urine may contain free hemoglobin, and in chronic intravascular hemolytic states, contains the iron-containing compound *hemosiderin.*

Chemical and Toxic Agents

Thermal Damage: Severe burns cause thermal damage to red cells circulating at the time of injury. As many as 20–30% of the red cells may be lysed within the first 24–48 hours, leading to massive hemoglobinemia and hemoglobinuria. Clinically, this may be disasterous because it contributes to the renal damage initiated by the blood pressure changes, fluid loss, and circulation of other cellular breakdown products, in particular myoglobin.

Drugs and Chemicals: Most drug-related hemolysis has an immune basis (see Chapter 8), or produces hemolysis in glucose-6-phosphate dehydrogenase-deficient patients (discussed earlier). Some agents, however, damage red cells directly. Accidental introduction of distilled water into the circulation causes rapid osmotic lysis. Arsene gas, sometimes generated during industrial processes, causes severe hemolysis, as do copper salts.

Oxidizing drugs, notably nitrites, nitrates, and aromatic amino and nitroso compounds cause methemoglobinemia, and in severe cases red cell destruction as well.

Hemolysis Associated with Infection

Malaria is the most dramatic and most common infectious cause of intravascular hemolysis. The protozoan ruptures red cells as part of its life cycle. The periodic chills and fever that characterize the disease occur as parasitized erythrocytes burst to release a new generation of organisms. The attachment of the parasite to erythrocytes, and its subsequent ability to enter the red cell, depends on normal cell membrane structures, in particular glycophorin, and the Duffy antigen system (see Chapter 8). Erythrocytes lacking the Duffy antigen fail to be parasitized by *Plasmodium vivax* (malarial infection is also discussed in Chapter 13). Hemolytic anemia in malaria occurs because of mechanical rupture by the parasite, but can also occur in association with immunologic mechanisms *(Blackwater fever).*

Hemolysis can also occur due to parasitization by the protozoan *Babesia,* which has been reported from Nantucket Island off the New England coast of the United States (babesiosis). Other infectious diseases causing hemolytic anemia include clostridial infections in which lecithinase enzymes damage the lipids of the red cell membrane and may lead to massive hemolysis, sometimes complicating fatal septic episodes. Hemolysis is also produced by organisms such as the *streptococcus* species and *Hemophilus influenzae.* A toxin produced by the bite of the brown recluse spider produces acute hemolysis of a milder sort, possibly mediated through a hypersensitivity reaction.

Hypersplenism

The normal spleen destroys red cells as they age at the rate of 1/120 of the circulating cells each day. Abnormal red cells undergo accelerated destruction in passing through a normal spleen. An abnormally large spleen tends to destroy excessive numbers of red cells, even perfectly normal cells. Any condition that increases spleen size can shorten red cell survival; white cells and platelets may also be affected. These include liver disease with portal hypertension, chronic congestive cardiac failure, infiltrative diseases such as leukemias and lymphomas, and protozoal infections such as schistosomiasis, all of which may increase spleen size, leading to increased red cell sequestration and decreased red cell survival. The sequestration of cells by the spleen in conditions associated with an increasing spleen size is termed *hypersplenism.*

Systemic Disorders Associated with Nonimmune Hemolytic Anemia

Lipid Disorders: Alterations in blood lipid concentrations can produce abnormalities of the erythrocyte membrane lipid composition. This produces shortened red cell survival in a condition called *spur cell anemia.* The peripheral blood shows abundant, sharp, spiculated red cells occurring in association with hyperlipidemia and liver disease. This condition has been termed *Zieve's syndrome.* In another condition associated with lipid disorders, abetalipoproteinemia, or hereditary acanthocytosis, the red cells show multiple, blunted projections in association with a very low blood cholesterol due to the deficiency of the blood transport protein beta-lipoprotein. These individuals may have a concomitant hemolytic anemia.

Renal Disease: Abnormal capillaries in renal glomerular disease can cause mechanical distortion of red cells as they flow through these channels. Typically, in renal disease, the erythrocytes show burr cell formation. Fibrin deposition in the glomerular channels is associated with MAHA.

Immune-Mediated Hemolytic Anemia

Immune-mediated red cell destruction occurs as a result of specific antibody attack against the antigens on the erythrocyte membrane, and results in membrane damage and lysis of the cell. This hemolysis may occur *intravascularly* or *extravascularly,* depending on the nature of the immune antibody and whether or not complement is activated. The characteristics of anti-erythrocyte antibodies are discussed in Chapter 8; however, these compounds are gammaglobulin proteins that are produced by a stimulating antigen. Antibodies can be directed against antigens on red cells, white cells, platelets, or against protein constituents. These antibodies are capable of producing hemolytic disease, for example, when an individual with preformed natural antibodies or immune antibodies is exposed to foreign red cells, as occurs with an incompatible blood transfusion. When preformed antibodies are directed against erythrocytes from another member of the same species this process is called alloimmunity. The antibodies produced are termed *alloantibodies.* In a hemolytic transfusion reaction, antibodies in the recipient's circulation rapidly destroy transfused cells as they enter the blood stream. Antibodies against A and B antigens usually cause prompt intravascular hemolysis with rapid liberation of free hemoglobin. Rh antibodies against Rh antigens, and many other antibodies, attach themselves to the surface of circulating red cells, causing the antibody-coated cells to be removed in the spleen *(extravascular hemolysis).* Clinical complications from both types of hemolysis can induce shock, coagulation abnormalities, and renal failure, but the severity of clinical response varies astonishingly among different patients exposed to the same immunologic situations. Diagnosis depends on documenting that the transfused cells possess an antigen to which the patient has a specific antibody directed, thus causing RBC destruction (see Chapter 8). The types of immune hemolytic anemia are listed in Table 3–17.

Autoimmune Hemolytic Anemia (AIHA)

Autoimmune hemolytic anemia occurs when the patient develops antibodies directed against antigens present on the *patient's own erythrocytes,* producing shortened red cell survival. The reasons for this autodestructive phenomenon are not understood. The cell surface characteristics may be modified sufficiently by a virus or a drug that they appear "foreign" to the host's immune system. Autoimmune phenomena often accompany other diseases, notably collagen vascular diseases, chronic lymphocytic leukemias and lymphomas, and some non-hematologic solid tumor malignancies. In addition, autoantibodies may accompany several infectious processes such as infectious mononucleosis, mycoplasma, pneumonia, syphilis, and other viral syndromes such as rubella and varicella. The clinical conditions

Table 3–17. CLASSIFICATION OF THE CAUSES OF IMMUNE HEMOLYTIC ANEMIAS

	Antibody	Thermal range of antibody	Antibody specificity
Auto-immune			
Primary/Idiopathic	IgG	W	Panspecific
Infections			
Mycoplasma pneumoniae	IgM	C	Anti-I
Epstein-Barr viral syndrome (infectious mononucleosis)	IgM	C	Anti-i
Varicella, rubella	IgG	C/W	Anti-P
Syphilis	IgG	C/W	Anti-P
Neoplasms			
Carcinomas, lymphomas, and chronic lymphocytic leukemia	IgG	W	Panspecific (usually)
	IgM (occasionally)	C	I/i/other
Collagen vascular disease (lupus erythematosus, etc.)	IgG	W	Panspecific
Drugs			
Quinidine/quinine group	Immune complexes	W	Non-specific
Penicillin group	Haptenic IgG	W	Panspecific
Aldomet, L-Dopa	IgG	W	Panspecific
Alloimmune			
Hemolytic transfusion reactions	IgM & IgG	C or W	Specific*
Hemolytic disease of the newborn	IgG	W	Specific*

W = warm; C = cold.
*Differing specificities.

associated with autoimmune hemolysis may be classified as primary (idiopathic) where there is no apparent etiologic cause, and secondary (where associated diseases are present). In many instances, drugs may be incriminated in the development of autoantibodies directed to the red cell (see Table 3–17). The drug may complex with a preformed antibody in the patient's plasma-binding complement, which destroys the red cells by an *innocent bystander* or paraphenomenon. Complement is secondarily adsorbed onto the red cell membrane, which is subsequently destroyed. Drugs eliciting hemolysis through this mechanism include *quinidine* and *quinine* derivatives. Three types of drug-induced hemolysis may occur, and two of these are illustrated in Figure 3–6.

The drug may combine with the red cell membrane, and is itself altered or alters the erythrocyte membrane, rendering it foreign to the host *(hapten mechanism)*. An antibody response then is elicited against the erythrocyte, producing erythrocyte

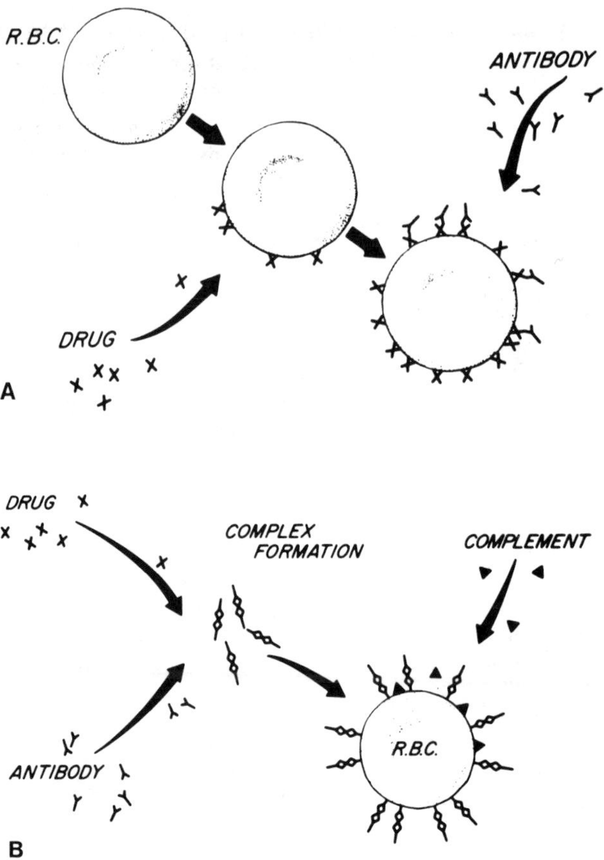

Figure 3–6. Two mechanisms of drug-induced hemolysis. (*A*) Drug absorption mechanism. Anti-drug antibody binds with drug bound to the red cell surface. Anti-drug antibody does not bind to "drug-free" red cells. (*B*) Immune complex mechanism. Complexes of the drug and anti-drug antibody attach to the red cell surface, where they initiate complement activation. (From AABB Technical Manual, ed 9. American Association of Blood Banks, 1985, pp 258–259, with permission.)

damage or sequestration. Drugs of the *penicillin* class are more commonly associated with this type of hemolytic mechanism.

Occasionally a true immune response against the drug occurs that in some way cross-reacts with the erythrocyte membrane antigens. The immune response does not require the presence of the drug once the antibody is formed, and a cycle of erythrocyte destruction can then ensue. This true immune type of drug-induced hemolysis occurs with the antihypertensive alpha-methyldopa (Aldomet) and L-dopa.

Thus, autoimmune hemolytic anemias may be classified according to the cause—namely, primary, secondary, and drug-induced. Another classification of immune-mediated red cell destruction is based on the *specific characteristics of the antibody.* It is customary to classify AIHA by the thermal optimum of the antibody as determined by serologic testing (see Chapter 8). *Warm antibodies* are usually clinically significant at temperatures greater than 30°C. *Cold antibodies* have a thermal optimum between room temperature (22°C) and 4°C.

Warm Autoimmune Hemolytic Anemia

Warm AIHA is more common and causes more severe problems than the cold variety. Intravascular lysis does not occur; instead, cells that are coated with antibody circulate and are prematurely removed by the spleen. The rate of splenic destruction varies with the specificity and concentration of the antibody, the presence or absence of complement attachment, and the functional capacity of the spleen. Autoimmune hemolysis can range from a mild, compensated condition with normal hemoglobin levels to a severe anemia compromising life. The laboratory findings in this condition would include a severe anemia, often an elevated mean cell volume reflecting a high percentage of young erythrocytes (reticulocytes), hyperbilirubinemia of the indirect or unconjugated variety, an elevated lactate dehydrogenase, and decreased haptoglobin. Hemoglobinemia and hemoglobinuria are extremely uncommon in warm autoimmune hemolytic anemia. The *antiglobulin test* will establish the presence of an antibody coating the red cells, and facilitate the diagnosis of an immune hemolysis. The nature of the antibody and the thermal characteristics are then evaluated, usually in the Blood Bank (see Antiglobulin Testing in Chapter 8). Diagnosis depends on demonstrating the presence of antibody or complement on the circulating red cells using the antiglobulin test. Antibody sometimes exists free in the serum, but this is not necessary to diagnose AIHA. The clinical syndromes associated with warm AIHA include the secondary causes discussed above, such as collagen vascular disease or lymphomas, drugs, and occasionally infections. Many cases of warm AIHA are idiopathic, where no associated disease is present. Occasionally a patient may develop a characteristic clinical syndrome of warm autoimmune hemolytic anemia; however, the direct antiglobulin test and serum screen are negative. In these patients suspected of having immune-mediated hemolysis, provided other conditions are excluded, a highly avid antibody may produce rapid clearance of red cells, and yet may be undetectable because of decreased sensitivity of the antiglobulin reagent. These cases of so-called *Coombs-negative immune-mediated hemolytic anemia* have been described.

In most instances of warm AIHA, corticosteroid treatment is usually instituted. Responses to treatment can be assessed by means of evaluation of an increasing hematocrit, decreasing reticulocyte count, bilirubin, and LDH. The direct antiglobulin test may remain positive well after the disease is under control.

The finding of a positive direct antiglobulin test in a patient who is otherwise clinically stable and is not anemic does not warrant treatment unless there are other laboratory parameters indicative of hemolysis, or, increasing symptomatic anemia. In Aldomet-associated positive AHG tests, despite the undoubted presence of immunoglobulin on the red cell surface, very few such patients have significant hemolysis, and fewer still become anemic. In most of the other drug-related hemolytic conditions, antibody is directed against drugs rather than against cells, and in these cases treatment is specifically aimed at elimination of the drug. Furthermore, hemolysis (if it occurs) is associated with the presence of the drug.

Cold Autoantibody Hemolytic Syndromes

Antibodies reactive only at low temperatures cause no clinical problems at the usual body temperatures. Cold autoantibodies that cause clinical illness may work best at 25°C, 18°C or 4°C, but retain some activity at 37°C. These cold antibodies may also be of clinical importance in patients undergoing heart procedures with the use of cold solutions for cardioplegia. Most cold antibodies activate the complement sequence when they combine with antigen, and it is complement that actually damages the circulating cells. Very rarely, powerful cold-reacting antibodies cause agglutination in the cooler, superficial parts of the vascular bed such as the fingers and toes, or with open heart procedures. This phenomenon may produce the clinical syndrome of acral cyanosis, and may be associated with ischemia to the hands and vasospasm (Raynaud's phenomenon). Cold antibody-induced hemolysis may be chronic or episodic, but hemoglobin levels rarely fall below 8 or 9 g/dl, and often remain within the normal range. Symptomatic cold AIHA is relatively rare, usually occurring after *viral infections,* in particular in association with *Mycoplasma pneumoniae* (anti-I antibody) or *infectious mononucleosis* (anti-i antibody) (see Table 3–17). Spontaneous or idiopathic cold agglutinin disease sometimes occurs in elderly people. It may be necessary for them to wear gloves, avoid cold exposure, or move to warmer climates, but the disease is usually not life threatening.

Cold Agglutinin Disease: This disorder is due to monoclonal auto-antibody directed against erythrocyte antigens and reactive at low temperatures. The antibody is usually an IgM antibody, and more commonly exhibits the kappa light chain type. This syndrome may be idiopathic or secondary, particularly in association with lymphoproliferative disorders. Hemolysis is usually mild and self-limiting. The direct antiglobulin test usually shows the presence of *complement only* on the erythrocyte membrane, and hemolysis, when it occurs, is usually intravascular. Occasionally chronic intravascular hemolysis may occur, producing hemosiderin in the urine and even iron deficiency anemia.

Paroxysmal Cold Hemoglobinuria: This condition is caused by an IgG antibody that is more reactive in the cold temperature. In actual fact this antibody has a dual thermal optimal reactivity, reacting with erythrocytes and binding complement in the cold temperature, and then completing the complement binding at body temperature, resulting in intravascular hemolysis. This type of antibody syndrome is seen, particularly in viral infections, and was formerly more commonly seen in association with syphilis. Hemolysis may be severe, producing hemoglobinemia and hemoglobinuria following cold exposure on return into the warm temperatures. The direct antiglobulin test usually shows the presence of *complement only* on the red cell membrane, and the *biphasic nature* of the antibody and antibody characteristics can be demonstrated by the Donath-Landsteiner test. Usually these *IgG antibodies* have specificity for the *P blood group system* (see also Chapter 8 for serologic techniques and a description of the antiglobulin test).

ERYTHROCYTOSIS

The foregoing discussion concentrated on erythrocyte disorders where the ultimate effect was a decrease in erythrocytes in the circulating blood. Certain conditions are also associated with an excess production of red cells, termed *erythrocytosis.* Erythrocytosis may be unregulated and inappropriate where an uncontrolled growth of red cells produces an excess for no apparent purpose, and this is called primary erythrocytosis. The main condition associated with this problem is *polycythemia vera,* which will be discussed under Myeloproliferative Disorders in Chapter 4. In other instances, an excess erythroid mass is appropriate since it is stimulated by erythropoietin because of decreased oxygen tension. Conditions such as chronic hypoxia, respiratory or cardiovascular disease, living at high altitudes, or high-affinity hemoglobins that fail to deliver oxygen to the tissues may all stimulate excess red cell production. This is considered an appropriate response since there is

Table 3–18. DIFFERENTIAL DIAGNOSIS OF ERYTHROCYTOSIS

Primary polycythemia
  Polycythemia vera

Secondary polycythemia
  Appropriate increase in erythropoietin secondary to tissue hypoxia
    High altitude
    Chronic pulmonary disease
    Cyanotic congenital heart disease
    Low cardiac output states
    Hypoventilation syndromes (neuromuscular disease, pickwickian syndrome, sleep apnea)
    High-affinity hemoglobin variants
    Methemoglobin variants
    Carboxyhemoglobinemia

  Inappropriate increase in erythropoietin
    Neoplasms (hypernephroma, hepatoma, uterine myoma, cerebellar hemangioblastoma, pheochromocytoma)
    Renal artery stenosis
    Renal transplantation
    Renal cysts
    Hydronephrosis

Relative erythrocytosis
  Dehydration and other secondary causes of volume depletion
  Gaisböck's syndrome (stress erythrocytosis)

From Pittiglio, DH and Sacher, RA: Clinical Hematology and Fundamentals of Hemostasis. FA Davis, Philadelphia, 1987, p 183, with permission.

an increased demand for red cells due to a deficiency in oxygen delivery. These will also be mentioned in Chapter 4. Table 3–18 lists the differential diagnosis of erythrocytosis.

DISORDERS OF HEME SYNTHESIS: PORPHYRIAS

Porphyrin metabolism has been discussed in the section on heme synthesis (Chapter 2). *Porphyrins* are an integral part of the hemoglobin molecule, and there are four porphyrin rings between which iron is suspended to produce *heme*. *Porphyrias* are diseases in which there is usually a genetically acquired inborn error of metabolism associated with impairment or deficiencies of enzymes involved in the porphyrin–heme biosynthetic pathway. Deficiencies of these crucial enzymes are associated with an excessive build-up of the precursor compounds, which produce the biochemical abnormalities and clinical features characteristic of this group of diseases. The major precursors that accumulate and are excreted in excess include the compounds *delta-aminolevulinic acid* (ALA) and *porphobilinogen* (PBG), or the later porphyrin compounds *(uro-, copro-* and *protoporphyrin)*. Increased levels of these compounds can be detected variably in the plasma, in the urine, or in the stools, either between or during attacks. The patterns of excretion of these compounds are useful in the diagnosis of the different porphyrias; however, it is the clinical expression of these syndromes that is most important in diagnosing the type of porphyria. Table 3–19 is a list of these disorders and the compounds that are at present in excess in asymptomatic periods and during the acute attacks. The clinical manifestations may be neurologic and include excruciating pain and other neurologic symptoms, cutaneous (particularly cutaneous blisters and solar sensitivity), or hepatic in nature. Major clinical syndromes are called *acute intermittent porphyria* (*AIP*), *porphyria variegata* (*PV*), and *porphyria cutanea tarda* (*PCT*). The latter is an acquired porphyria, particularly seen in alcoholics (see later in this section). Other unusual types are the *erythropoietic porphyrias* and *hereditary coproporphyria.*

One of the major implications of diagnosing these disorders is that the clinical features can be prevented, since the acute attacks are precipitated by exposure to certain drugs. Drugs, particularly of the barbiturate and sulfonamide classes, are some of the drugs that can precipitate these acute attacks. Individuals with a history of porphyria must not be given these drugs.

Laboratory evaluation is usually performed in patients who have unusual neurologic manifestations, particularly of unexplained abdominal pain or cutaneous blisters. Often a family history warrants laboratory assessment for the presence of abnormal or excess porphyrins. Assays of these porphyrin compounds are not available in smaller laboratories and are often done by a reference laboratory. The assay systems are fairly simple, using either Ehrlich's reagent (hydrochloric acid and a benzaldehyde indicator), which turns a magenta color with porphyrins, or the fluorescent properties of these compounds. During the *acute attack,* the urinary concentrations of ALA and PBG increase in AIP and PV. In PV, excessive amounts of coproporphyrins are present in the stools of affected patients (see Table 3–19). These porphyrins produce a characteristic reddish-brown (port wine) color to the urine when they are present in excess quantities. They also give a characteristic *pinkish fluorescence* in the presence of ultraviolet light. The diagnosis may be made on a 24-hour collected urine sample that shows excessive amounts of these porphy-

Table 3–19. CLASSIFICATION OF DISORDERS OF PORPHYRIN METABOLISM

	Erythrocyte			Urine				Feces		
	UP	CP	PP	ALA	PBG	UP	CP	UP	CP	PP
Acute intermittent porphyria (AIP)	N	N	N	LI	LI	I	I,N	N	N	N
Hereditary coproporphyria	N	N	N	I	I	N	I	N	I	N
Variegate porphyria (acute attacks)	N	N	N	I	I	I,N	I,N	N	I	LI
Congenital erythropoietic porphyria	LI	LI	I	N	N	LI	I	N	I	N
Erythropoietic protoporphyria	N	N	LI	N	N	N	N	N	I	I
Symptomatic porphyria	N	N	N	N	N	LI	I	N	I,N	I,N
Lead poisoning	N	I,N	I	I	I,N	N	I	N	N	N

UP= uroporphyrin; CP = coproporphyrin; PP = protoporphyrin; N = normal; I = increased; LI = large increase; I,N = increase or normal.

From Henry, JB: Clinical Diagnosis and Management by Laboratory Methods, ed 17. WB Saunders, Philadelphia, 1985, p 144, with permission.

rin pigments in the urine. Reference values for urinary ALA are 1.5–7.5 mg/24 hours and for PBG, <1.0 mg/24 hours. Stools should contain <500 μg of coproporphyrin per 24-hour collection (see also Chapter 19).

Acquired Disturbances of Porphyrin Metabolism

Acquired disturbances of porphyrin metabolism may occur with lead poisoning. This has already been discussed in the section dealing with sideroblastic anemias (see also Table 3–6). Lead interferes with several enzymes in the porphyrin biosynthetic pathway, and the precursor porphyrin accumulates in excess. Typically, elevated levels of ALA occur in the plasma and are excreted in the urine. In addition, urinary coproporphyrins are also present in excess in a 24-hour collected sample. In the acquired porphyria, termed porphyria cutanea tarda, alcohol is also associated with acute exacerbations of these attacks. Alcohol is believed to interfere with enzymes later on in the porphyrin biosynthetic pathway and is associated with an excessive build-up of some of the earlier porphyrins.

REFERENCES

1. Adamson, JN and Finch, CA: Hemoglobin function, oxygen affinity and erythropoietin. Ann Rev Physiol 37:351, 1975.
2. Annotation: Pure red cell aplasia. Br J Haematol 54:331, 1983.
3. Beck, WS: The megaloblastic anemias. In Williams, WJ, et al (eds): Hematology, ed 3. McGraw-Hill, New York, 1983.
4. Berlin, N and Berk, PD: Quantitative aspects of bilirubin metabolism for hematologists: A review. Blood 57:983, 1981.
5. Bessman, JD, Gilmer, PR, and Gardner, FH: Improved classification of anemias by MCV and RDW. Am J Clin Pathol 80:322, 1983.
6. Beutler E: Energy metabolism and maintenance of erythrocytes. In Williams, WJ, et al (eds): *Hematology,* ed 3. McGraw-Hill, New York, 1983, p 331.
7. Bothwell, TH, et al: Iron Metabolism in Man. Blackwell Scientific Publications, Oxford, 1979.
8. Camitta, BM, Storb, R, and Thomas, ED: Aplastic anemia: Pathogenesis, diagnosis, treatment and prognosis. N Engl J Med 306:645, 1982.
9. Chanarin, I: The Megaloblastic Anemias, ed 2. Blackwell Scientific Publications, Oxford, 1979, p 324.
10. Crosby, WH: Structure and function of the spleen. In Williams WJ, et al (eds): Hematology, ed 3. McGraw-Hill, New York, 1983, p 89.
11. Finch, CA: Erythropoiesis, erythropoietin, and iron. Blood 60:1241, 1982.
12. Golde, DW, et al: Polycythemia: Mechanisms and management. Ann Intern Med 95:71, 1981.
13. Harrison, BDW and Stokes, TC: Secondary polycythemia: Its causes, effects and treatment. Br J Dis Chest 76:313, 1982.
14. Herbert, V: Folic acid and vitamin B12. In Rothfield B (ed): Nuclear Medicine in Vitro. JB Lippincott, Philadelphia, 1983, p 337.
15. Hillman, RS: Acute blood loss anemia. In Williams, WJ, et al (eds): Hematology, ed 3. McGraw-Hill, New York, 1983, p 609.
16. Hillman, RS and Finch, CA: The Red Cell Manual, ed 5. FA Davis, Philadelphia, 1985.
17. Hoak, HL, et al: Acquired aplastic anemia in adults. Acta Haematol (Basel) 58:339, 1977.

18. Kellermeyer, RW: General principles of the evaluation and therapy of anemias. Am Clin North Am 68:533, 1984.

19. Lee, GR: The anemia of chronic disease. Semin Hematol 20:61, 1983.

20. Liebhaber, SA and Manno, CS: Update on hemoglobinopathies. In Cotsonas, N (ed): Dis Mon 29:1, 1983.

21. Lindenbaum, J: Status of laboratory testing in the diagnosis of megaloblastic anemia. Blood 61:624, 1983.

22. Lux, SE and Glader, BE: Disorders of the red cell membrane. In Nathan, DG and Oski, FA (eds): Hematology of Infancy and Childhood, ed 2. WB Saunders, Philadelphia, 1981, p 456.

23. Weatherall, DJ and Clegg, JB: Thalassemia Syndromes, ed 3. Blackwell Scientific Publications, Oxford, 1981.

24. Wood, WG and Weatherall, DJ: Developmental genetics of the human haemoglobins: A review. Biochem J 215:1, 1983.

CHAPTER

4

DISEASES OF WHITE BLOOD CELLS

OUTLINE

TESTS

CHAPTER

4

DISEASES OF WHITE BLOOD CELLS

CLASSIFICATION OF NONCLONAL AND CLONAL LEUKOCYTE DISEASES

An approach to classification of leukocyte disorders is presented here. The classification is not meant to be all-inclusive; however, it is organized to allow for an easier understanding of these complex disorders. Any classification is arranged so that the disorders are in categories that have a similar derivation, natural history, prognosis, and therapy. Leukocytes are heterogeneous cells that have markedly different functions. Despite this, they are derived from a common stem cell that differentiates (matures) to allow these functions to be performed. The disease presentation of many of the disorders of white cells depends on which cellular precursor is involved and the degree of differentiation of the cells. There is naturally a spectrum of clinical presentations that may overlap considerably. Since common cell lines are often involved, there are similar presenting symptoms; e.g., failure of bone marrow function causing anemia, infection, and thrombocytopenic bleeding. Also, since leukocytes migrate to many areas of the body, their presentations may be focal, involving specific organ systems, or a more diffuse disease. An understanding of the classification of the disorders of white blood cells is made easier by referring to Figure 2–2 on page 24, which outlines normal leukocyte differentiation.

White cell diseases may be classified according to whether they are clonal or nonclonal (see Table 4–1 for classification of white cell diseases). The clonal disorders are derived from a single precursor cell with all the affected cells (progeny) showing features of derivation from the precursor cell. The conditions included in this category are the *acute and chronic myeloproliferative disorders,* the *myelodysplasias,* and the *acute and chronic lymphoproliferative disorders.* Tissue macrophages, although ultimately derived from bone marrow, participate in nonhematologic conditions such as lipid and carbohydrate storage diseases, and also participate in the lymphoreticular disorders, notably lymphomas and certain leukemias. Similary, lymphocytes and plasma cells are intimately involved in immunologic functions, and diseases of these cells may occur that are also clonal diseases.

These conditions will be considered under the heading of *immunoproliferative disorders.*

The other major category of disorders of white cells are the *non-clonal* conditions. These include *growth regulation abnormalities* (cyclic and constitutional neutropenias), and *leukemoid reactions* (increased proliferative responses to various stimuli), and include bone marrow aplasia and hypoplasia: and the *qualitative leukocyte disorders* (inherited or acquired), characterized by deficiencies of *leukocyte function* involving the differentiated cells. Acknowledging that no classification is ideal, we can attempt to schematize white cell disorders as is shown in Table 4–1. Laboratory studies identifying functional impairment of leukocytes often are still available only in the research setting or specialized laboratory. However, identification of quantitative reduction of cell populations or morphologic abnormalities reflecting clonal expansion are readily appreciated by routine hematologic testing (CBC). Marker studies identifying the cells of origin and whether or not these disorders are clonal are becoming routine.

NONCLONAL DISEASES OF LEUKOCYTES

Disorders of Leukocyte Function

NEUTROPHILS

Neutrophils are especially effective defenders against microbiologic agents, principally bacteria. Granulocytes are motile, accumulating at sites of injury in response to chemotactic stimuli (as was discussed in Chapter 2). Their range of functional activities includes phagocytosis, enzymatic reactions inside the cell, and release of enzymes to the extracellular environment. Antibacterial defense requires that there be adequate numbers of neutrophils, that there be effective mechanisms to attract them to the site of invasion *(chemotaxis),* and that the neutrophils be able to engulf *(phagocytosis)* and destroy the invaders. Any defects in neutrophil numbers, in chemotaxis, or in bacterial killing activity will render the host abnormally susceptible to infection. Table 4–2 lists some of the constitutional and acquired problems that affect neutrophil activity.

Defective Chemotaxis

Chemotaxis is the ability of neutrophils to be attracted to areas of inflammation and infection. This function allows the defender cells to be drawn to areas where they are most needed to fight infection or to remove debris. Deficient numbers of neutrophils at these sites are most commonly associated with neutropenia, which is discussed later. In some conditions there is either failure of attraction due to deficient attractants (e.g., complement deficiencies), or a failure of neutrophil response to these attractants, as may occur with several primary or secondary disorders. Some of these are listed in Table 4–2.

Tests that assess chemotaxis can be performed *in vivo* and *in vitro.* The *REBUCK Skin Window Technique* is the *in vivo* method. The principle of this test is to superficially abrade an area of skin. A cover slip is then placed on the denuded area, and after a predetermined period of time the cover slip is removed and stained and the number of neutrophils is counted. The *in vitro* techniques assess the ability of isolated neutrophils to be attracted through a *semi-permeable membrane* by chemoattractants. After a set period of time, the *semi-permeable membrane* is removed

Table 4–1. CLASSIFICATION OF DISEASES OF WHITE BLOOD CELLS

Disorders of leukocyte function
Neutrophils
  Chemotaxis and phagocytosis
  Chronic granulomatous disease
  Chediak-Higashi syndrome
  Myeloperoxidase deficiency
Disorders of lymphocyte-monocyte and macrophage function

Nonneoplastic (nonclonal) quantitative disorders
Neutropenia
Agranulocytosis
Leukemoid reactions
Infectious mononucleosis

Clonal neoplastic disorders of leukocytes
Myeloproliferative disorders
  Acute myeloproliferative disorders (acute nonlymphocytic leukemias) (see Table 4–7)
  Chronic myeloproliferative disorders (see Table 4–8)
  Myelodysplastic syndromes (see Table 4–9)
Lymphoproliferative disorders
  Acute lymphoblastic leukemia
  Leukemic chronic lymphoproliferative disorders
  Non-Hodgkin's lymphoma
  Hodgkin's lymphoma
Immunoproliferative diseases
  Waldenstrom's macroglobulinemia
  Multiple myeloma
  Monoclonal gammopathy of undetermined significance
  Amyloidosis
  Heavy chain disease

and stained and the number of neutrophils adherent to the membrane is quantitated.

Before granulocytes can phagocytize particles, they must accumulate in the area and attach to the particles that they are about to engulf. *Surface adherence* is enhanced if antibodies or complement proteins or both coat the foreign particles. This process is also called *opsonization*. Patients with constitutional or acquired hypogammaglobulinemia lack antibodies and experience depressed neutrophilic antibacterial activity. Low complement, especially of components 3 and 5, also impairs immune adherence and response to chemotactic stimuli.

Hodgkin's disease and cirrhosis are often associated with the depressed neutrophilic function involving chemotaxis. Both of these conditions are characterized by increased incidence of infections. Exposure to alcohol, aspirin, prednisone, and nonsteroidal anti-inflammatory agents *reduces adherent properties* of granulocytes. Aspirin, prednisone, and the nonsteroidal anti-inflammatory agents are potent inhibitors of inflammation, and reduced adherence is only one of their many effects on the inflammatory process.

Defective Phagocytosis and Bacterial Killing

Phagocytosis may be assessed by exposing phagocytic cells to bacteria, fungi,

Table 4–2. DISORDERS OF NEUTROPHIL FUNCTION

Defective chemotaxis
- Abnormal generation of chemotactic mediators
  - Deficiency of C3 or C5
  - Hypogammaglobulinemia
  - Inhibitory effects of uremia
  - Cirrhosis
  - Hodgkin's disease
  - Hypocomplementemia in acute glomerulonephritis
- Abnormal cellular responses to chemotactic mediators
  - Job's syndrome
  - Diabetes mellitus
  - Rheumatoid arthritis
  - Wiskott-Aldrich syndrome
  - Myeloma
  - Chediak-Higashi syndrome
  - Lazy leukocyte syndrome
  - Hypophosphatemia

Defective phagocytosis and bacterial killing
- Defective opsonization or ingestion
  - Hypogammaglobulinemia
  - Complement deficiencies
  - Circulating immune complexes
  - Hyperosmolar states (diabetes mellitus, alcohol)
- Defective lysosomal function
  - Chronic granulomatous disease
  - Severe G-6-PD deficiency
  - Chediak-Higashi syndrome
  - Myeloperoxidase deficiency

latex beads, and antibody- or complement-coated particles. The engulfed particles or bacteria are then counted.

Microbial killing by phagocytic cells may be determined in the laboratory by a number of techniques. Some of these were discussed in Chapter 2. Defects may initially be appreciated by examination of a *peripheral blood smear,* where morphologic abnormalities such as toxic granulation, Döhle bodies, intracellular organisms, vacuolization, and granule deficiency may be appreciated. The composition and functional characteristics of the granules can be assessed by a variety of cytochemical techniques (see Chapter 2) and functional assays. The respiratory burst with oxidative metabolism is an important component of bacterial killing and can be assessed by the *Nitroblue Tetrazolium (NBT) Test,* as was discussed in Chapter 2. Briefly, phagocytic cells are exposed to endotoxin, which subsequently activates oxidative metabolism, stimulating the respiratory burst. A positive test is conversion of the yellow NBT dye to a black formazan pigment. Alternative tests of assessing the respiratory burst include *chemiluminescence* (light emission associated with generation of ATP). More specialized and research laboratories can precisely determine the amount of oxygen-free radical compounds (peroxide, superoxide) released following and associated with phagocytosis. The three best-characterized disorders of microbicidal function are *chronic granulomatous disease, Chediak-Higashi syndrome,* and myeloperoxidase deficiency.

Chronic Granulomatous Disease (CGD)

This disorder is an X-linked inherited disease characterized by severe recurrent infections caused particularly by staphylococci and gram-negative bacteria in which the affected tissues show a granulomatous type of inflammatory process. The tissues contain lipid-filled macrophages and small abscesses. These patients have normal neutrophil counts, neutrophil morphology, and chemotaxis. Phagocytosis is also normal; however, bacterial killing is defective. The primary defect is the inability to generate superoxide and peroxide, which are essential components for bacterial killing. Consequently, organisms proliferate and grow inside the phagocytic cells, emphasizing the intracellular bactericidal defect. These patients have abnormal nitroblue tetrazolium reduction and chemiluminescence.

Chediak-Higashi Syndrome

This condition is also discussed in Chapter 2, and is associated with the morphologic appearance of giant lysosomal granules in cells. These abnormal cells are readily seen on peripheral blood smears. These patients have defective microbicidal activity as well as defective chemotaxis.

Myeloperoxidase Deficiency

Bacterial phagocytosis requires, as a last step, interaction of hydrogen peroxide with an intracellular enzyme myeloperoxidase. A variant syndrome of CGD occurs if myeloperoxidase activity is congenitally absent. Acquired deficiency of myeloperoxidase occurs in granulocytic leukemia, a fact that may contribute to the increased infection rates that occur in leukemia. Severe bacterial infections depress bactericidal efficiency. Laboratories equipped to perform histochemical studies in circulating white cells can stain neutrophils directly for myeloperoxidase activity.

DISORDERS OF LYMPHOCYTE, MONOCYTE, AND MACROPHAGE FUNCTION

When lymphocytes are deficient in number or function, the patient suffers from immunodeficiency. This may either be inherited or acquired. Table 4–3 lists some of the more common immunodeficiency syndromes. See Chapter 2 for a discussion on the normal lymphocyte subpopulations and their functions. See also Cellular Immunology, Chapter 8. Inherited immunodeficiency syndromes are rare, but have an importance out of all proportion to their frequency because of the insight they reveal about normal immune functioning. Acquired deficiency states are increasingly common. The acquired immunodeficiency syndrome (AIDS) is an acquired immune deficiency state produced as a result of infection with a human immunodeficiency virus (HIV). This virus preferentially attacks helper T-lymphocytes, markedly depleting their numbers (see Chapter 8). Impairment of cellular proliferation or protein synthesis can also depress lymphocyte and plasma cell activity. Cytotoxic therapy for malignant diseases, adrenal corticosteroids, and negative protein balance are common predisposing conditions.

Blood monocytes and tissue macrophages are the same cells in different locations. The circulating monocyte is probably a young or de-differentiated form. Once in the tissues, macrophages develop organelles and enzymes that permit phagocytosis and lytic activity. The cells that line the sinusoids and spleen, liver, and lymph nodes are also derived from the same monocyte-macrophage pool. Tissue macrophages recruit new members by local cell reproduction and by repletion from bone marrow precursors. Macrophages exist as inconspicuous histiocytes in most tissues, becoming obvious only when they engage actively in phagocytosis. When there is substantial local demand for macrophages, as in tuberculosis and other granulomatous in-

Table 4–3. IMMUNODEFICIENCY DISORDERS

Primary immunodeficiency diseases
- T Cells
  - Severe combined immunodeficiency
  - Di George's syndrome
  - Wiskott-Aldrich syndrome
  - Chronic mucocutaneous candidiasis
- B Cells
  - Selective IgA deficiency in combination with various states
  - X-linked agammaglobulinemia
  - Common variable hypogammaglobulinemia
  - Selective IgM deficiency
  - IgG subclass deficiency

Secondary immunodeficiency diseases
- Viral infections
  - Acquired immunodeficiency syndrome (Human immunodeficiency virus)
  - Measles
  - Cytomegalovirus
  - Epstein-Barr virus
- Splenectomy
- Burns
- Immunosuppressive drugs
  - Antimetabolites
  - Corticosteroids
- Radiation
- Prematurity
- Hematologic disorders
  - Lymphomas
  - Leukemia
  - Myeloma
  - Aplastic anemia
  - Sickle cell disease
- Miscellaneous
  - Diabetes
  - Protein-losing states
  - Nephrotic syndrome
  - Enteropathies
  - Aging

Adapted from Graziano, FM and Bell, CL: Normal immune response. Med Clin North Am 69:439, 1985.

flammatory diseases, bone marrow and blood monocyte turnover increases and monocytes accumulate in substantial numbers (see Chapter 2).

Normal macrophages have enzyme systems capable of synthesizing and degrading sphingolipids, compounds important in biologic membranes and especially prominent in the nervous system. Several different inherited defects involve specific enzymes necessary for lipid breakdown. In these deficiency states, lipid products accumulate in those parts of the cells that normally degrade recycled lipids. These diseases are not primarily hematologic conditions, although the macrophages of the marrow, spleen, and liver become overloaded with these metabolic precursors. The major effects of this are enlargement of the reticuloendothelial organs, and numerous lipid-laden histiocytes present in the bone marrow. Some of these cells have distinctive morphologic features that characterize the disorders *Gaucher's disease* and *Niemann-Pick disease.* Pseudo-Gaucher cells can also be seen in the myeloproliferative disorders. Other morphologic curiosities include the *Sea-Blue Histiocyte Syndrome,* in which marrow histiocytes are laden with a bluish staining material on Giemsa-Wright stains. These diagnoses are often made on the basis of family history, but also on the identification of the characteristic cells, particularly in the bone marrow. The enlarged spleen often serves as reservoir for maldistribution of the peripheral blood cells, and therefore leads to hypersplenism. Many patients require splenectomy for symptomatic cytopenias.

Non-neoplastic Quantitative Disorders

Total and differential white counts are useful but nonspecific diagnostic signs in many physiologic and pathologic states. A discussion of neutropenia and immune deficiency syndromes has preceded, and is also mentioned in Chapter 2. Changing counts may indicate that an abnormal condition exists and the body is responding; however, changes in white cell levels may also reflect conditions that directly affect blood-forming organs (see also Chapter 2).

Neutropenia

Neutropenia is a decrease in the absolute neutrophil count below 2,000/μl. Neutropenia may be classified as mild (a neutrophil count of between 1000 and 2000/μl), moderate (a neutrophil count of 500–1000 μl), or severe or agranulocytosis (a neutrophil count of less than 500/μl). This classification is useful in that it predicts the likelihood of infectious events. Individuals with severe neutrophil depletion are susceptible to bacterial infection, particularly with the organisms *Klebsiella, Escherichia, Pseudomonas,* and *Staphylococcus.* Neutropenia may occur as a result of many primary bone marrow diseases or acquired disorders (see Table 4–4). Thirty percent of the black population may normally have a neutrophil count of less than 2000/μl, and this is termed *constitutional neutropenia.*

Evaluation of an absolute reduction in neutrophil count starts with an examination of the *peripheral blood smear.* A *differential count* is useful in assessing the degree of quantitative impairment as well as the percentage of immature cells present. Analogous to the reticulocyte count in anemia, the evaluation of bands in neutropenia can be helpful, and suggests increased neutrophil turnover. *Bone marrow examination* is important in categorizing the nature of the neutropenia. If the bone marrow is hypercellular and shows many normal neutrophil precursors in the presence of peripheral neutropenia, this suggests a peripheral destructive cause for the neutropenia. Normal neutrophil counts in the presence of increased bone marrow activity occurs when there is maldistribution of the neutrophil pools—e.g., change in the distribution between the marginating and the circulating pool, or in conditions associated with hypersplenism (where a large percentage of the circulating neutrophil pool is sequestered in the spleen). Neutrophils may also be consumed in the peripheral blood by increased destruction that can be immune- or non-immune-mediated. Unfortunately, there is no simple test like the Anti-Human Globulin Test for anemia; however, autoimmune neutropenia should be considered when all other conditions have been excluded and the marrow shows an increased number of normal neutrophil precursors in the absence of an enlarged spleen. Anti-neutrophil antibodies can be detected using immunofluorescence and other immunologic techniques. However, these tests are not readily available in routine laboratories.

The commonest cause of neutropenia, however, is bone marrow suppression or failure. This may occur with the primary marrow diseases or particularly associated with secondary suppression from drugs, medications, irradiation, and infections. Some of these conditions are listed in Table 4–4.

Another unusual disorder in which *cyclic neutropenia* occurs is characterized by periodic and often marked depletion of total neutrophil counts in the peripheral blood. Individuals with this disorder show an increased cyclic susceptibility to infection, characterized by cyclic fever and oral infections. These cycles may occur regularly, often at 21-day intervals. It is felt that this disorder is due to a defect in control of granulocyte differentiation, maybe related to cyclic disappearance of controlling colony-stimulating factors.

In several rare constitutional conditions, granulocytopenia occurs as part of the spectrum that may also include defective granulocyte differentiation, decreased gammaglobulins, the presence of inhibitors to granulopoiesis, or the presence of leukoagglutinating antibodies. Moreover, the range of symptoms is wide. In familial benign chronic neutropenia, the condition may be discovered by chance, whereas in infantile genetic agranulocytosis, death from infection usually occurs before the first birthday.

Investigation of suspected constitutional neutropenia should begin with observation of the bone marrow cellularity and maturational pattern. These individuals may also have defects in leukocyte chemotaxis and bacterial killing (discussed above). A search should also be made for simultaneous abnormalities of lymphocytes, of immune activity, and of red cell and platelet development. In addition, the patient's family should be studied to detect a possible familial incidence.

AGRANULOCYTOSIS

Agranulocytosis is a severe, acute neutropenia characterized by the disappearance of neutrophil precursors in the bone marrow and a severe depletion of the granulocyte count in the peripheral blood. The differential white count shows an absence or less than 500/μl of neutrophils or granulocytic cells. This may occur suddenly in an otherwise normal individual, and more especially occurs as an idiosyncratic drug reaction. It can also occur in association with autoimmune diseases and with some infections. Drugs sometimes affect the granulocyte levels without affecting the other marrow elements, but often red cells and/or platelet numbers are reduced as well. Antibodies may affect white cells only, but drug antibodies that damage cells through the "innocent bystander" effect (see Chapter 3) sometimes affect all three cell types in the blood as well.

Most of the agents and pathophysiologic conditions that cause anemia can depress granulocytes. Agranulocytosis is characterized clinically by the presence of fever and a severe throat infection, often with a white plaque-like membrane on the pharynx.

Most patients recover spontaneously following discontinuation of the offending drug. Antibiotic therapy is invariably given for those patients who are infected. The earliest signs of marrow recovery are associated with an *increased number of monocytes,* and subsequently bands, in the peripheral blood. In the early stages of marrow recovery, there is a predominance of promyelocytes, which can mimic the morphology of acute promyelocytic leukemia.

With some drugs there is a dose-related depression of white cells. In particular, drugs such as *carbamazepines (Tegretol)* are associated with gradually declining

Table 4–4. NEUTROPENIA

Definition
Neutrophil count <2000/μl

Classification

Mild	PMN count 1000–2000/μl
Moderate	PMN count 500–1000/μl
Severe	PMN count<500/μl

Causes
- Constitutional (normal in certain populations, e.g., blacks)
- Deficiency in production
  - Constitutional
    - Familial benign neutropenia
    - Cyclic neutropenia
    - Infantile genetic agranulocytosis
    - Many rare genetic conditions
  - Acquired
    - Nutritional deficiency (Vitamin B_{12}, folic acid, copper)
    - Leukemia
    - Aplastic anemia
    - Response to infection (typhoid, hepatitis, infectious mononucleosis, tuberculosis)
    - Cytotoxic drugs (cancer chemotherapy, immunosuppression)
    - Drug reactions (chloramphenicol, phenothiazines, propylthiouracil, phenylbutazone, phenytoins, carbamazepines)
- Excessive destruction
  - Immune-mediated
    - Autoimmune neutropenia (idiopathic or associated with collagen-vascular diseases, lymphoproliferative diseases, or drugs)
    - Acute granulocytotoxicity or leukoagglutination associated with blood transfusions
    - Neonatal alloimmune granulocytopenia
    - Antidrug antibodies
  - Nonimmune
    - Splenomegaly (portal hypertension, storage diseases, leukemias, lymphomas, rheumatoid arthritis)
    - Extracorporeal circulation (heart–lung machines, renal dialysis)
    - Disorders of pulmonary microcirculation
- Abnormal distribution
  - Splenomegaly
  - Margination shifts (see Fig. 2–3)
- Cyclic neutropenia

neutrophil counts. In some of these patients, this may herald the onset of agranulocytosis; however, in many others if the dosage is decreased, the white cell count improves. Periodic monitoring of patient's counts who are on these medications is important. Phenothiazines, phenytoins, some sulfonamides, and some antithyroid drugs depress leukocyte production as well. Neutropenia persists for several weeks after therapy ceases, but granulopoiesis resumes when the drug is stopped. Chloramphenicol-induced marrow depression, however, may last for months or years.

Diagnosis depends on careful evaluation of total and differential white counts. If agranulocytosis causes necrotizing mouth infections, prostration, and fever, it may be difficult to distinguish between drug-induced agranulocytosis, acute leukemia, and the granulocyte-suppressive effects of massive infection. Evaluation must include meticulous inquiry about drugs and food additives and about exposure to materials involved in industrial, domestic, recreational, and environmental activities. It is important to evaluate red cell and platelet numbers and bone marrow cellularity. Aplastic anemia may present with features of agranulocytosis. With pure agranulocytosis, the total white count is low, and mature lymphocytes are virtually the only leukocytes in the circulating blood. Red cell and platelet levels, both in blood and in bone marrow, are normal. Pure agranulocytosis is relatively rare, since many exogenous agents also tend to depress red cell and platelet production. In leukemias, the marrow usually has an increased proportion of blasts and immature cells, and the marrow is often hypercellular despite low levels of circulating cells. A list of the more common drugs associated with neutropenia is shown in Table 4–5.

Leukemoid Reactions

Reactive leukocytosis assumes florid proportions, with immature as well as mature white cells flooding the circulation. Because the blood picture resembles chronic leukemia, this event is called a "leukemoid reaction." It is not a primary marrow disorder, and is usually secondary to some other condition. Granulocytes are most often involved, but striking monocytosis can occur in tuberculosis, whereas leukemoid lymphocytosis has been reported in tuberculosis, whooping cough, and infectious mononucleosis.

Granulocytosis of leukemoid proportions may accompany malignant tumors with or without metastases to the bone, severe pyogenic or tuberculous infection, heavy metal poisoning, sickle cell crises, or severe metabolic disturbances involving the kidney or liver, and also diabetic ketoacidosis. A patient recovering from agranulocytosis or from recent chemotherapy may have an intense white cell overproduction that suggests a leukemic proliferation, but leukopoiesis seldom continues at this rate for longer than a week.

When a leukemoid reaction is secondary to some obvious, underlying condition, distinction from leukemia is not difficult. It should be remembered, however, that leukemia can coexist with other diesases. Leukemia and tuberculosis, for example, can occur together, and each exacerbates the other. If the primary condition is not apparent, the picture alone may suggest the presence of leukemia. Features that distinguish a leukemoid reaction from chronic myelogenous leukemia are shown in Table 4–6.

Infectious Mononucleosis

Infectious mononucleosis (IM) is also discussed in Chapter 14. It is, however, not uncommonly associated with a marked elevation in the total white cell count, and in particular in the lymphocyte differential count. The white count may be low when the disease begins, but by the end of the first week, leukocytosis of 10,000–30,000/μl is usual. There is an absolute increase in lymphocytes, many of which are large (see Color Plate 22) and atypical (Downey cells). These are transformed T-lymphocytes. These cells are reacting to the infected B-lymphocytes that are invaded by the Epstein-Barr virus, which is the cause of the IM syndrome. Circulating "virocytes" of this

Table 4–5. MORE COMMON DRUGS PRODUCING UNEXPECTED NEUTROPENIA AND AGRANULOCYTOSIS

Anti-inflammatory	Phenylbutazone, oxyphenbutazone
Antimicrobials	Chloramphenicol, sulphonamides, Co-Trimoxazol
Anticonvulsants	Phenytoin, carbamazepine
Tranquilizers	Phenothiazine group
Antithyroid	Thiouracil group
Hypoglycemia agents	Tolbutamide
Miscellaneous	Allopurinol, chlorothiazides, cimetidine, gold, isoniazid, ibuprofen

appearance are not unique to IM. In other viral diseases as well, circulating T-lymphocytes manifest these reactive changes to viral infections of other cells or tissues. In IM, the atypical lymphocytes are prominent during the second to the fourth weeks of the illness.

CLONAL LEUKOCYTE DISORDERS

Myeloproliferative Disorders

The myeloproliferative disorders are a group of clonal, neoplastic diseases that involve the pleuripotent hemapoietic stem cells. In these conditions there is unregulated and uncontrolled growth and proliferation of the ancestral progeny of multipotent cells that exhibit differing degrees of differentiation. These disorders can be further divided into the *acute* and *chronic types.* The *acute myeloproliferative disorders* are the *acute nonlymphocytic leukemias,* and are characterized by unregulated

Table 4–6. COMPARISON OF LEUKEMOID REACTION WITH CHRONIC MYELOGENOUS LEUKEMIA

Leukemoid Reactions	Chronic Myelogenous Leukemia
WBC usually $<50{,}000/\mu l$	WBC usually $>50{,}000/\mu l$
Toxic granulation and Döhle bodies	Toxic granulation $\pm$ – 0
Basophilia absent	Greater basophil count (usual)
Bands prominent	All stages, myelocytes particularly
Elevated leukocyte alkaline phosphatase (LAP) >100	LAP <10
Spleen usually not palpable	Spleen usually enlarged
Philadelphia chromosome not present	Philadelphia chromosome present in 90% of cases

growth with limited or no differentiation. The *chronic myeloproliferative diseases* include a group of disorders where there is unregulated and excessive proliferation of cells with substantial differentiation, usually producing an excess of the mature, differentiated hemapoietic cells. Tables 4–7 and 4–8 are classifications of the *acute* and *chronic myeloproliferative diseases.*

Another variant of these clonal nonlymphocytic disorders is the group of diesases termed the *myelodysplastic syndromes,* in which there is unstable and unregulated growth of cells with varying degrees of differentiation, and which differ from the above disorders in that they cannot be classified as acute leukemias because their clinical course is generally more benign and the cell populations are more mature. However, a substantial number of these disorders may transform into the leukemic stage after a variable latent period. It is because of this potential for leukemic transformation that these disorders have been called *preleukemia syndromes.* They should, however, be broadly grouped together with the myeloproliferative diseases. Because of their propensity for unstable growth, they are classified in a subcategory called the myelodysplasias. Table 4–9 is a list of these diseases grouped together as the *myelodysplastic syndromes.*

Figure 2–2 is a comprehensive diagram showing the differentiation of marrow elements from the pleuripotent stem cell. This cell is capable of proliferating and differentiating into progenitor cells that can give rise to granulocytes, erythrocytes, and platelets. Evidence supporting the clonal nature of these disorders has been derived from both cytogenetic and isoenzyme studies, using glucose-6-phosphate dehydrogenase isoenzymes, in black female heterozygotes. In these women, if a tumor is of clonal origin, only a single isoenzyme will be found in the tumor cells. Tumors with a multicentric origin would show both isoenzymes in these heterozygous women.

Despite their apparent homogeneity, in terms of specific cell types and morphology, the myeloproliferative disorders are probably extremely heterogeneous and may exhibit a markedly differing array of cell surface types, which may explain why some patients have a more aggressive course than others. Studies of various oncogenes may also lead to an understanding of the pathogenesis of these disorders and their differing growth patterns.

The Acute Myeloproliferative Disorders

Acute nonlymphocytic leukemia (ANLL) may be subdivided into *seven subtypes* on the basis of morphology. A classification system proposed by the French, American, British (FAB) Cooperative Group provides the morphologic and cytochemical standards for grouping these acute leukemias into the differing categories. As can be seen from Table 4–7, there are seven variants of ANLL that may be derived from the pleuripotent or multipotent stem cells, or from clonal proliferation of cells committed toward myeloid, erythroid, and megakaryocytic lines. Consequently, some of these leukemias may present with morphologic features of myeloid and monocytic characteristics, or erythroblastic characteristics. Presumably, the predominant morphologic type depends on where the clonal neoplastic event occurs in the development of the nonlymphocytic cells.

The importance of identifying these cell types is to separate them from the acute lymphoblastic leukemias. This distinction is important since specific therapy and prognosis are different. Table 4–10 outlines some of the features that distinguish ANLL from the acute lymphoblastic leukemias (ALL). In clinical usage, the FAB classification numbers have not replaced the descriptive diagnostic terms that are routinely employed in common practice. *Acute myeloblastic leukemia* (M1 or M2)

Table 4–7. CLASSIFICATION OF ACUTE MYELOPROLIFERATIVE DISORDERS

Preferred Name	Abbreviation	FAB	Alternate Names
Acute myeloblastic leukemia	AML	M1, M2	Acute myelocytic Acute granulocytic leukemia Acute nonlymphocytic leukemia
Acute promyelocytic leukemia	APL	M3	Acute progranulocytic Hypergranular promyelocytic
Acute myelomonocytic leukemia	AMML	M4	Naegeli-type leukemia
Acute monoblastic leukemia	AMoL	M5	Schilling-type
Erythroleukemia	EL	M6	DiGuglielmo's disease Erythremic myelosis
Megakaryocytic leukemia	ML	M7	Acute myelofibrosis

Table 4–8. CLASSIFICATION OF CHRONIC MYELOPROLIFERATIVE DISORDERS

Preferred Name	Abbreviations	Common Synonyms
Chronic myelogenous leukemia	CML	Chronic myelocytic leukemia Chronic myeloid leukemia Chronic granulocytic leukemia
Polycythemia vera	P. vera	Erythrocytosis Erythremia True polycythemia
Agnogenic myeloid metaplasia	AMM	Myelofibrosis Idiopathic myelofibrosis Osteomyelosclerosis Myelosclerosis
Essential thrombocythemia	ET	Primary thrombocythemia Hemorrhagic thrombocythemia Primary thrombocytosis

Table 4–9. MYELODYSPLASTIC SYNDROMES

FAB: Myelodysplastic Syndromes	Other Terms
Refractory anemia (RA)	Chronic erythemic myelosis Refractory megaloblastic anemia
RA with ring sideroblasts	Acquired idiopathic sideroblastic anemia
RA with excess blasts (RAEB)	Acute myeloproliferative syndrome
RAEB in transformation	Primary acquired panmyelopathy with myeloblastosis (PAMP)
Chronic myelomonocytic leukemia	Subacute myelomonocytic leukemia

From Pittiglio and Sacher,[10] p 240, with permission.

and *myelomonocytic leukemia* (M4) are the two most common subtypes. *Acute megakaryocytic* (M7) and *acute monoblastic leukemia* (M5) are the two more unusual categories of ANLL.

Epidemiology and Clinical Presentation

Acute, nonlymphocytic leukemia tends to be a disease of adults, whereas in contrast, acute lymphoblastic leukemia is primarily a disease of children. Only 10% of ANLL is found in children, and there is an increasing incidence with advancing age. It is more common in whites than blacks, and men than women. The M:F ratio is 3:2. Most of the acute myeloproliferative syndromes present with varying degrees of bone marrow failure. Consequently, clinical symptoms associated with anemia, leukopenia, and infection or thrombocytopenia predominate in varying degrees. Special presenting symptoms may occur in the *acute promyelocytic leukemias* (M3), which cause a disseminated intravascular coagulation syndrome and substantial bleeding manifestations. *Acute myelomonocytic leukemia* (M4) and *acute monocytic leukemia* (M5) in particular may present with gum hypertrophy due to monocytic invasion into the gum tissues. Fatigue and fever, however, are nearly universal. The actual white count is unpredictable. About 25% of patients have white blood cell counts above 50,000/μl. Another 25% have subnormal counts below 5,000/μl. About 15% have normal white cell counts (5,000–10,000/μl), but these are morphologically abnormal and immature cells. About half the patients with newly diagnosed acute leukemia have high serum uric acid levels, and elevated lactate dehydrogenase (LDH) levels. The M4 and M5 subtypes may also have decreased serum potassium and serum calcium due to marked liberation of lysozyme, which passes out in the urine and may damage the renal tubules. This produces an excess urinary loss of calcium and potassium in these types of leukemia. The laboratory effects of therapy are discussed below. Table 4–11 outlines possible etiologic factors that have been associated with acute leukemia.

Laboratory Diagnosis of Acute Leukemia and Differentiation of Subtypes

Diagnosis of acute leukemia is made on the basis of the following:

1. Demonstration of immature cells in the peripheral blood with confirmation of immature cells in the bone marrow. Usually the bone marrow contains greater than 20% "blastic" morphology.

Table 4–10. DISTINGUISHING CYTOLOGIC FEATURES BETWEEN ACUTE NONLYMPHOBLASTIC LEUKEMIA AND ACUTE LYMPHOBLASTIC LEUKEMIA

	AML Myeloblast	ALL Lymphoblast
Differences in blast morphology		
Blast size	Large blast	Small blast
Cytoplasm	Moderate	Scant
Chromatin	Fine, lacy	More dense
Nucleoli	Prominent (usually more than 2)	Indistinct (usually 2 or less)
Auer rods	Present in 10–40% of cases of AML	Never present
Cytochemical differentiation		
Sudan black/peroxidase	+ (monoblast ±)	–
Nonspecific esterase	– (monoblast +)	–
TdT	–	+

Modified from Perkins, ML: Introduction to leukemia and the acute leukemias. In Pittiglio and Sacher,[10] p 232.

2. Categorizing the leukemic cells as acute nonlymphocytic leukemia or acute lymphoblastic leukemia.
3. Categorizing the cell type enables placement within the FAB classification (see Color Plates 34–38 and 41–43).

In ANLL, the blasts that overrun the marrow have finely dispersed or granular chromatin, several or numerous nucleoli, delicate regular nuclear membrane, and modest amounts of cytoplasm, although the cell outline usually is regular. Although maturation is minimal, promyelocytes are present and often numerous, particularly in the M3 variant. Auer rods often can be seen in the cytoplasm (see Color Plate 33). In ANLL, cytochemical stains are positive for the peroxidase reaction and positive with Sudan black stains. Esterase stains are variable, as was discussed in Chapter 2.

Nucleated red cells and diffuse polychromatophilia tend to be more conspicuous in ANLL than in ALL. Platelet depression is often less extreme than in ALL; nearly half of ANLL patients present with platelet counts in the 30,000–100,000/μl range. Coagulation abnormalities are particularly prevalent in *acute promyelocytic leukemia* (M3), where the prothrombin time, partial thromboplastin time, and thrombin time are all prolonged (see Chapter 5). In addition, in this variant, fibrin degradation products are markedly elevated, and fibrinogen values are decreased (see Disseminated Intravascular Coagulation, Chapter 6). In *acute myelomonocytic leukemia* (M4) and *acute monocytic leukemia* (M5), monocytic cells proliferate in addition to myeloblastic cells. In the M4 variant, equivalent numbers of these cells may be seen; however, in the M5 type the majority of cells are monoblastic types and morphologically show twisted or indented nuclei, fine chromatin patterns, and

Table 4–11. ETIOLOGIC FACTORS ASSOCIATED WITH ACUTE LEUKEMIA

Inherited
- Down's syndrome
- Fanconi's syndrome
- Bloom's syndrome
- Ataxia telangiectasia
- Oncogenic activation

Acquired
- Drugs and chemicals
  - Benzene
  - Alkylating drugs (nitrogen mustard, melphalan, chlorambucil, cyclophosphamide, procarbazine)
- Radiation
- Viruses
  - Human T. leukemia virus type 1 (HTLV-1)—Jamaica, Japan
  - Epstein-Barr virus (Burkitt's lymphoma—L3)
- Oncogenes
  - C-abl, C-sis (CML)
  - C-myc (Burkitt's lymphoma—L3)
- Chromosomal instability
  - Translocations
    - t9:22 (CML)
    - t4:11 (ALL)
    - t8:21 (AML)
    - t8:14 (Burkitt's lymphoma)
  - Inversions
    - inv 16 (AML)
  - Deletion
    - 5q- (myelodysplasia, preleukemia)
    - Monosomy 7

a positive, nonspecific esterase stain. As already mentioned, in these types there is an increase in urinary lysozyme levels, presumably reflecting an increased turnover of these cells, liberation of the enzyme into the blood, and filtration through the kidney into the urine. Color Plates 34 to 38 show some of the morphologic variants of the different cells seen in the acute nonlymphoblastic leukemias.

In *erythroleukemia (FAB M6),* the erythropoietic precursors predominate in the marrow and exceed 50% of all the marrow elements. The morphology of these erythroid cells closely resembles that of a megaloblastic type of picture, described in Chapter 2 (see Color Plate 26). However, in addition, there are usually more than 30% myeloblasts and promyelocytes present in the bone marrow. The disease, therefore, is a neoplastic, malignant, clonal proliferation of cells with capabilities of expressing erythroid and myeloid, as well as monocytic, markers. Megakaryoblasts may also be abnormal in morphology if present. In the unusual variant M7 *(acute megakaryoblastic leukemia),* the blast cells contain platelet peroxidase rather than myeloperoxidase. The marrow may also show intensive fibrosis, which is coexistent with the blasts. The prognosis is particularly poor in this variant.

Cytogenetic abnormalities are also found in several of these leukemias. The most consistent abnormality is found in acute promyelocytic leukemia (M3) in which the majority of cases exhibit a translocation between chromosomes 15 and 17. Other abnormalities found in these leukemias include a translocation between chromosomes 21 and 8, found more particularly in ANLL, and the inverted chromosome 16 variant, which is found in acute myelomonocytic leukemia (M4), particularly with a prominence of eosinophil precursors in this variant.

Laboratory Effects of Treatment

The aim of treatment in acute, nonlymphocytic leukemia is to eradicate the malignant clone and allow normal hematopoiesis to reestablish itself. The first objective is to induce remission with *remission-induction chemotherapy.* Once remission is induced, the remission is consolidated with further chemotherapy, and current chemotherapeutic regimens using intensification treatment with subsequent courses of mixed chemotherapy are the rule. Two drugs, *cytosine arabinoside* and *daunomycin,* are the main drugs used. Other regimens call for intensive combinations of additional drugs. In 70–75%, an initial remission is induced; however, the median duration of remission is between 12 and 16 months.

With more intensive regimens, five-year survival figures are improving, with approximately 25% of patients alive after five years.

The intensive chemotherapy markedly suppresses total blood counts, which remain at a low level for two to three weeks. During this time patients require transfusion support with red blood cells for severe symptomatic anemia, and platelet transfusions for both prophylaxis against bleeding and the treatment of thrombocytopenic bleeding. White cell transfusions are generally unhelpful. Initial chemotherapy is associated with massive destruction of leukemic cells, with liberation of chemicals from inside of the cell to the plasma. This is associated with the syndrome termed the *tumor lysis syndrome,* which produces a marked elevation of uric acid, an increased serum potassium and phosphate, and a marked increase in serum LDH. Because of the propensity of uric acid crystals to precipitate in the urine, compounded by an excessive secretion of phosphate, renal function must be carefully monitored. For septic episodes during the periods of marked pancytopenia, in particular marked neutropenia, blood cultures need to be taken and infecting organisms identified. The usual organisms associated with infection during the chemotherapy phase include gram-negative organisms and opportunistic fungal infections (see Chapter 13). The use of the antifungal agent amphotericin B is associated with potassium wasting, which also needs to be monitored during this phase.

Therapy for acute promyelocytic leukemia during the initial induction phase requires close monitoring of coagulation parameters, including the prothrombin time, partial thromboplastin time, and fibrinogen levels, and may require the use of heparin and replacement of coagulation factors (see Laboratory Monitoring of Disseminated Intravascular Coagulation in Chapter 6).

Chronic Myeloproliferative Syndromes

Table 4–8 is a list of the chronic myeloproliferative diseases. These conditions are clonal disorders of the hemapoietic stem cell that are associated with unregulated growth and proliferation of multipotent cells that are capable of differentiation to maturity. Depending on the predominant cell lines involved and the predominant cell type found in the peripheral blood, these conditions may be classified as is shown in Table 4–8. These conditions comprise several disorders that have some common clinical and hematologic features. They are usually diseases of adults, and in particular elderly adults. Chronic myelogenous leukemia usually occurs in the

Table 4–12. DISEASES PRODUCING MASSIVE SPLENOMEGALY

Chronic myelogenous leukemia
Agnogenic myeloid metaplasia
Lymphomas
Chronic lymphocytic leukemia
Visceral leishmaniasis (Kala-Azar)
Gaucher's disease
Schistosomiasis (bilharziasis)
Malaria

40–60-year age group, polycythemia vera in the 50–60-year age group and agnogenic myeloid metaplasia and essential thrombocythemia in the 50–70-year age group. Patients may present with symptoms of disturbed marrow functioning including anemia and recurrent infections, bleeding, or thrombotic tendency. On clinical examination, the majority of patients have an enlarged spleen and often the spleen is massively enlarged. There are very few conditions that give rise to massive splenomegaly, and these are listed in Table 4–12. Common laboratory studies may be the finding of a normochromic, normocytic anemia (except in polycythemia vera), diffuse polychromatophilia, teardrop poikilocytosis (especially marked in agnogenic myeloid metaplasia—myelofibrosis), high blood uric acid levels, elevated serum vitamin B_{12} levels, and usually an *elevated leukocyte alkaline phosphatase,* except in *chronic myelogenous leukemia,* where it is *decreased.* Specific cytogenetic abnormalities may be found in some of these disorders. The consistent chromosomal abnormality found in chronic myelogenous leukemia is the *Philadelphia chromosome (translocation of chromosome 22 to 9).* Marrow fibrosis (myelofibrosis) may complicate any of these myeloproliferative disorders; however, it is usually more evident in agnogenic myeloid metaplasia.

Chronic Myelogenous Leukemia (CML)

Chronic myelogenous leukemia, also called chronic granulocytic leukemia (CGL), is a disorder characterized by unregulated growth, proliferation, and differentiation of myeloid precursors committed toward granulocytic development. As a consequence, all stages of granulocytic development are markedly increased. In addition, other granulocytic cells, including eosinophils and basophils, may be abundant. Leukemia literally means "white blood," and in CML white cell counts may be so high that the blood actually assumes a greyish hue. White cell levels are characteristically between 50,000 and 250,000/μl, but can go even higher. This condition is usually a disease of older adults. It accounts for 15% of all leukemias, and only occasional cases are seen in persons below 20 years of age.

The condition usually begins insidiously. Patients may present with symptoms of hypermetabolism due to the numerous, dividing, metabolically active cells, and complain of malaise, fatigue, abdominal fullness, or low-grade fever. There is usually only a mild anemia, with hematocrit between 25 and 35%. Thrombocytopenia is uncommon. Red cell and platelet levels vary independently of the white cell count. More than half of CML patients have platelet counts above 450,000/μl. There may, however, be abnormal bleeding despite the elevated platelet counts due to qualitative platelet defects. The spleen is almost always enlarged, sometimes to such an extent that it virtually fills the abdominal cavity. Hepatomegaly is common, but less impressive. Bone marrow tenderness is frequent, especially over the sternum: this is probably related to excessive marrow volume and activity. Serum uric acid levels are elevated and there may be urate kidney stones or clinical gout. Serum vitamin B_{12} and vitamin B_{12} binding proteins usually are above normal. Values for serum potassium often are high and glucose levels low, but these are artifactual findings, the result of prolonged contact between serum and huge numbers of metabolizing white cells and platelets. If serum is separated promptly, glucose and potassium levels are normal in the clinically stable state. There are *three main clinical stages* of the disease: *the stable, chronic phase* as described above, *the phase of metamorphosis* and *the acute leukemic phase.* Chronic myelogenous leukemia is a true preleukemia in that nearly all cases evolve into an acute blastic transformation. During this phase of evolution, the mature cells become dedifferentiated and there are many more immature cells seen. At this stage, patients may present with more profound symptoms, and thrombocytopenia may predominate and produce marked bleeding manifestations.

White Cell Findings

The blood and bone marrow look much alike in CML (see Color Plate 40). Vast numbers of granulocytes are present in all stages of maturation, but an interesting peculiarity is that there are more myelocytes and metamyelocytes. Chronic myelogenous leukemia granulocytes retain bactericidal capacity, and increased susceptibility to infection is rare at the time of diagnosis. The *leukocyte alkaline phosphatase* (LAP) is nearly always low and can be zero. Occasionally, the LAP may increase in patients who are infected or in those who are in the metamorphosis or blast transformation stage. The pathognomonic feature of chronic myelogenous leukemia is the finding of the *Philadelphia chromosome,* which occurs in 90% of patients with CML.

Phildadelphia Chromosome

The Philadelphia chromosome is a translocation of genetic material from the long arm of chromosome 22 to another chromosome, most usually chromosome 9. Other translocations can occur but are unusual. Standard nomenclature defines the short arm of a chromosome as p and the long arm as q. The Philadelphia chromosome, then, is t($9q^+$; $22q^-$) (see Fig. 2–12). The finding of this chromosomal translocation is diagnostic of CML. The genome of the translocation has been studied intensively, and it has been shown that it involves two human sequences of homologous retroviral transforming genes (the proto-oncogenes (C-abl and C-sis), which are located on chromosomes 9 and 22, respectively, at the sites of the breakpoint translocations. The V-abl is the viral sequence of the transforming gene that causes leukemias in mice. The molecular studies of the translocation in CML have shown that the translocation of chromosome 9, C-abl to chromosome 22, involves not only C-sis but a region called the *breakpoint cluster region (BCR).* This rearrangement produces recombinant genetic material that is capable of synthesizing marker proteins. Several marker proteins can be identified in different types of CML. Further analysis of these proteins may identify heterogeneity of CML. Future advances in laboratory technology will facilitate not only the understanding of the pathogenesis of this disorder, but also will provide more precise diagnostic and prognostic categories (of better and worse prognostic CML subtypes). It is highly likely that in the future, recombinant DNA technology and genetic probes may refine the diagnosis of a disease once thought to be homogeneous, into different subtypes.

Accelerated Phase and Acute Leukemic Phase of CML

The initiating event causing the chronic, stable disease to accelerate into an acute transformation is unknown. Whether this involves activation of the proto-oncogene sequences or whether another inciting stimulus promotes the unregulated, undifferentiated growth, this event is the almost inevitable termination of CML. Certain laboratory findings may herald the onset of the unstable phase and accelerated growth. Apart from the apparent clinical manifestations of increasing spleen size, increasing bone pain, and symptoms of anemia or hypermetabolism, the peripheral blood shows increasing basophilia and blasts, and the leukocyte alkaline phosphatase may rise. Cytogenetic studies performed during the accelerated phase may show *multiple* cytogenetic abnormalities, including double or triple Philadelphia chromosomes. Another feature is the cytochemistry staining on the blasts, which in approximately 25% of cases shows lymphoblastic markers. This may represent a de-differentiation, or imply that the primary disease is one of an immature stem cell with capabilities of exhibiting myeloid and lymphoid characteristics. The lymphoblastic marker terminal deoxynucleotidyl transferase (TdT) may be present in these blasts. Approximately 60–70% of patients will have a myeloblastic transformation.

The median duration of chronic, stable CML is 40 months. Following this, the accelerated phase with blastic acute leukemia develops, and untreated there is progression to death within 1–6 weeks. The median duration of survival of treated patients with acute transformation of CML is also dismal, and is approximately 3 months. Interestingly, patients with the lymphoid markers treated with vincristine and prednisone may have a higher rate of remission; however, long-term survival is only marginally better.

Philadelphia Chromosome-Negative CML

Patients with all the clinical features of chronic myelogenous leukemia who do not demonstrate a Philadelphia chromosome on cytogenetic study occur in about 10% of cases. This group of Ph-negative patients are generally older, and have lower initial white counts and platelet counts. The median duration of survival is only 8 months, compared with the usual 40 months for Ph-positive CML. These patients, then, may fit into an even poorer prognostic CML category.

There are some laboratory findings that may be interpreted as having especially poor prognostic implications. These include leukocytosis greater than 100,000/μl, blast count of greater than 1% in the peripheral smear and 5% in the marrow, a basophil count of greater than 15–20%, a platelet count of greater than 700,000/μl or a platelet count of less than 150,000/μl, or the presence of additional Philadelphia chromosomes or other cytogenetic abnormalities.

Polycythemia Vera

Polycythemia literally means "many blood cells," but usually it refers to increased red cell mass. A better term for this is erythrocytosis or erythremia. When red cells increase to meet a recognizable physiologic stimulus, the condition is called secondary or reactive polycythemia. Spontaneous or seemingly unprovoked increase in red cell production and blood volume is called *polycythemia vera* or *"true polycythemia."* The *secondary polycythemias* or *erythrocytosis* is discussed in Chapter 3. Polycythemia vera (PV) belongs to a group of myeloproliferative cell disorders characterized by unregulated growth and proliferation of hemapoietic precursors with excessive erythrocytic proliferation. Since this involves a clonal, multipotent stem cell, other marrow elements may also be present in excess (leukocytosis in 75% of cases, thrombocytosis in 50% of cases). Polycythemia vera occurs in older adults, in men slightly more often than in women, usually with an insidious onset easily confused with other causes of erythrocytosis from which it must be excluded (see Chapter 3).

The clinical presentations of PV are those of excessive red cell proliferation, and patients may present with *a ruddy complexion* or symptoms of hyperviscosity such as headaches, visual disturbances, or thrombotic events. There is a higher incidence of peptic ulcer disease in these patients. They may also present with symptoms of increased blood histamine (released from basophils) including itching, particularly after a hot shower. Physical examination usually reveals an individual with a plethoric cherub face and, in 75% of cases, they have splenic enlargement. The differential diagnosis involves exclusion of all the causes of secondary erythrocytosis discussed in Chapter 3. Laboratory diagnosis of this disorder aims at establishing that the red cell mass is increased and is not simply an elevated hematocrit or red cell count, since these may be increased due to contracted plasma volume. There should be a normal PO_2, or blood oxygen, to exclude those conditions where the red cell mass is appropriately increased due to erythropoietin stimulation and splenomegaly may also be present. These three features are major diagnostic criteria used in establishing the clinical diagnosis of PV. Several minor diagnostic criteria are also useful, and include those listed in Table 4–13. Clearly, the minor diagnostic criteria are features that are seen in many of the other myeloproliferative disorders. These criteria were originally introduced by the Polycythemia Vera Study Group for the purpose of classifying patients with PV. They have since been retained by many clinicians to standardize the diagnostic criteria of PV. To establish a diagnosis of PV, either all three diagnostic criteria from category A, or an elevated red cell mass and normal arterial oxygen saturation in addition to two criteria from category B must be present (see Table 4–13). The red cell count, hemoglobin concentration, and hematocrit are all elevated unless there is significant associated iron deficiency. Examination of the peripheral smear reveals normochromic, normocytic red cells with hypochromic, microcytic cells if iron deficiency exists. Myelocytes and metamyelocytes are occasionally seen in the peripheral blood smear, and the basophil count may be elevated. Platelets are often morphologically abnormal, and platelet aggregation studies may reveal functional defects.

Examination of the bone marrow usually shows a hypercellular marrow with an abundance of all cell lines and normal maturation. Stainable iron is often reduced or absent.

Table 4–13. CRITERIA FOR ESTABLISHING DIAGNOSIS OF POLYCYTHEMIA VERA

Category A (major criteria)
- Elevated red cell mass
- Normal arterial oxygen saturation
- Splenomegaly

Category B (minor criteria)
- Leukocytosis
- Thrombocytosis
- Elevated leukocyte alkaline phosphatase score
- Increased serum vitamin B_{12} or vitamin B_{12}-binding proteins

To establish a diagnosis of polycythemia vera, either all 3 diagnostic criteria from Category A or an elevated red cell mass and normal arterial oxygen saturation in addition to 2 criteria from Category B must be present.

The disease usually progresses in a relatively indolent fashion, and prolonged survival is common. Treatment is aimed at reducing the red cell mass by frequent, therapeutic bloodletting (phlebotomy), and this usually controls thrombotic and hemorrhagic complications. However, approximately one third of patients will suffer these complications during the course of the illness. After a variable period (average, 10 years), the proliferative, erythrocytic phase of the disease evolves into the *"spent phase"* in approximately 15–20% of subjects. The clinical picture of this phase is associated with progressive anemia and striking hepatosplenomegaly. This syndrome resembles *agnogenic myeloid metaplasia* (see below) in many respects, with an abundance of teardrop poikilocyte red cells and nucleated red blood cells in the peripheral blood (see Color Plate 39). The bone marrow biopsy shows extensive marrow fibrosis and bone marrow aspirate is usually a dry tap—that is, unobtainable. Patients present with symptoms of increasing splenic enlargement or liver enlargement. Life expectancy in this phase is less than three years. Polycythemia vera can terminate in acute leukemia in as many as *15%* of patients, in those patients who have received alkylating drug therapy (otherwise, less than 5% in patients treated only with phlebotomy).

Agnogenic Myeloid Metaplasia

Agnogenic myeloid metaplasia, also called *myelofibrosis* or *idiopathic myelofibrosis,* is a clonal disorder of the hemapoietic stem cell characterized by unregulated proliferation of hemapoietic precursors within the bone marrow and within extramedullary sites. The two major clinical components of this disorder represent expansion of reticuloendothelial organs, including the liver, the spleen, and, more rarely, lymph nodes, as well as replacement of the bone marrow by fibrous tissue. The clinical presentations are anemia with tiredness, fatigue, and palpitations, hypermetabolism with fever and weight loss, and splenomegaly producing abdominal fullness, splenic pain, and fever. The enlarged spleen may also serve as a reservoir sequestering white cells, red cells, and platelets. Many times the platelets are malfunctional and, despite the high levels that can occur in this disorder, a bleeding tendency may predominate. Studies using the G-6-PD isoenzyme marker have shown that the clonal proliferation involves the hemapoietic precursors in the marrow and extramedullary sites; however, the fibrosis in the marrow is nonclonal, indicating that it is not derived from the abnormal clone. It is believed that the fibroblastic proliferation occurs as a result of liberation of platelet-derived growth factor from the abnormal platelets.

Laboratory Data

Most patients develop a normochromic, normocytic anemia; however, some patients may have a macrocytic anemia and, in patients with chronic bleeding tendency, iron deficiency occurs and produces hypochromic, microcytic anemia. Red cell morphology is strikingly abnormal on the peripheral smear, showing the presence of abundant teardrop poikilocytes, which are always prominant in this disorder (see Color Plate 12). Nucleated red blood cells are also evident, as are many other morphologic variations in the red cell series, including the presence of inclusion bodies such as Howell-Jolly bodies. Again, the other features consistent with a chronic myeloproliferative syndrome such as an elevated LDH, increased uric acid, and increased vitamin B_{12} binders, are also present. The leukocyte alkaline phosphatase in this condition is usually raised. Platelets are often morphologically very abnormal on the peripheral smear and megakaryocytic fragments may also be seen. The leukocytes may show hypersegmentation with other immature precursors also being evident; however, blasts are not a conspicuous feature. The typical blood picture is termed a *leukoerythroblastic reaction* (see Color Plate 39). The differen-

Table 4–14. CAUSES OF LEUKO-ERYTHROBLASTIC REACTION

	26%	Solid tumors and lymphomas
63%	24%	Myeloproliferative disorders including CML
	13%	Acute leukemias
	3%	Benign hematologic conditions
37%	8%	Hemolysis
	26%	Miscellaneous, including blood loss

Data are from Weick, JK, Hagedorn, AB and Linman, JW: Leukoerythroblastosis: Diagnostic and prognostic significance. Mayo Clin Proc 49:110, 1974.

From Henry, JB: Basic methodology. In Nelson and Morris (eds): Clinical Diagnosis and Management by Laboratory Methods, ed 17. WB Saunders, Philadelphia, 1984, p 611, with permission.

tial diagnosis of a leukoerythroblastic reaction is shown in Table 4–14. Bone marrow aspiration is usually a dry tap and biopsy shows the presence of extensive fibroblastic replacement with numerous bizarre, atypical, and dysplastic megakaryocytes. Patients may also develop osteosclerosis, which may be evident on bone roentgenographic examination as increasing bone density. Cytogenetic abnormalities are not consistent; however, if abnormalities are found, this tends to impart a worse prognosis.

Clinical Course

If patients are asymptomatic at presentation, they tend to remain stable for approximately five years. When symptoms develop, particularly those of increasing transfusion dependency and symptoms referable to increasing cytopenia (anemia, decreased white cell count, and decreased platelet count) or enlarging splenic size with painful symptoms of splenic infarction, these patients may require splenectomy or palliative drug or radiation therapy. In most patients, however, once the disease progresses, the median duration of survival is less than a year. Some patients terminate with acute leukemia.

Essential Thrombocythemia

Essential thrombocythemia is a clonal disorder of the pleuripotent stem cell characterized by excessive proliferation of cells of the megakaryocytic lineage with the production of excess numbers of platelets. The condition is associated with an unexplained elevation in the platelet count, usually to levels greater than 1 million/μl. This condition, however, usually has a much more benign course than the other conditions classified as chronic myeloproliferative syndromes. The condition may occur at a younger age, and often presents itself in otherwise asymptomatic patients. Some patients may present with thrombotic or thromboembolic symptoms, and others with bleeding tendency despite the excessive numbers of platelets. The reason for this is that these platelets may be functionally abnormal. The gastrointestinal tract is the commonest site of bleeding; however, patients may present with mucous membrane bleeding as well. These patients may have more substantial bleeding with trauma or surgery. Approximately 50% of patients may also have splenomegaly, which is usually mild. In the younger patients, the prognosis is excellent; however, older patients do present with more hemorrhagic and thrombotic problems. Of all the myeloproliferative syndromes, essential thrombocythemia has the lowest potential for termination in acute leukemia.

Laboratory Features

The hallmark of this condition is the elevated platelet count, which is usually greater than 1 million/μl. The peripheral blood smear usually shows normochromic, normocytic red cells; however, teardrop poikilocytes may be present. The most striking features are the abundant platelets and megakaryocytic fragments with abnormal morphology. Bone marrow aspirate may be a dry tap; however, it is usually cellular and shows a marked abundance of megakaryocytes and platelet debris. Bone marrow biopsy may show the presence of increased fibrous tissue. Many of the megakaryocytes present appear of abnormal morphology. Iron is often absent in the bone marrow. In keeping with some of the other myeloproliferative disorders, the white cell count is usually elevated in the 10–20,000/μl range. Chromosomal findings are not consistent; however, the Philadelphia chromosome is absent. Platelet function studies are usually abnormal, but coagulation tests (see Chapter 6) are usually normal. Table 4–15 lists the major distinguishing features of the chronic myeloproliferative disorders.

MYELODYSPLASTIC SYNDROMES

These syndromes are a heterogeneous group of disorders in which there is clonal, unregulated, and unstable growth characterized by disturbed maturation, refractoriness to standard vitamin and iron therapy, and a propensity to develop acute leukemia. Because of this last feature, these conditions have previously been termed the pre-leukemic syndromes, a term that is inaccurate since the majority of them do not evolve into acute leukemia. Only about 25–35% of them do, and there are certain clinical and laboratory features that may herald this transformation. The classification of these disorders is presented in Table 4–9, which gives the French, American, and British nomenclature for the myelodysplastic syndromes. These conditions were also discussed under the refractory anemias (Chapter 3). The hallmark of these conditions is ineffective hematopoiesis, which includes erythroid development, granulopoietic development, and platelet production. The unstable growth may affect any combination of these major cell lines of maturation. The ineffective growth is characterized by bone marrow hypercellularity, but cytopenia in the peripheral blood of varying degrees. This occurs because of intramedullary cell death. The major clinical presentations of these disorders are anemia unresponsive to standard hematinic treatment (vitamins and iron), fever, recurrent infections, or a bleeding tendency. Splenomegaly usually is not a feature of the myelodysplastic syndromes as it is with the chronic myeloproliferative disorders. Patients may, however, present with other clinical features of a hypermetabolic state, including fever and weight loss. They may also present with features of increased cellular turnover such as gout due to the hyperuricemia or bone pain due to marrow expansion.

Refractory Anemia

This condition is the most benign of the myelodysplastic syndromes, and has the least likelihood of transformation into acute leukemia (<10%). It occurs more commonly in elderly people and is associated with a normochromic, normocytic anemia, or a macrocytic anemia, in the presence of a hypercellular marrow that shows megaloblastic features, and blasts are fewer than 5% of marrow cytology. Cytogenetic findings are unusual. Repeated marrow aspirates are often needed to follow these patients.

Refractory Anemia with Ringed Sideroblasts

This condition, also called *acquired idiopathic sideroblastic anemia,* is typically associated with an elevated serum iron and percentage iron saturation (see Chapter

Table 4–15. COMPARISON OF CELLULAR PROLIFERATION, LAP, AND CYTOGENETIC FINDINGS IN CHRONIC MPD*

Diagnosis	RBC	Granulocytes	Platelets	Fibroblasts	LAP	Chromosomal Abnormality
Chronic granulocytic leukemia	0–↓	4+	0–3+	0–2+	↓	$Ph^1$90%
Polycythemia vera	4+	1–2+	1–3+	0–2+	↑↑↑	Aneuploidy 25%
Agnogenic myeloid metaplasia	0–↓	↓1–2+	↓0–3+	2–4+	N–↑	Monosomy or trisomy; group C chromosomes
Essential thrombocythemia	0–1+	0–1+	4+	0–2+	N–↑	Normal
Cellular proliferation	Clonal	Clonal	Clonal	Nonclonal	—	—

From Jacobson RJ. Myeloproliferative Disorders, In Pittiglio and Sacher,[10] p 262, with permission.
*Key: 0 = unchanged from normal. 1+ to 4+ represent various degrees of cellular proliferation.

2). Patients also usually present with a hypochromic, microcytic anemia; however, a dimorphic blood picture showing some cells hemoglobinized with other cells underhemoglobinized is common. The white cell count and platelet count are *usually* normal. A bone marrow is *usually* hypercellular due to erythroid hyperplasia that shows megaloblastic features; however, the pathognomonic finding in this condition is the presence of numerous positive iron granules arranged in a ring or partial ring around the nucleus on an iron stain (see Color Plate 15A). At least 15% of developing erythroid cells must contain these ring forms to be classified as this disorder. Blasts constitute <5% of the marrow cytology. The inability to utilize iron is felt to be due to a defect in iron incorporation from mitochondria into developing erythroid cells (see Chapter 2 and Fig. 2–4). This condition also has a relatively chronic course; however, it may transform into acute leukemia in approximately 10% of cases.

Refractory Anemia with Excess Blasts (RAEB)

The hallmark of this condition is a normochromic or macrocytic anemia in the presence of a hypercellular marrow that shows between 5–20% myeloblasts; however, Auer rods are absent. This condition has also been called a smoldering leukemia or subacute leukemia. Circulating peripheral mononuclear cells may show abnormal granulation, hypersegmentation or the pseudo-Pelger-Huet anomaly. This condition transforms into ANLL in 30% of cases; however, the majority of patients remain stable for many months or even years.

RAEB in Transformation

This condition represents a more advanced stage of RAEB, with a greater percentage of blasts developing in the marrow in association with a severe anemia. The features are intermediate between cells with normal differentiation and evolution into acute leukemia. This condition is more refractory to chemotherapy than ANLL presenting *de novo.*

Chronic Myelomonocytic Leukemia

This condition is characterized by an increased peripheral blood absolute monocyte count in the absence of a secondary stimulus such as tuberculosis or chronic inflammation. Many of the monocytes appear atypical or immature, and may show nucleoli. The bone marrow may also show an abundance of cleaved and clefted cells with horseshoe-shaped nuclei characteristic of monocytic precursors. These patients may also have an elevated lysozyme, a feature that is seen in acute monocytic leukemia. Typically, there is no gum infiltration by these abnormal cells. This condition also carries a high likelihood of transformation into acute myelomonocytic or monocytic leukemia (M4 or M5).

Chromosomal Abnormalities in the Myelodysplastic Syndromes

Cytogenetic abnormalities in this condition usually impart a worse prognosis with a greater likelihood of leukemic transformation. Transformation into acute leukemia is more commonly associated in these syndromes with the $5q^-$ chromosomal abnormality, which represents a loss of the long arm of chromosome 5. The $5q^-$ abnormality appears more commonly in secondary leukemia developing from previous alkylating drug therapy. Other cytogenetic abnormalities may also occur, such as loss of chromosomes (hypodiploidy) or excess chromosomes (hyperdiploidy). These are generally thought to be associated with a poorer prognosis or a greater likelihood of leukemic transformation.

Lymphoproliferative Disorders

These conditions represent unregulated growth and proliferation of cells of the lymphoid lineage. These disorders are also classified into the *acute lymphoproliferative disorders* where there is little or no differentiation to terminal maturity, and the *chronic lymphoproliferative disorders* where there is an unregulated growth *with differentiation* and an abundance of mature cells. These conditions are also clonal in origin, representing expansion of a single clone of cells, all exhibiting the same phenotypic markers as the parental cell. These lymphoproliferative disorders may be subclassified in terms of their functional characteristics into the *T cell disorders* (disorders of lymphocytes programmed or under the influence of the thymus) and the *B cell disorders* (disorders programmed or influenced by the bone marrow). Finally, lymphoproliferative disorders may be subcategorized according to their anatomic distribution into those diseases predominantly involving the bone marrow and peripheral blood, called *the leukemias,* and those disorders predominantly involving the reticuloendothelial organs (lymph nodes, spleen, and liver) called collectively *the lymphomas.* These conditions are further defined on the basis of these various criteria into distinct types that will be individually discussed. In the diagnosis of each of the subtypes, the differentiation, functional characteristics, and distribution are all considered.

It is important to refer to Chapter 2 for the outline of normal lymphoid differentiation and functional classification. Conceivably, since these disorders involve a *neoplastic clonal change* somewhere along their development and maturity, excess growth and proliferation of cells frozen at a specific stage in differentiation can occur, and these cells may be defined by the clinical laboratory.

Understanding the clinical presentation involves an appreciation that lymphoreticular cells can be either fixed or mobile. *B-lymphocytes* and their plasma cell progeny constitute a mobile, or potentially mobile, population, even though at any one time most B cells reside in the lymphoid tissues. *T-lymphocytes* are in continuous movement between tissue sites, blood, and lymph fluid. The *monocyte-macrophage-histiocyte* population is less conspicuous in body fluids, the cells spending most of their active life within the tissues. Since there is a continual exchange between the tissue sites, blood, and bone marrow, all of these sites may be involved in one or another stage of a lymphoproliferative disease.

The Acute Lymphoproliferative Disorders

There are three types of acute lymphoproliferative disorders, 1) *acute lymphoblastic leukemia* (ALL) (a notable characteristic is that acute lymphoblastic leukemia is the commonest acute leukemia of childhood), 2) *undifferentiated leukemia,* and 3) *lymphoblastic transformation of chronic myelogenous leukemia.* Since all of these disorders may present in a similar way, they will be discussed together. Acute lymphoblastic leukemia occurs in approximately 15% of adult leukemias, and many of these cases may be the initial presentation of an acute transformation of chronic myelogenous leukemia. The major distinction in this disorder is the demonstration of the Philadelphia chromosome.

Acute Lymphoblastic Leukemia

Acute lymphoblastic leukemia is the major childhood leukemia, accounting for nearly all leukemias before age 4, and more than half of the leukemias through puberty. It is rare in patients over the age of 30. Clinically, ALL and acute myeloblastic leukemia (AML) have similar features, but the onset of ALL tends to be strikingly acute. There is almost never a smoldering or preleukemic phase in ALL. Lymph node enlargement and hepatosplenomegaly occur more often in ALL than in AML, as do bone pain and bone lesions. Leukemic meningitis can occur late in the disease, but does, however, tend to be a sanctuary site for relapse in this leukemia and must be specifically treated despite an apparent blood and bone marrow remission. Consequently, because of this problem, prophylactic treatment consisting of chemotherapy and radiation therapy is routinely given to the central nervous system in all cases of ALL. Table 4–16 represents the French-American-British classification of lymphoblastic leukemias. According to this classification, there are three morphologic categories of lymphoblastic leukemia, termed L1, L2, and L3. The lymphoblastic leukemias are separated from the myeloblastic leukemias on the basis of morphology and cytochemical staining. The morphologic differences are listed in Table 4–10, and as can be seen in the Table, these differences are confirmed additionally by cytochemical staining patterns using *myeloperoxidase, Sudan black,* and *nonspecific esterase stain* (see Chapter 2), which stain the myeloblastic leukemias, and the *PAS and TdT* stains, which are positive in the acute lymphoblastic leukemias. The FAB classification defines cytologic differences. They also define prognostic categories; L1 having the best prognosis, L2 intermediate, and L3 the worst. Consequently, the nature of aggressive chemotherapy can be planned accordingly. L1–ALL consists of a monotonous population of uniform cells with a high nucleo-cytoplasmic ratio and very scanty cytoplasm. There are usually two or less nucleoli that are fairly well defined (see Color Plate 41). The nucleus is usually regular in shape.

L2–ALL is characterized by more heterogeneity, in that both small and large cells can be seen replacing the bone marrow and in the peripheral blood. The larger cells often show nuclear clefting, prominent nucleoli, and abundant cytoplasm (see Color Plate 42).

L3, or Burkitt's type, consists of a uniform population of uncleaved immature cells with both nuclear and cytoplasmic vacuolization. The cytoplasm is usually basophilic and may be abundant (see Color Plate 43).

Blood and Bone Marrow Findings

Very few recognizable neutrophils circulate in ALL, and even in the bone marrow normal red and white cell elements may be hard to find. The predominant cell, both in blood and in the marrow, is a blast that may have morphologic characteristics as mentioned above under the FAB types. However, the blasts usually have scant cytoplasm, contain no Sudanophilic granules, no peroxidase-reactive granules, and no Auer rods. The few neutrophils that are present have normal leukocyte alkaline phosphatase scores. Anemia is usually pronounced, with few reticulocytes and a very low platelet count.

A marrow aspirate shows the marrow spicules to be almost totally replaced by blasts. Very few normal marrow elements are in evidence. Culturing marrow for chromosomes usually shows no distinct chromosomal abnormalities; however, a translocation of chromosome *4 and 11* is sometimes seen in *infantile ALL,* a *9–11 translocation* is occasionally seen in ALL in children; and in *adults* presenting with an ALL, Philadelphia chromosome may be detected representing *de novo* presentation of the blastic phase of CML.

Cell Surface Markers

Acute lymphoblastic leukemia can be subdivided into different cells of origin using surface antigens as markers. This allows more vigorous evaluation of treatment regimens and epidemiologic features than is possible if all cases of ALL are considered together. These markers may subcategorize the FAB types.

Table 4–16. CELL CHARACTERISTICS IN ACUTE LYMPHOBLASTIC LEUKEMIA (FAB CLASSIFICATION)

Cell Characteristics	L1	L2	L3
Cell size	Predominently small cells, homogeneous	Large, heterogeneous	Large, homogeneous
Nuclear chromatin	Homogeneous in any one case	Heterogeneous	Stippled, homogeneous
Nuclear shape	Regular, round, occasional clefting	Irregular, clefting	Regular, round to ovoid
Nucleoli	Inconspicuous	One or more, may be large	One or more, prominent
Cytoplasm	Scanty	Variable, moderately abundant	Moderately abundant, strongly basophilic
Cytoplasmic vacuolation	Variable	Variable	Prominent

Adapted from Bennett et al.[9] and from Maslon, WC, et al: Practical Diagnosis: Hematologic Disease. Houghton Mifflin, Boston, 1980, p 332. From Perkins, ML: Introduction to leukemia and the acute leukemias. In Pittiglio and Sacher,[10] p 234, with permission.

The majority of ALL (approximately 70%) involves cells that lack features characteristic of either B- or T-lymphocytes (see Chapter 2). These neoplastic cells possess a distinctive surface membrane marker called the *common ALL antigen (CALLA)*; this form of leukemia is called *common ALL.* In addition, these cells also stain positive for the marker TdT (see Chapter 2). This type of ALL usually has the best prognosis and presents with low white cell counts and is the usual FAB L1 category. There are three other types of ALL also identified on the basis of immunologic markers. These are B cell ALL, T cell ALL, and a type that stains negative for both B and T as well as CALLA, called null or undifferentiated ALL. The prognosis appears to be worse for both B and T types, as well as the undifferentiated type. These types are usually subjected to more aggressive chemotherapy. The immunologic classification of acute lymphoblastic leukemia is shown in Table 4–17.

The next most common type (20–22% of ALL) is *T cell ALL.* These cells are capable of forming rosettes with sheep red blood cells and also stain positive with monoclonal T cell markers. Other characteristics are listed in Table 4–17. This form tends to affect older patients and has unfavorable clinical findings, including occurrence in men with mediastinal tumors and a white cell count of greater than 50,000/μl. The most significant adverse prognostic feature for all types of ALL is a white cell count of greater than 50,000/μl. Although T cell ALL responds well to initial therapy, remissions tend to be shorter and long-term prognosis is much less favorable than in common ALL. As it becomes possible to distinguish helper T cells from suppressor T cells routinely, different subsets of T cell leukemia may emerge and enable further categorization of the more aggressive or better prognostic types. A rare type of T cell ALL is becoming recognized that is associated with hypercalcemia and previous exposure to the retrovirus HTLV-I (Human T Cell Leukemia virus 1 Type 1). This condition has a higher prevalence in Jamaica and Japan.

B cells are responsible for 1–3% of ALL, and also tend to carry a poorer prognosis. These cells show surface immunoglobulins and receptors for F_c and complement characterizing the circulating cells, which resemble cells from the center of germinal follicles and are morphologically similar to the cells of Burkitt's lymphoma (for a description of immunoglobulins and complement, see Chapter 7).

Still poorly characterized is a moderately large group of ALL patients in whom common ALL antigen is present, but the cells also have immunoglobulin (IgM or its heavy chain) in their cytoplasm. This is considered a pre-B-cell leukemia. It has a better prognosis than the B cell leukemia, resembling that of common ALL (see Development of B-Lymphocytes).

Treatment

Before 1950, 80% of children with ALL were dead eight months after diagnosis. By 1970, 5–10% of children with ALL could expect long-term survival of five years or longer, and most had disease-free intervals of one to two years. At present, 50% of children newly diagnosed as having ALL can anticipate long-term survival and complete cessation of therapy (cure).

Certain features at diagnosis have favorable prognostic significance. The most favorable category is diagnosis between the ages of two and nine, peripheral white cell count no higher than 20,000/μl at diagnosis, little or no organ involvement, and normal immunoglobulin status. The L2- and L3-type morphology, a male gender, and the presence of central nervous system leukemia are relatively poor prognostic signs.

The strategy in treating ALL is to attempt to eradicate every malignant cell so that none remain to cause recurrent disease. Combination chemotherapy employs agents that exert different kinds of damaging effects to the multiplying cells and is directed

Table 4–17. IMMUNOLOGIC CLASSIFICATION OF ACUTE LYMPHOBLASTIC LEUKEMIA

		Immunologic Features						
Types	Morphology	E	T	SIg	CIg	cALLA	TdT	HLA-DR
Undifferentiated ALL	L1/L2	–	–	–	–	–	+	+
Common ALL	L1/L2	–	–	–	–	+	+	+
Pre-T-ALL	L1/L2	–	+	–	–	±	+	–
T-ALL	L1/L2	+	+	–	–	–	+	–
Pre-B-ALL	L1/L2	–	–	–	+	+	+	+
B-ALL	L3	–	–	+	+	–	–	+

ALL = acute lymphoblastic leukemia; cALLA = common ALL antigen; CIg = cytoplasmic immunoglobulin; E = receptors for sheep erythrocytes; HLA-DR = Ia-like antigen; L1, L2, L3 refer to the FAB classification; SIg = surface immunoglobulin; T = T-cell antigen; TdT = terminal deoxynucleotidyl transferase.

From Pittiglio and Sacher (eds.), Clinical Hematology and Fundamentals of Hemostasis. FA Davis, Philadelphia, 1987, with permission.

toward damaging cell growth at different stages. The three common drugs used are vincristine, prednisone, and L-asparaginase. Central nervous system prophylaxis is usually accomplished by the administration of methotrexate into the spinal fluid and courses of cranial irradiation. Maintenance chemotherapy is also continued for between two and three years with 6-mercaptopurine and methotrexate. Patients receiving these drugs need to have regular blood counts checked for bone marrow suppression and liver function studies to evaluate liver toxicity. The principles of therapy and the requirements of transfusion support, vigorous antibacterial therapy, and microbiologic searches for causes of sepsis are the same as were discussed under the treatment of acute myelogenous leukemia. A comparison of the features of acute myelogenous leukemia and acute lymphoblastic leukemia are listed in Table 4–10.

Leukemic Chronic Lymphoproliferative Disorders

These conditions are characterized by unregulated clonal growth of differentiated cells, each expressing individual immunologic characteristics, either B subtypes, T subtypes, or undifferentiated subtypes. These disorders are broadly grouped into the leukemic chronic lymphoproliferative disorders and the lymphomas. The major diseases in the former category are *chronic lymphocytic leukemia, prolymphocytic leukemia,* and *hairy cell leukemia* (see Color Plates 44 and 45).

Chronic Lymphocytic Leukemia

Chronic lymphocytic leukemia (CLL) differs from the other leukemias in that it runs a typically indolent course over many years in most cases. It occurs almost exclusively in adults over the age of 40. In most CLLs, the proliferating cells are B-lymphocytes, which have normal surface characteristics and no detectable immunologic activity. Leukemic B cells survive as long as five years, compared with one-year survival for normal "long-lived" B-lymphocytes. Because the lymphocyte production rate also increases as much as tenfold, the net result is massive cellular accumulation. The accumulating cells are immunologically inert, and their presence crowds out normally reactive B cells. The spleen, lymph nodes, and bone marrow are overrun by these cells, which interfere with the movement of normal granulocytes, monocytes, and erythrocytes across vascular membranes.

Clinical Findings

Chronic lymphocytic leukemia always develops gradually. Often it is discovered incidentally during a blood count performed for other reasons. The white cell count runs between 10,000/μl and 100,000/μl; 95% of the circulating white cells are small lymphocytes of normal appearance (see Color Plate 44). Granulocytes, although sparse in the differential count, are present initially in normal absolute numbers. As the lymphocytes overrun the marrow, platelet counts and red cell production may decline, but intrinsic erythropoietic and thrombopoietic capabilities are normal. Since these lymphocytes are functionally inert, both humoral and cell-mediated immunity is defective, and individuals are at risk for infections with bacterial and opportunistic microbes.

Chronic lymphocytic leukemia adversely affects immune function. Half of the CLL patients have decreased immunoglobulin levels, especially IgM, at some time during their disease. One third of patients experience autoimmune manifestations and have a positive direct antiglobulin test (Coomb's Test) (see Chapter 8). This may be associated with an autoimmune hemolytic anemia, whose effect may be profound since the marrow cannot mount an appropriate response due to the overcrowding by lymphocytes (see Autoimmune Hemolytic Anemia, Chapter 3). The

Table 4–18. CLINICAL STAGES OF CHRONIC LYMPHOCYTIC LEUKEMIA

Stage 0	Bone marrow and blood lymphocytosis only
Stage I	Lymphocytosis with enlarged nodes
Stage II	Lymphocytosis with enlarged spleen or liver or both
Stage III	Lymphocytosis with anemia (hemoglobin <11 g/dl)
Stage IV	Lymphocytosis with thrombocytopenia (platelets $<100{,}000/mm^3$)

clinical stages of chronic lymphocytic leukemia are listed in Table 4–18.

Some patients in stages 0–2 may live for 10–20 years, whereas for those with stages 3 and 4, the median survival is less than five years. Some untreated persons survive for years with a CLL. Symptomatic anemia and thrombocytopenia are indications for therapeutic intervention. If red cells and platelets remain adequate, however, patients may never need therapy and may succumb to other cardiovascular problems and diseases of old age. Many patients, however, experience a progressively more aggressive course. As organ infiltration progresses, CLL and well-differentiated lymphocytic lymphoma become difficult to distinguish both clinically and histologically. Indeed, the need to distinguish between these two disorders may only be technical, since therapy would generally be the same. In the terminal phase of CLL, increasing immunologic impairment, anemia, hemorrhagic complications, and infection develop. An unexplained observation is the finding that patients with CLL have solid cancers more often than age-matched controls; skin and colon are especially common sites.

In treating CLL, it is impossible to eradicate all malignant cells because, by the time disease becomes apparent, leukemic proliferation is widespread, longstanding, and massive. Chlorambucil and cyclophosphamide are drugs used to control disease proliferation. Therapy seeks mainly to prevent bone marrow replacement and alleviate symptoms or bulk disease arising from splenomegaly or lymph node enlargement. Agents useful in treating acute leukemia are generally ineffective in combating the accelerated terminal phase of CLL. There is current interest in exploring the biologic response modifiers, such as interferon, in influencing the course of this disease.

Prolymphocytic Leukemia

This represents a more aggressive and de-differentiated form of chronic lymphocytic leukemia, where the proliferating cells have a more rapid growth potential, more abundant cytoplasm with very *prominent nucleoli* (of which there are usually less than two), and patients usually present with a *markedly enlarged spleen.* This course tends to be more aggressive, and patients may have an elevated blood calcium (note T cell ALL and HTLV-I and hypercalcemia in the previous section).

Hairy Cell Leukemia

This condition is a clonal proliferation of morphologically distinct cells that are characterized by the presence of fine, cytoplasmic projections, a distinctive nuclear pattern (salt and pepper chromatin), the presence within the cells of a specific isoenzyme of acid phosphatase (that is *tartate-resistant; TRAP test*; see Color Plate 46), and *clinical splenomegaly.* This disorder may present with increased numbers of these cells in the peripheral blood, and may mimic chronic lymphocytic leukemia,

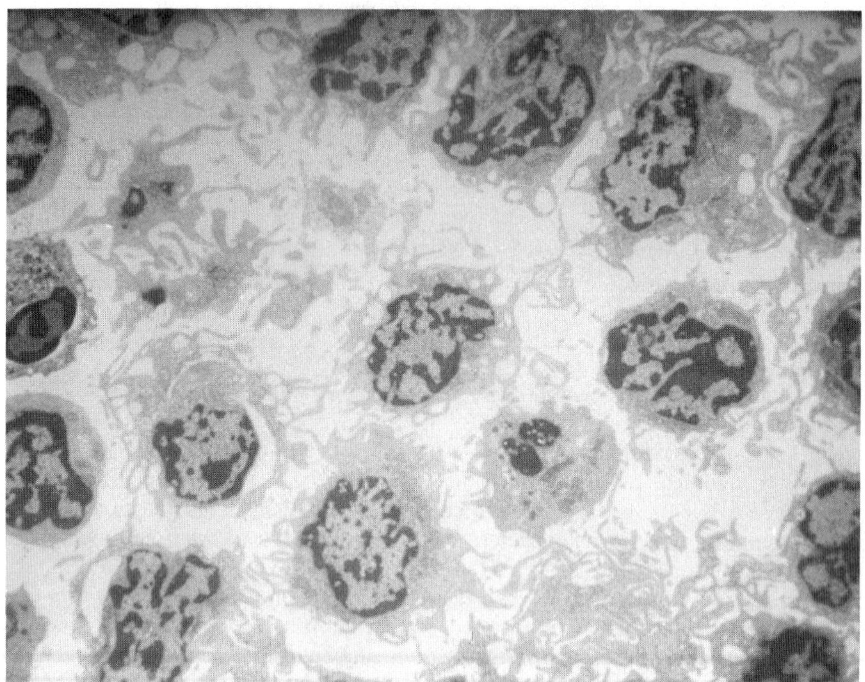

Figure 4–1. Electron micrograph of hairy cells from a patient with hairy cell leukemia.

but *pancytopenia* is common. Another distinctive differentiating feature is the fact that, in most cases, a bone marrow aspirate performed on these patients is usually a dry tap. Bone marrow biopsy shows a characteristic eosinophilic interdigitating material that looks very much like fibrous tissue but is negative for fibrous stains. Also, characteristically the electron microscopy of the cells shows the hairy projections, and abnormal ribosomal lamellar complexes. The differentiation of this disorder from CLL is extremely important, since therapy is distinctly different. This disorder may be well controlled using interferon treatment or 2-deoxycoformycin. Another name for this disorder is *leukemic reticuloendotheliosis.* Fig. 4–1 shows the characteristic morphology of these cells. The patients also characteristically have a severe peripheral pancytopenia (see also Color Plate 45).

THE LYMPHOMAS

Lymphomas are malignant neoplasms of the lymphoid organs characterized by autonomous neoplastic growth of cells committed toward lymphoid differentiation. These tumors primarily affect lymphoid tissues, particularly lymph nodes and spleen, but may involve other lymphoreticular sites, including the liver, gastrointestinal tract, nasopharyngeal tissues, and the lungs. Diagnosis is by tissue biopsy; laboratory data are, at best, suggestive or confirmatory. Because of the close association of lymphomas with the hematologic and immunologic diseases already considered, a brief discussion of diagnosis and classification will be presented.

Hodgkin's Disease

Lymphomas are categorized as one of the lymphoproliferative disorders. Lym-

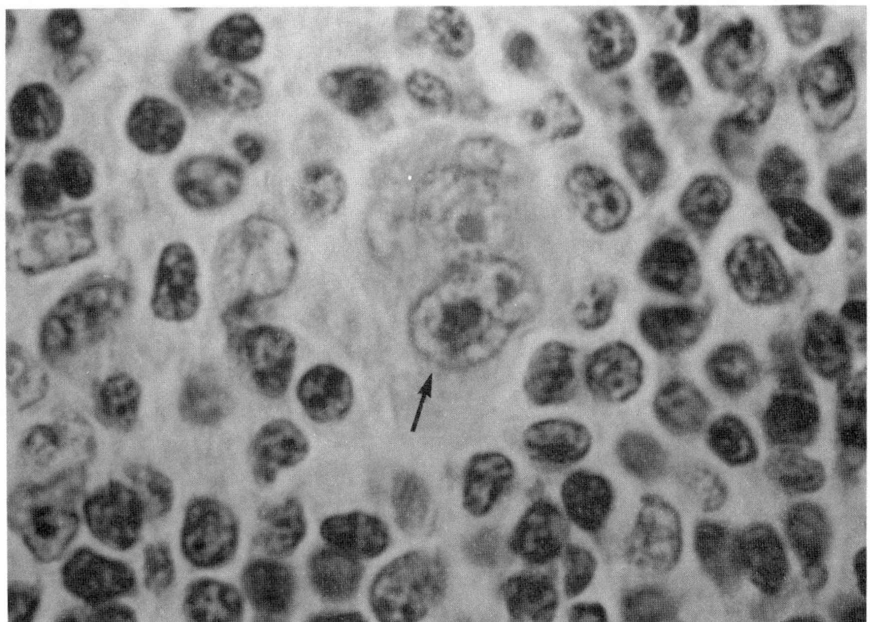

Figure 4–2. Reed-Sternberg cell (arrow) from a lymph node biopsy in Hodgkin's disease. (From Pittiglio, DH and Sacher, RA: Clinical Hematology and Fundamentals of Hemostasis. FA Davis, Philadelphia, 1987, with permission.)

phomas fall into two major categories: *Hodgkin's disease* and the *non-Hodgkin's lymphomas*.

Classification

Hodgkin's disease is classified separately because the neoplastic cell has not yet been fully determined, and furthermore, the prognosis and therapy are distinctly different from non-Hodgkin's lymphomas. Hodgkin's disease is further subclassified into *four major subtypes,* all of which have the presence of the pathognomonic cell called Reed-Sternberg cell (Fig. 4–2). The subtypes of Hodgkin's disease are classified according to the preponderance of lymphocytes and larger transformed cells or Reed-Sternberg cells. Table 4–19 is a breakdown of the subtypes of Hodgkin's disease. Hodgkin's disease almost invariably originates in the lymph nodes and spreads from one chain of nodes to adjacent ones in a regular progression. The diagnosis of Hodgkin's disease is made by tissue histology and the finding of the characteristic Reed-Sternberg cells. These Reed-Sternberg cells are giant cells with characteristic mirror-image nuclei and prominent nucleoli-owl's eye nucleus. The precursor of the pathognomonic cell remains controversial. The lymphocytes are clearly of T cell origin, but they may not be the distinctive neoplastic element. Controversy also surrounds the etiology of the disease; epidemiologic features suggest infection as a contributing cause, but no specific agent has been implicated and it is obvious that other unknown considerations critically influence the development of the disease.

Clinical Features

Since the disease initially involves lymph nodes, painless asymmetric swelling of

Table 4–19. CLASSIFICATION OF HODGKIN'S DISEASE

Pattern	General Age Group	Description	Presence of Reed-Sternberg (RS) Cells	Frequency (*% of Cases*)	Prognosis
1. LP (lymphocyte predominant)	Young individuals	Characterized by a diffuse infiltrate of mature lymphocytes mixed with variable numbers of histiocytes.	Few in number	5–10	Best
2. NS (nodular sclerosis)	Young individuals (often females)	Represents a distinct entity with a different epidemiology and biologic significance from the other 3 patterns. Unique to this pattern are 2 characteristics: 1. biopsy specimen characterized by birefringent bands of collagen, which traverse the lymph node, enclosing nodules of normal and abnormal lymphoid tissue; and 2. presence of a Reed-Sternberg cell variant called a lacunar cell, which looks like a Langhans' giant cell that sits in a lacunal space.	RS variant (lacunar cells present)	35–60	Second best

3. MC (mixed cellularity)	Middle-aged (30 yr old)	Characterized by a diffuse infiltrate of lymphocytes, histiocytes, eosinophils, and plasma cells, which obliterate the underlying nodal architecture.	Usually plentiful	30–50	Third best
4. LD (lymphocyte depletion)	Middle-aged	Characterized by a paucity of lymphocytes and diffuse fibrosis.	Few in number	1–5	Worst

From Forlenza, TJ and Pittiglio, DH: Malignant Lymphomas. In Pittiglio and Sacher,[10] p 299, with permission.

the lymph nodes is the commonest presenting feature. Patients may present with constitutional symptoms that include night sweats, fever, and weight loss. The constitutional symptoms impart an adverse prognostic consideration, and are termed "B" symptoms. The disease can then be classified on the basis of the presence or absence of these symptoms into A or B types.

Laboratory Findings

Table 4–20 lists the laboratory findings often associated with Hodgkin's disease. The peripheral blood may show a normochromic, normocytic anemia, and monocytosis and eosinophilia may also occur. The platelet count is often increased, with an elevated sedimentation rate reflecting increased cell turnover and inflammation. The sedimentation rate serves as a useful, nonspecific marker of the disease activity. Disease involvement of other organs may show specific chemical abnormalities; e.g., abnormal liver function.

Another feature of this disorder is decreased cell-mediated immunity, reflecting abnormal T cell function. A common finding is the *absence* of skin reactivity following intradermal injections of common antigens such as candida, mumps, and streptokinase. This failure to elicit a skin reaction is termed *cutaneous anergy.*

Therapeutic response and long-term prognosis correlate not only with the morphologic type but also with the extent of the disease at the time of diagnosis. Table 4–21 indicates the staging of Hodgkin's disease. In stage I disease, the least extensive at the time of diagnosis, only a single lymph node group or a single extranodal site is involved. Stage IV disease, the most widespread, involves many lymph node groups and also nonlymphoid organs like bone marrow, liver, and spleen. At any given stage, patients without constitutional symptoms like fever, weight loss, and night sweats do better than those with symptomatic disease. In recent times, combination chemotherapy and/or radiation therapy has proved very successful in the management of Hodgkin's lymphoma, and in better than 85% of cases complete and durable long-term remission has been achieved. Patients are generally followed

Table 4–20. LABORATORY FINDINGS IN HODGKIN'S DISEASE

Early in course
Mild normochromic, normocytic anemia from depressed erythropoiesis
Moderate leukocytosis with eosinophilia to 10%
Normal or increased platelet count
Increased ESR
Decreased serum iron and iron-binding capacity, normal or increased marrow iron
Decreased cell-mediated immunity; antibody activity normal
Later in disease
Lymphopenia
More severe anemia
Coombs'-positive hemolysis (relatively rare)
Thrombocytopenia
Mild hypoalbuminemia, hyperglobulinemia
Hypercalcemia
Hyperuricemia
Low serum zinc, high serum copper

Table 4–21. CLINICAL STAGING OF LYMPHOMAS

Stage I	One group of lymph nodes involved with disease, either above or below the diaphragm.
Stage II	Two different groups of lymph nodes involved with disease, both being either above or below the diaphragm.
Stage III*	Two different groups of lymph nodes involved with disease, one on each side of the diaphragm.
Stage IV	Extranodal involvement in areas not contiguous with lymph nodes (includes bone marrow or liver involvement).†

*Stage IIIA is subdivided into 1 and 2.
†E classification indicates extension from a lymph node area.
From Forlenza, TJ and Pittiglio, DH: Malignant lymphomas. In Pittiglio and Sacher,[10] p 300, with permission.

up at regular intervals by monitoring complete blood counts, a chemistry profile screen, and a sedimentation rate. The presence of cytopenias and an elevated sedimentation rate may herald the onset of relapse.

Non-Hodgkin's Lymphomas

Non-Hodgkin's lymphomas are disorders characterized by autonomous proliferation of lymphoid cells that are classified according to their *histopathologic morphology (nodular* or *diffuse),* the *cell type (small cells, large cells-lymphocytic-histiocytic-mixed),* and *cytologic differentiation (well differentiated, poorly differentiated).* Because of the complexity of lymphocyte differentiation and lymphocyte subtypes, several classifications have been developed of varying complexities. The most practical classification is that of *Rappaport,* which, although it is not accurate in terms of functional types, certainly has prognostic and therapeutic implications. More recently, a *"working formulation"* of international experts has categorized the non-Hodgkin's lymphomas into *low grade, intermediate grade, high grade,* and other types, as is listed in Table 4–22. The working formulation represents a compromise classification that reconciles the advantages of the various classifications. For the purpose of discussing the laboratory features in non-Hodgkin's lymphomas, the Rappaport classification will be used.

Well-Differentiated Lymphocytic Lymphoma

This condition is analogous to chronic lymphocytic leukemia developing within the B-lymphocytes of the lymph nodes. There is a clonal expansion of well-differentiated small lymphocytes replacing the normal architecture of the lymph node. This produces lymph node swelling and may spill over into the peripheral blood, producing a leukemic-like picture. The morphology of this leukemia is like chronic lymphocytic leukemia, and the clinical features and stages are very similar. A Coomb's positive autoimmune hemolytic anemia and thrombocytopenia may also coexist in this disorder.

Poorly Differentiated Lymphocytic Lymphoma

This type may be subclassified into the *diffuse* and *nodular types.* The nodular poorly differentiated lymphocytic lymphoma is more common. It usually presents with asymmetric enlargement of lymph nodes and other clinical features of non-Hodgkin's lymphoma, such as splenomegaly. The leukemic phase of this disorder is

Table 4–22. CLASSIFICATION OF NON-HODGKIN'S LYMPHOMAS (WORKING FORMULATION AND RAPPAPORT TYPE)

Low-grade malignant lymphoma	*High-grade malignant lymphoma*
Small, lymphocytic (CLL, WDL)	Large cell, immunoblastic (DHL)
Follicular, predominantly small, cleaved (NPDL)	Lymphoblastic (undifferentiated/lymphoblastic)
Follicular, mixed small, cleaved and large cell (NML)	Small, noncleaved (Burkitt's)
Intermediate-grade malignant lymphoma	Miscellaneous
Follicular, predominantly large cell (NHL)	Composite
Diffuse, small, cleaved (DPDL)	Mycoses fungoides (+ Sezary)
Diffuse, mixed small and large cell (DML)	Histiocytic (malignant histiocytosis)
Diffuse large cell (DHL)	

Key for abbreviations:
CLL = chronic lymphocytic leukemia
WDL = well differentiated lymphoma
NPDL = nodular poorly differentiated lymphoma
NML = modular mixed lymphoma
NHL = nodular histiocytic lymphoma
DPDL = Diffuse poorly differentiated lymphoma
DML = Diffuse mixed lymphoma
DHL = Diffuse histiocytic lymphoma

characterized by the appearance of cleaved or clefted lymphocytes in the peripheral blood and, depending on marrow involvement, there may or may not be leukopenia and thrombocytopenia. This type of morphology has been referred to as *lymphosarcoma cell leukemia.* Surface marker studis show the B-lymphocyte origin of these cells.

Histiocytic Lymphoma

This condition is an unregulated growth of transformed lymphocytes, usually of the B-lymphocyte type. These "immunoblasts" are really not histiocytes at all. Therefore, the Rappaport terminology is inaccurate. These cells are usually larger than those found in poorly differentiated lymphoma and have a vesicular nucleus and prominent nucleoli. This condition is termed large-cell lymphoma in the working classification (see Table 4–22).

Mixed Cell Type

Some lymphomas have features of both small and large cell types. These are termed mixed-cell lymphomas and may morphologically appear in a diffuse or nodular pattern. Occasionally abnormal cells may be seen in the peripheral blood in these disorders as well.

Lymphoblastic Lymphoma

This is a rare lymphoma that tends to occur in young men and is associated with an enlarged thymus and often an increased number of T-lymphoblasts in the peripheral blood. This condition may be considered the lymphomatous counterpart of acute lymphoblastic leukemia of the T-cell type.

Burkitt's Lymphoma

This is an aggressive, lymphoproliferative disorder that is associated with an infiltration of B-lymphocytes of noncleaved, uniform size producing a diffuse sea of closely packed cells with round to oval nuclei and frequent mitotic figures. Interspersed within this background are pale-staining histiocytes that produce a *starry sky appearance.* Epstein-Barr virus has been implicated in the pathogenesis of this disease. This condition may have a leukemic counterpart with "undifferentiated" lymphoblasts appearing in the peripheral blood. These cells fail to show any consistent staining characteristics and immunologic markers are usually negative. Another feature of this disorder is a markedly elevated serum LDH, and often an elevated serum calcium.

Adult T Cell Leukemia

See ALL—HTLV-I.

Other T Cell Lymphomas (Mycosis Fungoides; Sezary Syndrome)

This is a cutaneous T cell lymphoma characterized by reddening of the skin, *(erythroderma)* and shedding of the outer layers of the epidermis *(exfoliation).* The condition is the result of neoplastic T cells invading the skin, often producing a fungal-like elevated appearance (hence the name fungoides). The *Sezary syndrome* is the cutaneous condition associated with the finding of abnormal T-lymphocytes in the peripheral blood. These T-lymphocytes characteristically have a Sezary cell morphology. The classical morphology is one of an immature cell with a cleaved and convoluted nucleus termed cerebriform, or brain-like. Sezary cell counts can be performed on buffy coat preparations of peripheral blood to follow the course of cutaneous disease or the effects of systemic chemotherapy. These patients may also have associated lymphadenopathy. Electron microscopy of these cells is very diagnostic, showing the characteristic cerebriform convolutions.

Angio-Immunoblastic Lymphadenopathy

This is a rare disorder that mimics a lymphoma and is really a nonclonal proliferation of immunoblasts within the lymph nodes. The condition probably represents an immunologic malfunction and occurs particularly in elderly people. Laboratory features in this disorder are often consistent and comprise a *polyclonal hypergammaglobulinemia,* a *positive Coomb's test,* and occasionally the presence of circulating immunoblasts (transformed B cells) in the peripheral blood. This condition has a high likelihood of transforming to immunoblastic lymphoma.

Malignant Histiocytosis/Hemophagocytic Syndromes

Malignant histiocytosis is a true neoplasm of histiocytes (tissue monocytes), the phagocytic cells of the reticuloendothelial system. These phagocytic cells may produce a severe wasting disorder characterized by spiking fevers and enlargement of the liver and spleen. The condition can also be diagnosed in the presence of the clinical syndrome and the finding of abnormal, malignant histiocytes in the bone marrow that show phagocytosis of other marrow elements *(hemophagocytosis).* This *hemophagocytosis* is a characteristic finding in this disorder and produces peripheral blood pancytopenia. The indirect bilirubin is occasionally elevated as a result of the hemophagocytosis of the red cells. The Coomb's test is negative. This condition has a poor prognosis.

This condition must be distinguished from a viral associated hemophagocytic syndrome that has recently been described (VAHS). Again, hemophagocytosis, which may be demonstrated in the bone marrow aspirate, is the main element, and is associated with peripheral blood pancytopenia. Hepatosplenomegaly is also present. The 'reactive' histiocytes do not appear neoplastic. This condition has a poor prognosis and the viral syndromes it is associated with include infectious mononucleosis (EBV infection).

Clinical Laboratory Findings in the Lymphomas

Laboratory findings in non-Hodgkin's lymphomas are not consistent; however, depending on the degree of marrow involvement, a *leuko-erythroblastic* blood picture may be seen (see Color Plate 39). Occasionally, circulating abnormal lymphocytes may be found in the peripheral blood. A bone marrow biopsy and aspirate are useful in staging of the disorder. Approximately 40% of patients with lymphoma may have bone marrow involvement at the time of diagnosis. If marrow involvement occurs, there is a greater likelihood of central nervous system involvement.

Immunoproliferative Disorders and Plasma Cell Dyscrasias

The *immunoproliferative disorders* are a heterogeneous group of diseases characterized by the unregulated growth and proliferation of *B-lymphocytes* that may or may not be capable of *immunoglobulin production.* These disorders are also characterized by *disturbance of immunoglobulin secretion,* producing an excess of one immunoglobulin type called *monoclonal gammopathy,* or an absence or decreased gammaglobulin production termed *hypogammaglobulinemia.* The ability to secrete immunoglobulin and the type of immunoglobulin secreted depend on the timing of neoplastic transformation of these cells during the normal maturation sequence. Neoplastic change can occur at any stage during B cell development and immunoglobulin production (Fig. 4–3). Chronic lymphocytic leukemia is a proliferation of B cells that can fail to produce immunoglobulins and has been discussed earlier. In *Waldenstrom's macroglobulinemia* there is unregulated production of cells that are intermediate in transformation between mature B-lymphocytes and plasma cells. Characteristically, then, there is an excess of *plasmacytoid lymphocytes* that elaborate the initial immunoglobulin in immune stimulation, namely *IgM*

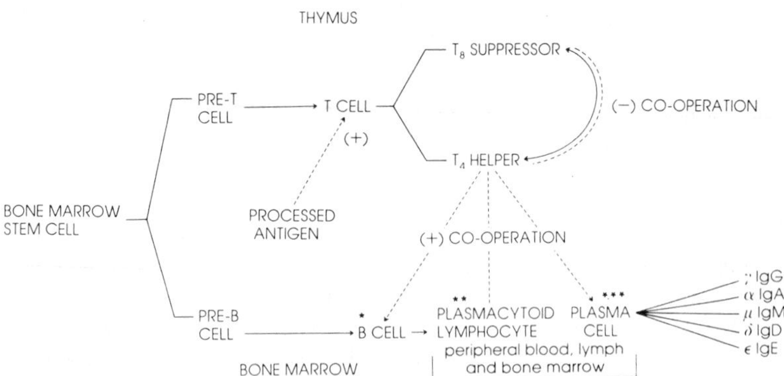

Figure 4–3. B-lymphocyte and plasma cell development with T-cell cooperation. Asterisks indicate the sites of immunoproliferative disorders: *chronic lymphocytic leukemia; **Waldenstrom's macroglobulinemia; ***multiple myeloma. (From Pittiglio, DH and Sacher, RA: Clinical Hematology and Fundamentals of Hemostasis. FA Davis, Philadelphia, 1987, p 268, with permission.)

(for a description of immunoglobulin structure and function, see Chapter 7). As a consequence, a monoclonal IgM is produced. This is termed *macroglobulinemia.* In *multiple myeloma,* the unregulated production of cells involves the *plasma cells,* which may or may not be capable of excess immunoglobulin proliferation. They are classified according to the *type of immunoglobulin* that they produce and their ability to manufacture whole immunoglobulins or components of the immunoglobulin molecules such as *light chains* or *heavy chains* (see Chapter 7). In *heavy chain disease,* proliferating abnormal cells cause a lymphoma-like syndrome in addition to unbalanced production of heavy chains that are not incorporated into the immunoglobulin molecules.

MONOCLONAL GAMMOPATHIES AND MULTIPLE MYELOMA—GENERAL FEATURES

The monoclonal gammopathies are a group of disorders that have one common denominator; they represent excessive production of an immunoglobulin molecule or parts of an immunoglobulin molecule caused by the uncontrolled proliferation of cells of the B-lymphocyte or plasma cell origin. These cells result from expansion of a single clone of B-lymphocytes, having undergone neoplastic transformation during the normal maturation sequence. Consequently, the term monoclonal refers to the cellular abnormality. The term gammopathy refers to the abnormal excess of immunoglobulin proteins—gammaglobulins. Table 4–23 is a classification of monoclonal gammopathies.

The Clinical Laboratory Evaluation of Immunoglobulin Disorders

Serum Protein Electrophoresis

Serum protein electrophoresis is the process whereby the patient's serum proteins are separated by electrical charge and molecular size when exposed to an electrical

Table 4–23. CLASSIFICATION OF MONOCLONAL GAMMOPATHY

Monoclonal gammopathy of uncertain significance (MGUS)
- Tumor-associated gammopathy
- Biclonal gammopathy
- Monoclonal gammopathy associated with miscellaneous disorders

Malignant monoclonal gammopathy
- Multiple myeloma
  - Smouldering myeloma
  - Nonsecretory myeloma
  - Plasma cell leukemia
- Plasmacytoma
  - Localized (solitary)
  - Diffuse
  - Extramedullary
- Monoclonal gammopathy associated with:
  - Lymphoproliferative disease
  - Malignant lymphoma
  - Waldenstrom's macroglobulinemia
- Heavy chain disease
- Primary systemic amyloidosis

current. The serum is placed on a support medium, most commonly agarose, suspended in an electrostatic medium. An electrical charge is applied to the medium and the serum proteins are made to migrate. Separation occurs because of their different charges and molecular weights. Figure 4–4 shows the major serum protein components separated into albumin and the globulin fractions. *Immunoglobulins* separate electrophoretically as the *gammaglobulins.* The separated protein bands are identified by staining with a protein stain, and the intensity of the stain reflects the amount of protein present. The density of the different bands is read by a *densitometer,* which translates the staining intensity into the amount of protein and gives a *tracing,* which is the familiar *serum protein electrophoresis profile.* Differing profiles are outlined in Figure 4–4. In the monoclonal gammopathies, an abnormal protein, the *monoclonal protein* or *M protein,* is identified. In this case, a single population of immunoglobulin-producing cells proliferates and secretes a single immunoglobulin type, which migrates in the same position on the serum protein electrophoresis, producing a single, dense band. The serum protein electrophoresis, therefore, differentiates a monoclonal paraprotein from polyclonal hypergammaglobulinemia, where there are several clones of immunoglobulin-producing cells, each producing different immunoglobulins migrating at different rates during protein electrophoresis. The serum protein electrophoresis will not identify the class of immunoglobulin, but indicates the relative percentage of the separated proteins.

Immunoelectrophoresis

Immunoelectrophoresis couples *electrophoretic separation* of the immunoglobulins with a two-dimensional *immunodiffusion* reaction, and is used to identify the specific immunoglobulin types. The process requires the placement of a serum sample in an agar gel, followed by subsequent electrophoresis. After the serum protein separation has occurred, the protein diffuses into the gel and then immunoprecipitates with an antibody of a known specific anti-heavy chain (gamma, alpha, mu, delta) or anti-light chain (anti-kappa or anti-lambda). If an immunoprecipitation line occurs following diffusion with the known antibody, then the protein is the specific corresponding immunoglobulin (Fig. 4–5; see Chapter 7). This technique enables the identification of the immunoglobulin type as well as the identification of single chains. It is, therefore, mainly a qualitative test and is only semiquantitative. The urine may also be analyzed using this method if protein excretion has occurred. The urine is concentrated prior to immunoelectrophoresis in an effort to identify the presence of light or heavy chains (see later section of text).

Immunoglobulin Quantitation

The method of immunoglobulin quantitation is discussed in Chapter 7. Briefly, however, the technique also uses an immunoprecipitation technique (but not electrophoresis) in an agar gel that is impregnated with a specific anti-immunoglobulin. The protein is allowed to diffuse into the gel in a radial fashion that will produce an immunoprecipitate in a ring around the application point. The diameter of the immunoprecipitation ring is proportional to the amount of immunoglobulin present. There are now immunochemical methods available for the quantitation of IgG, IgM, and IgA. The advantage of these over the immunodiffusion techniques is the speed of testing. Immunodiffusion is an overnight test, whereas the immunochemical methods give quantitative results in minutes (see also Chapters 7 and 15).

Urine—Tests for Light Chains

Urine immunoelectrophoresis is the definitive test that allows differentiation between kappa and lambda light chains in the urine.

The Sulfosalicylic Acid Test is the procedure used for quantitating the amount of

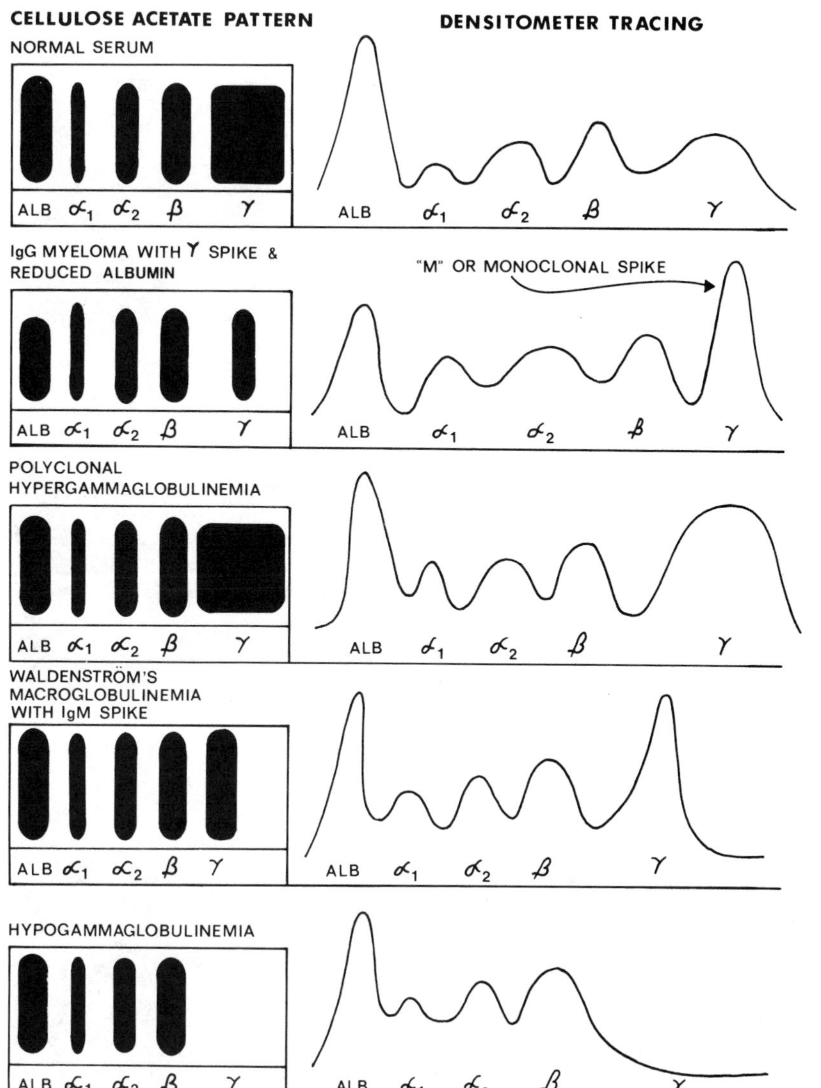

Figure 4–4. Serum protein electrophoretic profiles in differing medical conditions. (From Pittiglio, DH and Sacher, RA: Clinical Hematology and Fundamentals of Hemostasis. FA Davis, Philadelphia, 1987, p 272, with permission.)

protein excreted in a 24-hour period. It is a protein precipitation test.

The *Heat Precipitation Test* is based on the original test described by Bence-Jones for the detection of urine light chains. It is often called the *Bence-Jones Protein Test.* On heating a sample of urine to 56°C, Bence-Jones proteins (light chains) will precipitate, but will redissolve again at about 100°C.

CLASSIFICATION OF PLASMA CELL DYSCRASIAS

Table 4–23 is an outline of the classification of monoclonal gammopathies.

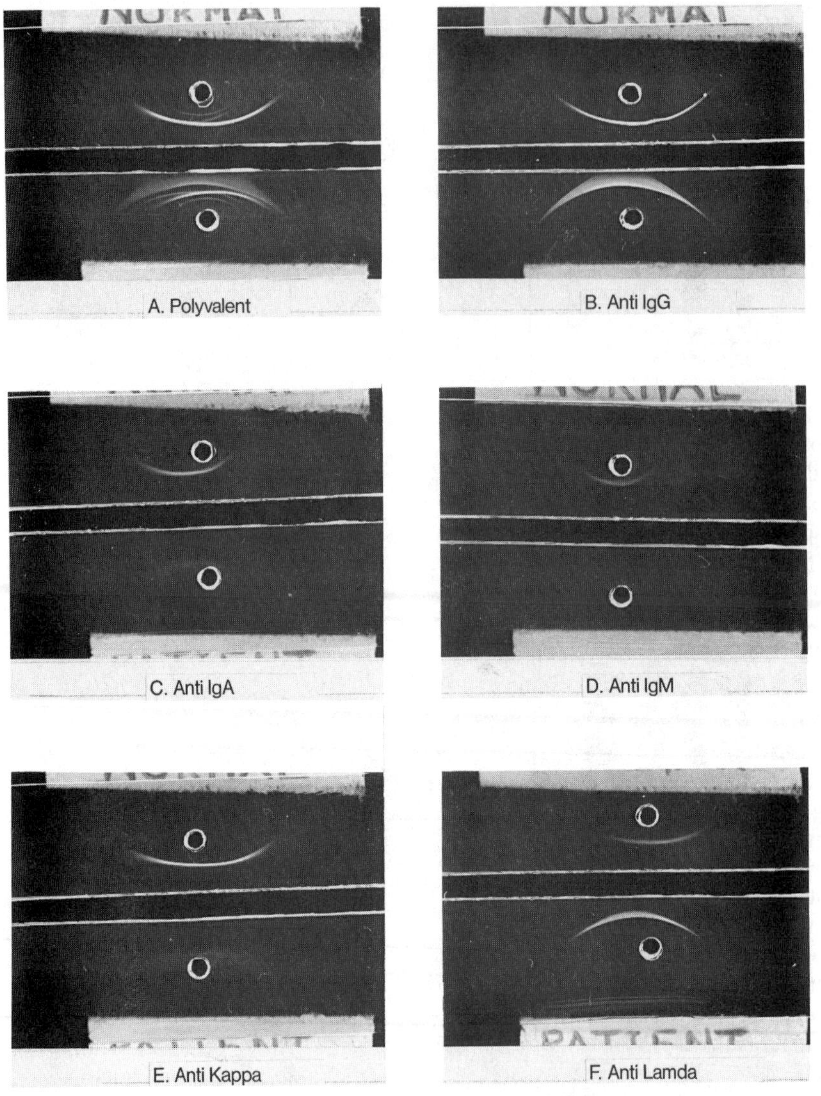

Figure 4–5. Immunoelectrophoretic serum patterns from a patient with IgG-lambda multiple myeloma. Each photograph shows a normal control sample (upper well) and patient sample (lower well). The antisera used for each analysis is specified on the lower border of each figure:

A - polyvalent	D - Anti IgM
B - Anti IgG	E - Anti Kappa
C - Anti IgA	F - Anti Lambda

The patient's serum protein is defined by a precipitation arc in the lower part of each figure. The most intense areas are IgG (Fig B) and lambda (Figure F).

Monoclonal gammopathies are classified according to the clinical course (benign or malignant), the proliferating cell type (the lymphomas-lymphocytes, macroglobulinemia-plasmacytoid lymphocytes, and multiple myeloma-plasma cells) and the nature of the abnormal immunoglobulin produced (IgG, IgA, IgM light chains).

Waldenstrom's Macroglobulinemia

This condition is an immunoproliferative disorder as described above, but is characterized by clinical features intermediate between a *lymphoproliferative disorder* and a *plasma cell dyscrasia* (see later). As a consequence, the clinical syndrome is one of lymph node enlargement with enlargement of the liver and spleen in addition to bone marrow involvement, but also associated with the production of excess IgM immunoglobulins. The clinical features may vary from a lymphoma-like condition—depending on whether lymphadenopathy or hepatosplenomegaly predominates—to a consequence of the excess production of the IgM macromolecule. IgM is a large molecule consisting of a pentamer of immunoglobulin chains attached by disulfide bridges (for a more detailed description of immunoglobulin types, see Chapter 7). Its size and abundance in this disorder produce sluggish flow and increased viscosity. If the latter predominates, the clinical features are those of the *hyperviscosity syndrome,* a disorder that is characterized by increased blood viscosity with symptoms of sluggish circulation, increased blood volume, and macroglobulin (IgM) excess, causing impairment of platelet function and hemostasis. Consequently, the major clinical features are those of neurologic impairment, congestive cardiac failure, and a bleeding diathesis characterized by nosebleeds, cutaneous bleeding, and other mucosal bleeding episodes. In addition, ocular effects occur and vision impairment is common.

Laboratory Findings

The peripheral blood smear shows *rouleaux formation* (see Color Plate 47A), and *plasmacytoid lymphocytes* may be seen in the differential leukocyte count. Depending on the degree of involvement of the plasmacytoid lymphocytes and the predominance of hypersplenism, a pancytopenia may be present. The sedimentation rate is variable but may be normal or low. The *serum viscosity,* which is the ratio of the flow of serum in a graduated tube compared with water, is usually elevated, often above 4 (the normal serum viscosity is 1.4–1.8) (see Color Plate 96). A bone marrow aspirate may show the presence of abundant plasmacytoid lymphocytes; that is, cells intermediate between lymphocytes and plasma cells. These cells have an eccentric nucleus with prominent basophilic cytoplasm, and a supranuclear halo similar to those seen in plasma cells may be found. The cytoplasm is not as abundant as occurs in typical plasma cells. Other clinical syndromes associated with this disease can involve other organ systems, including liver dysfunction, renal insufficiency, and nephrotic syndrome (see later in chapter). Immune globulin quantitation usually shows an increased level of IgM macroglobulin, often associated with decreased levels of IgG and IgA. Immunoelectrophoresis confirms the presence of an IgM of monoclonal type (Mu-heavy chain), and *either* kappa *or* lambda light chain (see above and Chapter 7).

Multiple Myeloma

This is a disorder that is characterized by the unregulated growth and proliferation of a clone of plasma cells that proceeds in a progressive manner, leading ultimately to the death of the patient. It is a disease of the elderly. The condition is characterized by a *diffuse, plasma cell infiltration* in the bone marrow, overproduction of either intact monoclonal immunoglobulins (IgG, IgA and, rarely, IgD) or light chains only. The disorder usually presents with a *diffuse* involvement of the marrow, but occasionally can present as *focal* tumor masses *(plasmacytomas),* which may be in the marrow or at an extramedullary site (usually the nasopharynx). There are several variant forms of multiple myeloma, including smoldering myeloma, nonsecretory myeloma, plasma cell leukemia, and plasmacytomas.

Multiple myeloma occurs more commonly in blacks than whites, and is one of the most common hematologic malignancies of the black population. It is seen in younger age groups in blacks than in whites.

Clinical Features

The clinical features and complications of multiple myeloma are shown in Figure 4–6. Patients may be asymptomatic at the time of presentation, but usually present with multiple symptoms, of which bone pain, infections, anemia, and renal insufficiency predominate.

The skeletal destruction and bone pain occur as a result of the elaboration of osteoclast-activating factor (OAF), which stimulates bone resorption and demineralization of the bone and lytic areas. A constellation of clinical features may be produced on the basis of the amount and type of abnormal protein released by the malignant plasma cells. These include hyperviscosity syndrome, cryoglobulins (proteins that precipitate on exposure to the cold), bleeding disorders due to interference with clotting factors and platelet function, and infiltration by abnormal plasma cells or abnormal parts of immunoglobulins deposited in tissues producing organ failure.

Laboratory Features

Hematologic: Patients usually present with a normochromic, normocytic anemia that can be macrocytic. The hemoglobin is usually below 10 g/dl and the hematocrit below 30%. Red cell morphology is usually unremarkable, with the exception of rouleaux formation. *Rouleaux formation* occurs as a result of protein coating the erythrocytes, which contributes also to a markedly elevated erythrocyte sedimentation rate (see Color Plate 47A). *Sedimentation rates* in excess of 100 mm/hour are common in multiple myeloma (see Chapter 2). Initially, the white cell count and platelet count are not decreased; however, pancytopenia may develop as the disease progresses or as chemotherapy is used. Some patients may show a *leukoerythroblastic* blood picture, and occasionally plasma cells may be seen on the peripheral smear (if in excess of 5%, termed plasma cell leukemia) (see Color Plate 47A).

A bone marrow aspirate usually shows a markedly hypercellular marrow with an abundance of *plasma cells* in all stages of maturity. Characteristically, the abnormal plasma cell has a *"punched-out"* nucleolus that is very prominent. Binucleate plasma cells may be seen. In multiple myeloma, the plasma cells constitute more than 20% of the marrow cell population; however, the marrow may be almost entirely replaced by malignant plasma cells.

Biochemical Parameters: If renal insufficiency occurs, levels of *blood urea nitrogen* and *creatinine* will be elevated in addition to *uric acid,* a purine nucleotide breakdown product. *Serum calcium* may be markedly increased because of bone resorption. A serum protein electrophoresis usually shows the presence of the monoclonal ("M") protein. Usually the M spike is greater than 2 g/dl; however, the level is dependent on what type of myeloma is present. Light chain myeloma is not associated with a serum M spike, but the monoclonal light chains are found only in the urine. Additional tests can be performed to demonstrate the presence of proteins that precipitate in the cold *(cryoglobulins)* or *hyperviscosity* (see below). The frequencies of monoclonal paraproteins in multiple myeloma are IgG—52%; IgA—

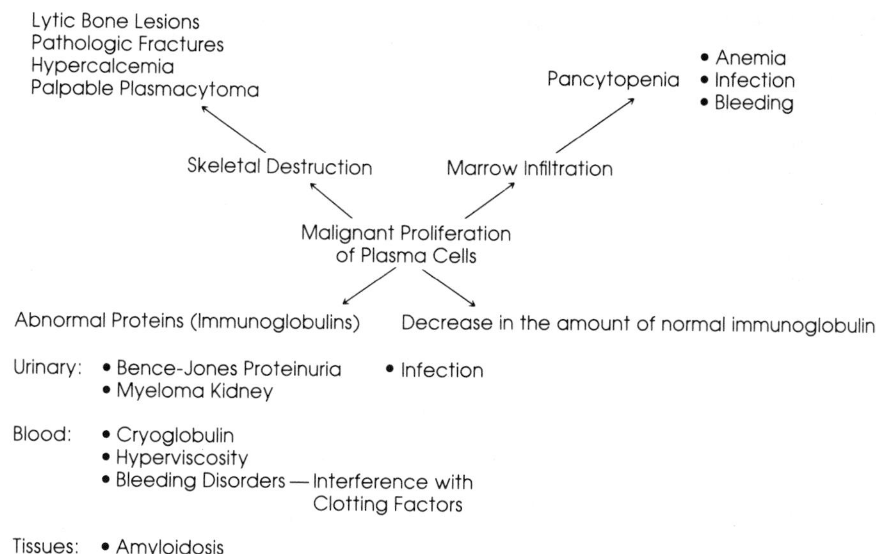

Figure 4–6. Diagram outlining the clinical features and complications in multiple myeloma. (From Pittiglio, DH and Sacher, RA: Clinical Hematology and Fundamentals of Hemostasis. FA Davis, Philadelphia, 1987, p 276, with permission.)

25%; Bence-Jones (light chain myeloma)—22%; others—1%. Identification of the type of protein and the absolute quantity of the immunoglobulin is performed, as already mentioned, by immunoelectrophoresis and immunodiffusion, respectively.

Protein may be identified in the urine and quantitated with a 24-hour urine specimen. Occasionally, protein levels in excess of 4 g/24 hours may be seen, and in this situation one must consider the possibility of light chain deposition in the tissues—*amyloidosis*—that is associated with the clinical syndrome called the *nephrotic syndrome.* Examination of *urine sediment* may reveal the presence of *hyaline protein casts* or *uric acid crystals.*

Monoclonal Gammopathy of Undetermined Significance (MGUS)

This category of disorders includes those patients who present with an *incidental finding* of a serum M spike on routine testing. The accumulation of this monoclonal protein usually occurs in the absence of any clinical disease or symptoms. In most instances, the patients are not aware of any problem and the M spike is discovered incidentally. This condition was formerly called "benign monoclonal gammopathy," a term that is misleading because a certain percentage of these disorders go on to the malignant variety, namely multiple myeloma. The problem is that the clinical or laboratory features at initial presentation cannot allow a distinction between those cases that will become aggressive and those that will not. There is a 10% likelihood of progression to hematologic malignancy. The monoclonal protein may result in expression of a complete immunoglobulin or light chains only. Patients with MGUS usually have less than 2 g/dl of monoclonal protein in the serum, and less than 5% plasma cells in the marrow. Monoclonal gammopathy of undetermined significance is frequent, and has been found in approximately 3% of persons

Table 4–24. PRINCIPLES IN DIFFERENTIAL DIAGNOSIS OF MONOCLONAL GAMMOPATHIES

Establish presence of a monoclonal gammopathy by documentation of an M spike.
  Serum protein electrophoresis
  Urine protein electrophoresis
  Serum immunoelectrophoresis
Establish nature of proliferating cell type.
  Bone marrow aspirate/biopsy
  Skeletal survey
Establish presence of entire or partial protein and activity of the protein.
  Urine light chains
  Quantitative analysis by radial immunodiffusion
Establish the degree of organ system involvement.

over the age of 70 years, and in 1% over 50 years. Since it is impossible to predict which patients are likely to evolve into the more malignant presentation, periodic examination of these patients is the only definitive way of evaluating incipient myeloma. Table 4–24 is an approach to the differential diagnosis of the monoclonal gammopathies.

Amyloidosis

This disorder includes a heterogeneous group of conditions characterized by the extracellular deposition of an amorphous, waxy-like material derived from different proteins by different mechanisms. The term "amyloid" is originally derived from the waxy, starch-like property of the material. The accumulation of this material within tissues and organs leads to a loss of function and organ enlargement. Diagnosis is usually made on tissue histology; however, patients with this disorder, particularly the type that occurs in association with multiple myeloma, may present with excess light chains in the urine and may produce excess loss of protein in the urine (nephrotic syndrome).

Heavy Chain Diseases

These disorders are characterized by an uncontrolled production of the heavy chain components of immunoglobulins. These proteins are elaborated by monoclonal B-lymphocytes. There are three main types, all of which are rare. These are *gamma chain disease, alpha chain disease,* and *mu chain disease.* The commonest of these three disorders is *alpha chain disease,* a condition that has also been referred to as *"Mediterranean lymphoma."* This condition more commonly afflicts younger individuals from the Middle East. The patients present, typically, with a *malabsorption syndrome* due to the deposition of plasma cells and lymphocytes in the mucous membrane of the small bowel. An excess amount of the abnormal component of immunoglobulin may be seen in the serum of any of these conditions.

REFERENCES

1. Cytogenetics symposium. Mayo Clin Proc 60:675, 1985.
2. Foon, KA and Todd, RF: Immunologic classification of leukemia and lymphoma. Blood 68:1, 1986.

3. Petersdorf, RG, et al (eds): Harrison's Principles of Internal Medicine, ed 10. McGraw-Hill, Philadelphia, 1983.
4. Hoffbrand, AV and Lewis, SM: Postgraduate Hematology, ed 2. Appleton-Century-Crofts, New York, 1981.
5. Jaffe, E and Cossman, J: Immunodiagnosis of lymphoid and mononuclear phagocytic neoplasms. In Rose, NR and Fahey, JL (eds): Manual of Clinical Immunology, ed 3. American Society of Microbiology, Washington, DC, 1986, p 779.
6. Koeffler, HP: Syndromes of acute non-lymphocytic leukemia. Ann Intern Med 107:748, 1987.
7. Lehrer, RI, et al: Neutrophils and host defense. Ann Intern Med 109:127, 1988.
8. McCullogh, EA: Stem cells in normal and leukemic hemapoiesis. Blood 61:1, 1983.
9. Cassileth, PA (ed): Symposium on hematology and hematologic malignancies. Med Clin North Am 68(3):675–788, 1984.
10. Pittiglio, DH and Sacher, RA: Clinical Hematology and Fundamentals of Hemostasis. FA Davis, Philadelphia, 1987.
11. Williams, WJ, et al: Hematology, ed 3. McGraw-Hill, Philadelphia, 1985.
12. Rai, KR, et al: Clinical staging of chronic lymphocytic leukemia. Blood 46:219, 1975.
13. Rosenberg, SA, et al: National Cancer Institute sponsored study of classification of non-Hodgkin's lymphomas. Summary and description of working formulation for clinical usage. Cancer 49:2112, 1982.

OUTLINE

TESTS

CHAPTER

5

HEMOSTASIS AND TESTS OF HEMOSTATIC FUNCTION

Hemostasis is the collective term for all the physiologic mechanisms the body uses to protect itself from blood loss. It is the process by which the body simultaneously stops bleeding from an injured site, yet maintains blood in the fluid state within the vascular compartment. Hemostasis involves synchronized cooperation between several interrelated physiologic systems.

Failure of hemostasis leads to *hemorrhage;* failure to maintain fluidity leads to *thrombosis*. Both hemorrhage and thrombosis are extremely common and dangerous clinical problems. Characterizing the defects that cause hemorrhage is, at present, easier than characterizing potentially treatable conditions that predispose to thrombosis.

NORMAL HEMOSTASIS

Hemostatic mechanisms comprise four main systems: 1) the vascular system, 2) platelets, 3) the coagulation system, and 4) the fibrinolytic system.

Vascular system: Blood vessels have one or more layers of smooth muscle surrounding endothelial cells that cover the luminal surface. When vessels are damaged, the muscle constricts, narrowing the path through which blood flows and sometimes halting blood flow entirely. This *vascular phase* of hemostasis affects only arterioles and their dependent capillaries; large vessels cannot constrict sufficiently to prevent blood loss. Even in small vessels, vasoconstriction provides only the briefest sort of hemostasis.

Platelets: Permanent repair requires that breaks in the vessel wall be plugged; the effective hemostatic plug consists of platelets and the gel-like protein *fibrin.* Platelets are nonnucleated fragments of megakaryocytic cytoplasm, but they are living entities with complex structure, active metabolism, and a reactive biologic constitution. Platelets may plug small holes in blood vessels and can form an effective primary hemostatic mechanism.

Coagulation System: Coagulation is a chemical process whereby plasma proteins interact to convert the large, soluble plasma protein molecule *fibrinogen* into the stable, insoluble gel called *fibrin.* The active compound is the enzyme thrombin, which preferentially converts fibrinogen (soluble) into fibrin (insoluble). There is a delicate balance between coagulation and maintaining blood in a liquid state. Imbalance in one direction can lead to excessive bleeding, whereas in the other it may lead to thrombosis.

Fibrinolysis: The fibrinolytic system is the system that limits coagulation to the sites of injury and wound repair and prevents coagulation from becoming more widespread and uncontrolled. The active compound of this system is the enzyme *plasmin.* Plasmin (derived from the plasma protein plasminogen) is a relatively nonselective enzyme that more preferentially digests fibrin and fibrinogen.

The relative importance of the hemostatic mechanisms vary with vessel size. Capillaries may rapidly seal injured sites by the formation of hemostatic plugs with little disruption of local blood flow. Larger vessels quickly become occluded by numerous fused platelets. Failure of the formation of hemostatic plugs allows small, pinpoint hemorrhages to occur that are called *petechiae.* Larger areas of bleeding into the tissues produce severe bruising and confluent hemorrhages called *ecchymoses,* which, when large, form confluent areas of *purpura.* The practical application of laboratory tests to evaluate clinical disorders of hemostasis and thrombosis requires an understanding of the organization of the coagulation and fibrinolytic systems. This may best be appreciated by considering the above four mechanisms responsible for normal hemostasis.

Tables 5–1 and 5–2 represent normal values for platelet and coagulation studies.

The Vascular System

The formation of the hemostatic plug is initiated by vascular and/or tissue damage, producing a sequence of orderly events. Vascular injury is usually associated with the contraction of blood vessels *(vasoconstriction),* contact activation of platelets with subsequent platelet aggregation, and contact activation of the coagulation pathway. Under normal circumstances, the endothelial lining of the blood vessels is smooth and uninterrupted. When this endothelial lining is damaged, this exposes

Table 5–1. NORMAL VALUES FOR PLATELET STUDIES

Bleeding time	
Ivy	3–6 min
Template	2–7½ min
Platelet count	150–450 × $10^3/\mu l$
Clot retraction	>40% retraction at 1 hr
Platelet aggregation	Results are compared against light-transmission of normal platelets
Von Willebrand factor	60–160% of normal activity

Table 5–2. COAGULATION FACTOR NOMENCLATURE AT A GLANCE

Factor	Synonym	Clotting Pathway	Molecular Weight	Site of Production	Plasma Concentration ($\mu g/ml$)	Half-life Disappearance (hr)	Minimum Hemostatic Level	Storage Stability	Active Form	Other Characteristics *(all factors are present in normal fresh plasma*
I	Fibrinogen	Both intrinsic, extrinsic, common pathway	340,000	Liver	2500 (250 mg%)	120	50–10 mg%	Stable	Protein	Activity destroyed during coagulation process/present in absorbed plasma
II	Prothrombin	Both intrinsic, extrinsic, common pathway	70,000	Liver—vitamin K-dependent	100	100	40% concentration	Stable	Serine protease	Consumed during coagulation process
III	Tissue thromboplastin	Extrinsic system only	45,000	Thromboplastic activity present in most tissues	0				Cofactor	
V	Labile factor proaccelerin	Both intrinsic, extrinsic, common pathway	330,000	Liver	5–12	25	5–10% concentration	Labile	Cofactor	Activity destroyed during coagulation process/present in absorbed plasma
VII	Stable factor proconvertin	Extrinsic system only	55,000	Liver—vitamin K-dependent	1	5	5–10 concentration	Stable	Glycoprotein	Present in serum
VIII/vWF	Antihemophilic factor (AHF)/von Willebrand factor	Intrinsic system only	1–2 million	Possibly endothelial cells & megakaryocytes	7	12	30% concentration	Labile	Cofactor	Activity destroyed during coagulation process/present in absorbed plasma
IX	Christmas factor, plasma (PTC), thromboplastin component	Intrinsic only	57,000	Liver—vitamin K-dependent	4	24	30% concentration	Stable	Serine protease	Present in serum
X	Stuart Prower factor	Both intrinsic, extrinsic, common pathway	59,000	Liver—vitamin K-dependent	5	40	8–10% concentration	Stable	Stable protease	Present in serum
XI	Plasma thromboplastin antecedent (PTA)	Intrinsic only	160,000	Liver	4	65	20–30 concentration	Stable	Serine protease	Present in serum and absorbed plasma
XII	Hageman factor/contact factor	Intrinsic only	80,000	Liver	29	60	0%	Stable	Serine protease	Present in serum and absorbed plasma
XIII	Fibrin stabilizing factor (FSF)	Both intrinsic, extrinsic, common pathway	300,000	Liver or platelets	10	150	1% concentration	Stable	Transglutaminase	Actively destroyed during coagulation process/present in absorbed plasma
Prekallikrein	Fletcher factor	Intrinsic only	80,000	Liver	50	?	?	?Stable	Serine protease	
High molecular weight kininogen	Fitzgerald factor	Intrinsic only	120,000	Liver	70	?	?	?Stable	Cofactor	

Note: Although not a coagulation protein or factor, calcium is sometimes denoted as factor IV.
From Pittiglio, DH and Sacher, RA: Clinical Hematology and Fundamentals of Hemostasis. FA Davis, Philadelphia, 1987, p. 342 with permission.

underlying collagen to which circulating platelets can adhere *(platelet adhesion)*. Recruitment of more platelets to "plug" the injured vascular site then occurs.

Platelets

Platelets serve two different functions: 1) they protect the vascular integrity of the endothelium, and 2) they initiate repair when blood vessel walls are damaged. This platelet–vessel wall interaction is termed *primary hemostasis*. Persons whose platelets are defective in number or function experience *petechiae* on skin and membrane surfaces; they are also unable to stem bleeding that occurs following accidental or induced injury to blood vessels.

Production and Structure

As was mentioned in Chapter 2, platelets are fragments of the cytoplasm of their parent, precursor cell, the *megakaryocyte*. Platelets vary in size from one to about four microns and circulate for approximately 10 days as disc-shaped, anucleate cells. Regulation of platelet production is ascribed to *thrombopoietin*, analogous to erythropoietin for erythrocyte production, but no single substance or activity has yet been characterized. With pronounced hemostatic stress or marrow stimulation, platelet production can increase seven- to eightfold. Newly generated platelets are larger and have greater hemostatic capacity than mature, circulating platelets. One third of the circulating platelet pool is normally sequestered in the spleen.

A diagrammatic representation of platelet structure is shown in Figure 5–1. The platelet membrane is rich in phospholipids, among them *platelet factor III*, which promotes clotting during hemostasis. This membrane phospholipid serves as a surface for interaction of plasma proteins involved in blood coagulation. The membrane of the platelet also becomes sticky, allowing for other essential platelet functions of adhesion and aggregation. The cytoplasm of the platelet contains *microfilaments*, which are composed of *thrombosthenin*, a contractile protein similar to *actinomyosin*, the contractile protein involved in muscle tissue contraction. *Microtubules*, which form an internal skeleton, are also found in the cytoplasm. They comprise a circumferential band of hollow, tubular structures similar to the microtubules of other cells and lie immediately beneath the platelet membrane. The microtubules and microfilaments forming the platelet cytoskeleton are responsible for platelets maintaining the normal discoid platelet shape and allow shape changes, as well as facilitating the platelet release reactions. Interspersed within the platelet cytoplasm are also platelet granules, of which there are two main types; *dense granules* contain adenosine diphosphate (ADP), adenosine triphosphate (ATP), ionized calcium and serotonin and *alpha granules*, which contain platelet-specific proteins, especially *platelet factor IV, beta-thromboglobulin, platelet-derived growth factor*, and, among others, *thrombospondin*. In addition, plasma proteins, in particular fibrinogen and von Willebrand factor (see factor VIII), are present in the alpha granules. The alpha granules are more numerous than the dense granules. The dense granules represent the storage pool of adenine nucleotides. Prostaglandin synthesis, which is also an integral part of normal platelet function, is believed to occur in an internal tubular system called the *dense tubular system*, which is another component of the cytoplasm of the platelet (Fig. 5–1). Platelet factor IV and beta-thromboglobulin are substances normally present only within intact platelets. The presence of these proteins in the circulating plasma indicates excessive platelet turn-

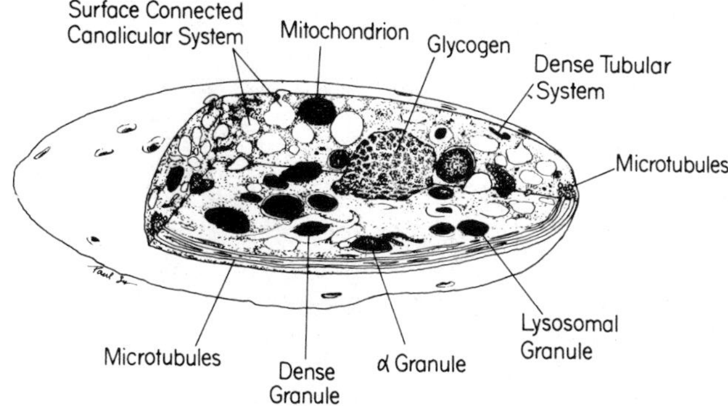

Figure 5–1. Platelet structure. Understanding platelet fine structure provides a morphologic basis for platelet function. The peripheral surface coat mediates the membrane contact reactions of adhesion and aggregation. Plasma membrane, which also contributes the phospholipid procoagulant activity, forms an invaginated, sponge-like open canalicular membrane system that represents an expanded reactive surface to which plasma hemostatic factors are selectively adsorbed. Submembranous filaments and other cytoplasmic microfilaments of the sol-gel zone appear to constitute the platelet's contractile actomyosin system. Residual endoplasmic reticulum, free of ribosomes, forms a calcium binding dense tubular membrane system. Microtubules form a circumferential cytoskeleton that maintains the discoid shape. Following stimulation, the microtubules undergo a concentric central shift with an inner clustering of organelles; concurrently, cytoplasmic pseudopods form on the periphery. Constituents from the α-granules, dense granules, and lysosomal granules are then released into the open canalicular system in association with contraction of the actomyosin filaments, which results in a fused impermeable platelet mass. Energy for these events is derived by aerobic metabolism in the mitochondria and anaerobic glycolysis utilizing glycogen granule stores. (From Thompson, AR and Harker, LA: Manual of Hemostasis and Thrombosis, ed. 3. FA Davis, Philadelphia, 1983, p 10, with permission.)

over or accelerated platelet destruction. Assays for these substances are available in reference laboratories.

FORMATION OF PRIMARY HEMOSTATIC PLATELET PLUG

For normal primary hemostasis to occur, and for the platelets to fulfill their role in forming the initial platelet plug, adequate numbers of circulating platelets must be present, and they must be functioning normally. Normal function requires their participation in an orderly manner, which is important in the formation of the primary hemostatic plug (Fig. 5–2). This involves, initially, platelet adhesion, platelet aggregation, and, finally, platelet release reaction with additional recruitment of other platelets.

Platelet Adhesion

Platelets become activated by exposure to subendothelial collagen and areas of tissue injury. Platelet adhesion involves an interaction between the platelet membrane glycoproteins and exposed or injured tissue. Platelet adhesion is dependent on a plasma protein factor called the *von Willebrand factor,* which has a complex and integral relationship with the plasma anti-hemophilic coagulant *factor VIII* and a

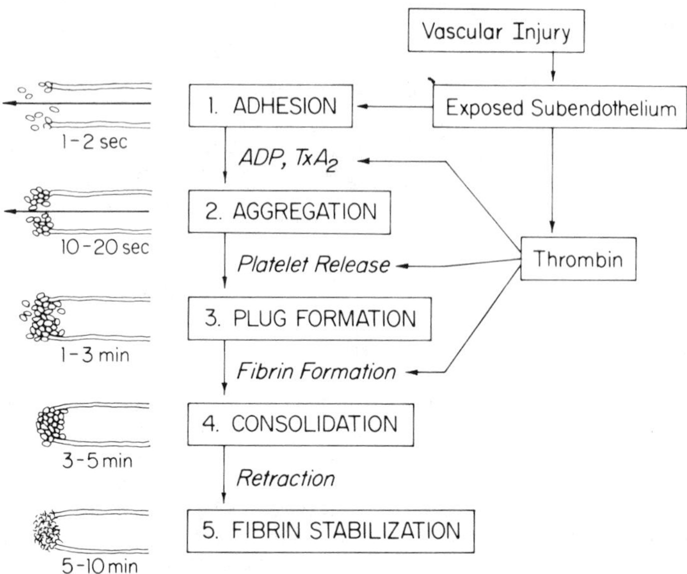

Figure 5–2. Hemostatic plug formation. The formation of a platelet plug proceeds through the sequence of: (1) platelet adhesion to exposed subendothelial connective tissue structures; (2) platelet aggregation by ADP, thromboxane A_2 and thrombin recruitment through transformation of discoid platelets into reactive spiny spheres that interact with one another through calcium-dependent fibrinogen bridges; (3) contribution of platelet procoagulant activity to the coagulation process which stabilizes the plug within a fibrin mesh; and (4) retraction of the platelet mass to form a dense thrombus. (From Thompson, AR and Harker, LA: Manual of Hemostasis and Thrombosis, ed. 3. FA Davis, Philadelphia, 1983, p 11, with permission.)

platelet receptor called the *platelet membrane glycoprotein Ib.* Individuals lacking either the von Willebrand factor or the platelet glycoprotein Ib have a defect in platelet adhesion that occurs in the disorders *von Willebrand's disease* (see later) and the rare *Bernard-Soulier syndrome.* Platelet adhesion is associated with an increase in platelet stickiness, which allows platelets to adhere to themselves as well as to adhere to the area of damaged endothelium or tissue. Thus, an initial or primary hemostatic plug is formed. Activation of the platelet surface and the recruitment of other platelets produces a sticky platelet mass and is facilitated by the process of platelet aggregation.

Aggregation

Aggregation is the ability of platelets to stick to one another to form a plug. Initial aggregation is produced by surface contact and release of ADP from other platelets adhering to the endothelial surface. This is termed the *primary wave of aggregation.* Subsequently, as more and more platelets are involved, more and more ADP is released, producing a *secondary wave of aggregation* with recruitment of additional platelets. Aggregation is associated with platelet shape changes from *discoid to spherical shape.* The secondary wave of platelet aggregation is an irreversible phenomenon, whereas the initial shape change and primary aggregation is reversible (Fig. 5–3 shows patterns of platelet aggregation as determined by a platelet aggregometer).

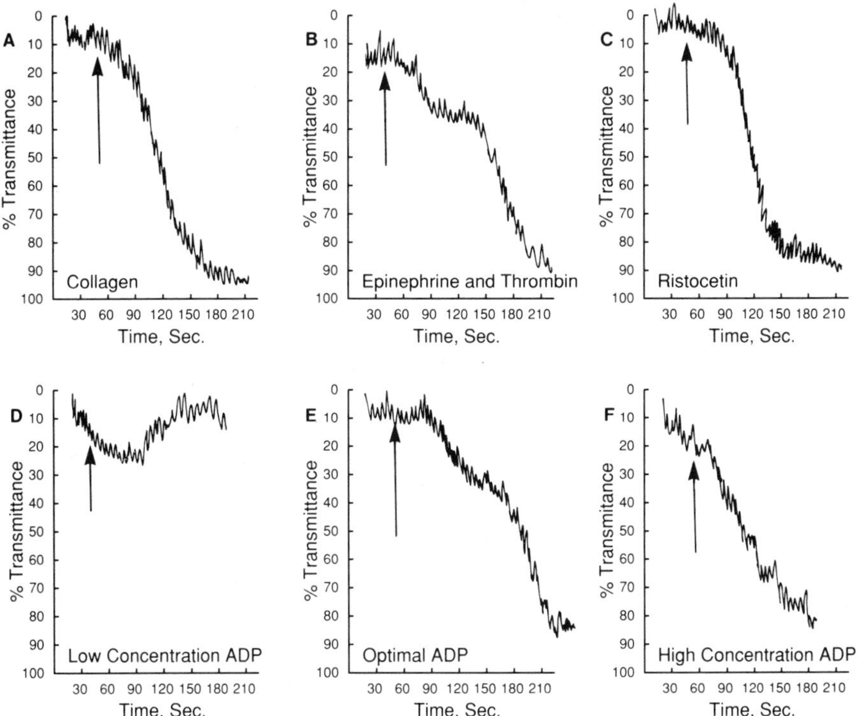

Figure 5–3. Patterns of platelet aggregation. Aggregation curves with various aggregating agents: *A,* Aggregation curve induced by collagen. Note the lag time before aggregation, followed by a single wave of aggregation. *B,* Aggregation curve induced with epinephrine and thrombin. Note the biphasic wave of aggregation. *C,* Aggregation curve induced by ristocetin. Note the generally single wave of aggregation.

Aggregation curves with various concentrations of ADP: *D,* Very low concentrations of ADP induce a primary wave of aggregation followed by disaggregation. *E,* The optimal concentration of ADP induces a biphasic wave of aggregation. *F,* High concentrations of ADP induce a broad wave of aggregation. Note: Arrow indicates point of application of aggregation inducer. (From Triplett, DA [ed]: Platelet Function: Laboratory Evaluation and Clinical Application. The American Society of Clinical Pathologists, Chicago, 1978, with permission.)

Binding of ADP released from activated platelets to the platelet membrane activates the enzyme *phospholipase,* which hydrolyzes phospholipids in the platelet membrane to produce *arachidonic acid.* Arachidonic acid is the precursor of very potent chemical mediators of both aggregation and inhibitors of aggregation involved in the *prostaglandin pathway.* Through this process, arachidonic acid is converted in the cytoplasm of the platelet by the enzyme *cyclo-oxygenase* to *cyclic endoperoxides,* PGG_2 and PGH_2. The potent stimulator of platelet aggregation, the compound *thromboxane* A_2, is produced by the action of the enzyme thromboxane synthetase on these cyclic endoperoxides (Fig. 5–4). *Thromboxane* A_2 is a very active, yet unstable, compound that degrades to its stable, inactive form *thromboxane* B_2. Thromboxane A_2 is also a very potent vasoconstrictor that further prevents blood loss from damaged blood vessels.

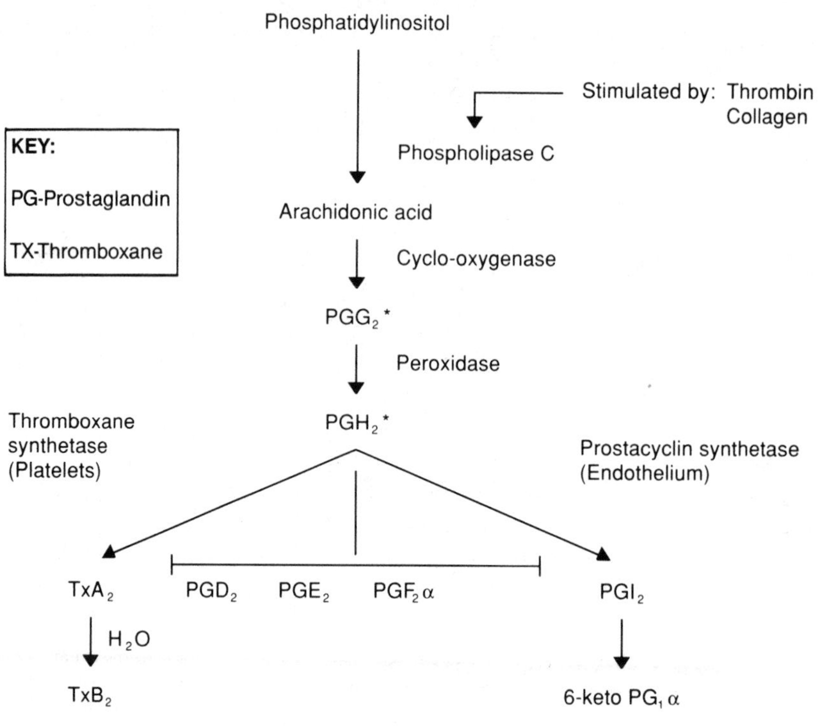

Figure 5–4. Prostaglandin pathway. (From Treating Hemostatic Disorders: A Problem Oriented Approach. American Association of Blood Banks, Arlington, Virginia, 1984, p 15, with permission.)

Release Reaction

During this process, *platelet factor III,* a compound that is released from the internal cytoplasm of the platelet, enhances the coagulation cascade (which is the next phase of hemostasis) and the formation of the secondary, or *stable, hemostatic plug*. Aggregation can be induced *in vitro* with reagents ADP, thrombin, epinephrine, serotonin, collagen, or the antibiotic ristocetin.

In vitro aggregation also occurs in 2 phases: 1) primary, or reversible, aggregation and, 2) secondary, or irreversible aggregation. Primary aggregation involves platelet shape change and is brought about by contraction of the microtubules. The secondary wave of platelet aggregation involves, predominantly, release of the chemical mediators contained within the dense granules. This, then, completes the third major function of platelets, namely the release reaction. Augmentation of the release reaction is facilitated by an increase in intracellular calcium, which produces further activation and release of thromboxane A_2.

Laboratory Tests Used to Assess Platelet Function

Patients experience defects in hemostasis if they either have too few platelets *(thrombocytopenia)* or platelets that function poorly *(thrombopathy)*. The clinical consequences of these platelet defects are small petechial hemorrhages, larger hemorrhages (ecchymoses), or bleeding from mucous membranes, the gastrointestinal tract, and also bleeding from venipuncture sites. Thrombocytopenia occurs a great deal more often than the thrombopathia. Causes of thrombocytopenia are discussed in Chapter 6. Table 5–1 is a list of normal values for platelet studies.

Platelet Count

The quickest and simplest, but least accurate, way to assess platelet number is to examine a stained blood film. This approach has the advantage of revealing platelet size and morphology, but the disadvantage that adherence to glass or uneven distribution within the smear can produce marked differences in the apparent degree of platelet concentration. A rule of thumb is that the platelet count is adequate if the smear contains one platelet per twenty red cells, or two–three platelets per oil immersion field.

Manual Platelet Count

The best manual counting method uses phase-contrast microscopy on a sample diluted 1:100 in ammonium oxalate. If the platelet count is known to be low, a lower dilution factor can be used. The major causes of error, besides technical conditions or inaccurate dilution, are inadequate mixing and the occurrence of adherence or aggregation. Very few platelets are seen and counted, and the total count is extrapolated from this initial data.

Electronic Counting

Several automated cell counters are able to directly measure platelet counts in addition to white cell counts and red cell values. Most of these use an ethylene diaminetetracetic acid (EDTA) blood sample. Most electronic counters count red cells and platelets together; however, they are differentiated on the basis of size. The smaller particles are counted as platelets and the larger particles are counted as red cells. With electronic particle counting, larger numbers of platelets are examined. This technique is subject to error if the white cell count is over 100,000/μl, if there is severe red cell fragmentation, if the diluting fluid contains extraneous particles, if the plasma sample settles too long during processing, or if platelets stick to one another.

Interpretation

Normal platelet counts are between 150,000 and 450,000/μl. The mean is about 250,000/μl. The blood must be drawn briskly through a clean, nontraumatic venipuncture, and it must be mixed promptly and adequately with anticoagulant. If the coagulation sequence is even minimally activated, platelet clumps occur and may adhere to the walls of the test tube. Excessive agitation should be avoided because this, too, causes adherence. A properly drawn specimen mixed with EDTA and kept at room temperature retains a stable platelet count for as long as 12 hours.

Clot Retraction

When blood first clots in the test tube, the entire column of blood solidifies. As time passes, the clot diminishes in size. Fluid (serum) is expressed, and only the red cells remain enmeshed in the shrunken fibrin mass. Platelets are necessary for the fibrin clot to retract and for serum to be expressed.

The speed and extent of clot retraction indicate roughly the degree of platelet adequacy. A normal clot, gently separated from the side of the tube and incubated at 37°C, shrinks to about one half its original size in an hour. The result is a firm, cylindrical fibrin clot that contains all the red blood cells and is sharply demarcated from the clear serum above. Patients with thrombocytopenia or abnormally functioning platelets have samples with scant serum and a soft, plump, poorly demarcated clot.

Clot retraction is a simple test that can be performed repeatedly by individuals without special technical training. Certain constraints are, however, present; if the patient has a low hematocrit, there is more abundant serum, and patients with polycythemia have poor clot retraction because the large numbers of captured red cells interfere with platelet contraction. If fibrinogen levels are low, the initial clot is fragile. If fibrinolysis is present because of markedly reduced fibrinogen levels, the incubated tube contains only cells and plasma, with no fibrin clot at all. If platelet activity is inhibited by drugs or antibodies, clot retraction is markedly diminished.

Platelet Aggregation

Platelet aggregation can be measured by bringing platelet-rich plasma into contact with known aggregation inducers. Most inducers such as collagen, epinephrine, and thrombin act through the effects of ADP that the platelets themselves release. Adding exogenous ADP causes aggregation directly. Aggregation is quantitated by determining whether turbid, platelet-rich plasma becomes clear as evenly suspended platelets aggregate and fall to the bottom of the tube. Aggregometers are spectrophotometers adapted to record changes in light transmission while maintaining constant temperature and gentle agitation of the platelet suspension.

After a normal curve of light transmission is obtained, the test platelets can be exposed to the various agents and to various conditions. Aspirin, other anti-inflammatory agents, and many phenothiazines markedly inhibit the aggregating ability of collagen and epinephrine, but do not interfere with the direct action of ADP. Constitutional disorders of platelet function differ from one another in the nature of the agents that fail to elicit aggregation. It is essential that patients suspected of these disorders abstain from all medications for at least a week before testing.

In performance of the tests, it is important that a clean (nontraumatic) venipuncture be obtained. The number of platelets used in the test must be standardized, since aggregation responses may vary with the platelet count. Consequently, patients with thrombocytopenia are difficult to evaluate. Aggregation studies should be performed within three hours of the sample collection. The samples must never be refrigerated, since this inhibits platelet function, and the test is consequently performed at 37°C. The anticoagulant used is sodium citrate, and the samples must never be collected in glass because this activates platelets. Hemolyzed and lipemic samples cannot be used because this may interfere with the interpretation of optical density.

Interpretation

The most commonly induced aggregating agents are ADP in varying concentrations, collagen, epinephrine, and ristocetin.

Low concentrations of *ADP* induce a biphasic aggregation containing a primary and a secondary wave (see Fig. 5–3). High concentrations of ADP induce only a single wave of aggregation. Patients with platelet release disorders fail to show a secondary wave of aggregation. Patients with Glanzman's thrombasthenia fail to aggregate to ADP at all.

Aggregation with *collagen* produces a latent period followed by a single wave of aggregation (see Fig. 5–3). Decreased aggregation to collagen occurs in patients taking aspirin and anti-inflammatory drugs.

Aggregation with *epinephrine* is usually biphasic. Epinephrine-induced aggregation is also defective in patients taking aspirin and anti-inflammatory agents (see Fig. 5–3). Similarly, *thrombin* aggregation is also biphasic and may be defective in certain intrinsic platelet defects.

The aggregation response produced by the antibiotic reagent *ristocetin* is normally monophasic. In patients with von Willebrand's disease, the platelets respond normally to epinephrine, collagen, and ADP, but fail to respond to ristocetin. Their platelets are normal; however, it is the plasma that fails to contain the von Willebrand factor (vWF). As mentioned previously, this factor is essential in encouraging platelet–vessel wall interaction. In the quantitative assay for vWF, the patient's plasma is compared against graduated dilutions of normal plasma by measuring ristocetin-induced aggregation of formalin-fixed platelets suspended in the different concentrates. Abnormal ristocetin-induced platelet aggregation may also occur in other disorders, in particular *Bernard-Soulier syndrome.* Correction of abnormal ristocetin aggregation in von Willebrand's disease can be induced by the addition of normal plasma, which provides the vWF.

Although congenital defects in platelet function are rare, many acquired conditions depress the release mechanisms. *Aspirin* is undoubtedly the commonest etiologic agent, but few patients develop severe enough bleeding that platelet testing becomes necessary. Patients with *uremia, severe liver disease,* or *advanced alcohol-related conditions* often develop a complex bleeding disorder that includes platelet dysfunction. These three conditions depress the release-inducing effect of collagen, epinephrine, or exogenous ADP added directly. *Myeloproliferative disorders* and *dysproteinemias* may create a similar problem.

Other Tests of Platelet Function

Platelet Retention

The quantitative determination of the number of platelets that adhere to glass beads can be determined. Platelet retention is abnormal in von Willebrand's disease and other rare, hereditary disorders. It is also abnormal in some acquired disorders, including myeloproliferative syndromes. This test is rarely performed these days.

Beta-Thromboglobulin and Platelet Factor IV

The assay of certain products of platelet release such as beta-thromboglobulin, platelet factor III, platelet factor IV, and prostaglandin intermediates can also be determined. These generally reflect increasing platelet sequestration and turnover, and have been used as tests that are predictive of intravascular coagulation or hypercoagulability. These will be discussed in the section on hypercoagulability.

Bleeding Time

The single best indication of functional platelet deficiency is prolonged bleeding after a controlled, superficial injury. The bleeding time is prolonged in *thrombocytopenia* of any cause, in *von Willebrand's disease,* in most *dysfunctional conditions,* and after *aspirin ingestion.* The bleeding time test is somewhat difficult to standardize and to use repeatedly for the evaluation of changing clinical conditions. Every operator performs it differently. The nature of the "standard" injury differs each time it is inflicted, and the results differ with different skin sites and external conditions. In addition, it is unpleasant for patients to be subjected to a standard skin incision time after time. Some patients may also exhibit excess scar tissue formation.

General Techniques and Interpretation. Capillaries subjected to a small, clean incision bleed until the defect is plugged by aggregating platelets. If blood accumulates over the incision, coagulation occurs and the overlying fibrin prevents additional bleeding. Welling blood must be removed, but gently so as not to disrupt the fragile platelet plug. After the incision is made, oozing blood is removed at 15-

second intervals by touching filter paper to the drop of blood without touching the wound itself. As platelets accumulate, bleeding slows and the oozing drop of blood gets smaller. The endpoint occurs when there is no fluid blood left to produce a spot on the filter paper. Some variation is inevitable; results of duplicate tests performed on the same individual should agree within two to three minutes at most.

The bleeding time is prolonged when platelet counts fall below 100,000/μl. Aspirin prevents platelet aggregation and prolongs the bleeding time for as long as five days after a single dose of 300 mg. Patients should be warned not to take aspirin or any over-the-counter pain remedies for five days before the test is scheduled. Congenital absence of fibrinogen and hereditary coagulation defects do not prolong the bleeding time, but acquired fibrinogen problems do. Bleeding time may be less prolonged than expected in some thrombocytopenic patients if all their circulating platelets are young, since young platelets have enhanced hemostatic capabilities. Such a condition may occur in sequestrative disorders associated with increased destruction, such as immune thrombocytopenic purpura (ITP).

IVY and Template Techniques. The bleeding time test is best done on the volar surface of the forearm, a site that is readily accessible, has a reasonably uniform superficial blood supply, is relatively insensitive to pain, and can easily be subjected to mildly increased hydrostatic pressure. The incision should be made at a cleansed site that is free of skin disease, and away from obvious underlying veins. A constant pressure of 40 mmHg should be applied throughout the test. In the IVY technique, incisions 3 mm deep are made freehand with the blood lancet. With the template method, it is possible to achieve a reproducible, precise incision every time. A normal IVY bleeding time is *3–6 minutes.* A normal template bleeding time is *6–10 minutes.* The Simplate II method is a standardized modification of the template procedure and employs a commercially available device. The device is disposable and makes a uniform incision in the forearm. The incision is 5 mm long and 1 mm deep. Bleeding time values of greater than 15 minutes in the absence of a low platelet count indicate a qualitative platelet disorder that needs further investigation (e.g., aggregation studies or factor VIII von Willebrand assay).

Following the activation of platelets and the release of platelet factor III (platelet phospholipid), activation of the coagulation cascade with formation of thrombin occurs. This sequence involves two major pathways: intrinsic coagulation with contact activation of blood clotting factors initiates the process of clot formation (Fig. 5–5), augmented by the platelet phospholipid factor III. Extrinsic coagulation, which is stimulated by tissue factors released from the damaged tissues, also leads to the development of the clot or thrombus.

Coagulation Cascade

The purpose of the coagulation system is to generate the active serine protease enzyme *thrombin,* which in turn acts selectively on the *soluble* plasma protein *fibrinogen,* converting it into *insoluble fibrin.* Fibrin is the visible end product of coagulation, and is a gelatinous protein easily identified in tissues or test tubes. Conversion of fibrinogen to fibrin is the last step in a highly complex series of protein reactions that are described schematically in Fig. 5–5. Official nomenclature uses Roman numerals to identify the coagulation factors. Some have descriptive or eponymic names as well. Almost all of these factors are present in circulating blood in an inactive, precursor, or zymogen form. The activated form that participates in this sequence is designated by an "a" after the Roman numeral number. Table 5–2 is a list of the coagulation factors and some of their synonyms. Fibrin, in essence,

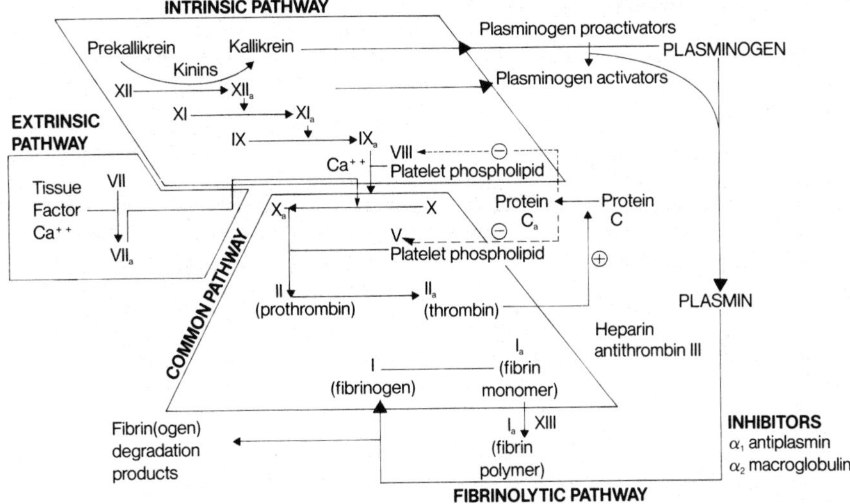

Figure 5–5. Diagram showing interrelationship between coagulation and fibrinolytic pathways.

acts as the cement substance to stabilize the initial primary platelet plug. Thrombin formation can be generated by the intrinsic coagulation pathway or the extrinsic coagulation cascade.

INTRINSIC COAGULATION PATHWAY

Activation of this pathway occurs through "contact" activation of circulating plasma proteins, the *contact coagulation factors* (XI, XII), which become activated by exposure to damaged vascular endothelium, tissue, or foreign surfaces. In an orderly manner, or cascade, the factors are sequentially activated to convert *prothrombin* into *thrombin. Thrombin (II)* preferentially converts *fibrinogen (I)* into *fibrin* through a process of enzymatic cleavage of certain *fibrinopeptides* to produce *fibrin monomer.* The fibrin monomer subsequently polymerizes into an insoluble *polymer,* which is then stabilized into the stable clot.

Contact Activation of Intrinsic Coagulation

An important aspect of the intrinsic coagulation sequence is the activation of the contact coagulation factors, factors XI and XII. Factor XII also serves as a key factor in linking several different physiologic pathways synchronously, as is shown in Fig. 5–5. Therefore, in addition to coagulation activation, humoral factors are released from complement activation which bring neutrophils and other cells to the area to help clean the debris. In addition, *kinins* are activated, and these compounds have very potent effects on smooth muscles that facilitate vessel constriction or dilatation to limit bleeding or to enhance the inflammatory response. Furthermore, the *fibrinolytic pathway* is activated, which is a check system to ensure that coagulation is kept under control through the breakdown or lysis of more extensive clots. Intrinsic coagulation begins when the contact with appropriate surfaces or materials activates *factor XII* (Hageman factor). *In vivo* activators include collagen and other subendothelial vessel wall constituents, and such other activators as gram-negative bacterial endotoxins, cell wall products from gram-positive organisms, fatty acids, and antigen-antibody complexes. In the laboratory, *factor XII* is activated by contact with glass, kaolin, or ellagic acid, but not with silicon or plastic surfaces. Activated *factor XII (factor* XII_a*)*, is assisted by a cofactor called high molecular weight *(HMW) kininogen* (Fitzgerald factor), which converts *prekallikrein* (Fletcher factor) to kallikrein that in turn serves to activate more *factor XII.* This is a self-amplifying system. *Factor XI* is converted to its active form by *factor* XII_a with *HMW kininogen* serving as the cofactor. As was mentioned above, contact activation of *factor XII* and *kallikrein* initiates more than just coagulation. It promotes conversion of plasminogen to the fibrin-dissolving agent *plasmin* (see Fibrinolysis). *Kallikrein* activates *bradykinin,* a vasodilating agent that causes increased vascular permeability and is responsible for acute inflammation. The contact system also initiates parts of the complement sequence (see Chapter 7, Fig. 7–2, p 247). *Kallikrein* may also be involved in the extrinsic coagulation system (see below). Since persons congenitally deficient in *factor XII, Fletcher factor,* or *HMW kininogen* suffer no apparent hemostatic abnormalities or defects in inflammation, the significance of contact activation remains mysterious. Absence of *factor XI,* however, does cause a bleeding disorder.

Activation of Factor X by the Intrinsic Pathway

The role of *factor XI-a* is to activate *factor IX* in a calcium-dependent, enzymatic cleavage. *Factor* IX_a*,* along with platelet factor III released from stimulated platelets, reacts with *factor VIII* to produce *factor X activator complex.* Ionized calcium is required, and thrombin, if present, enhances the process. *Factor* $X\text{-}_a$ and *phospholipid* can, by themselves, activate *factor X,* but *factor VIII* enhances the process a thousandfold. Congenital deficiencies of factor VIII and factor IX are called hemophilia A and B, respectively.

Extrinsic Coagulation Pathway

Products of damaged tissue cause fluid blood to coagulate. *Tissue thromboplastin* is the term used to describe the clot-promoting activity of lipoproteins present in all tissues. Tissue thromboplastin acts on *factor VII,* converting it to VII_a*,* which directly affects *factor X. Factor VII* can undergo activation in the presence of *kallikrein,* a suggestive link with the intrinsic phase of coagulation.

The physiologic significance of the entire extrinsic system is unclear. It seems to be an alternate route of the common goal of factor X activation, but in a clinical sense, the extrinsic and intrinsic pathways are not substitutes for one another. *Factor VII deficiency,* by itself, is very rare, but can cause severe bleeding. The hemorrhagic diathesis of *factor VIII* and *factor IX deficiency,* however, is far more severe.

In the laboratory, factor X can also be activated by exposure to the Russell Viper snake venom or to trypsin. This appears to be a direct proteolytic cleavage that does not require the presence of factor VII.

The Common Pathway

Both the intrinsic and extrinsic pathways converge to form the "common" pathway, which ultimately activates the plasma protein *prothrombin (II)* into its active form, *thrombin* *(*II_a*)*. Activation of *factor X* initiates the terminal phase of coagulation and, as described, can be activated by both intrinsic and extrinsic coagulation. The reaction of *factor* $X\text{-}_a$ with *prothrombin* requires *calcium ions* and *phospholipid* and is markedly enhanced by association with another plasma protein, *factor V.*

Thrombin is a proteolytic enzyme of tremendous potency and relatively little discrimination. The quantity of thrombin that evolves from a single milliliter of plasma, if released simultaneously throughout the circulation, could solidify the entire bloodstream. Under normal hemostatic conditions, only small amounts of thrombin develop at a time. Besides converting *fibrinogen* to *fibrin,* thrombin also enhances platelet release reactions as described above, and augments the activation of *factor V* and *factor VIII.* Under pathologic conditions, *thrombin* can cleave *fibrinogen* into *fragments* and split the peptide bonds in a wide range of other proteins.

Fibrinogen becomes *fibrin* when *thrombin* removes the tips of two pairs of peptide chains, releasing *fibrinopeptides A and B.* The resulting molecule, which consists of 97% of the original molecule, is *fibrin monomer. Fibrin monomer* polymerizes spontaneously to form a loosely adherent gel that quickly depolymerizes if exposed in the laboratory to 5M urea solution or a 1% monochloroacetic acid solution. *In vivo,* the fibrin monomer constitutes a bulky but fragile clot. Irreversible polymerization occurs when activated *factor XIII* causes the peptide bonds to cross-link. Thrombin is also responsible for activating *factor XIII.* Table 5–2 lists the properties of the various clotting factors.

The Clotting Factors

Table 5–2 shows the nomenclature of coagulation factors.

Factor I, always called *fibrinogen,* is a glycoprotein of 340,000 daltons and is composed of three pairs of polypeptide chains. Synthesized in the liver, it has a half-life of about 3.5–4 days. Fibrinogen levels increase with hemostatic stress, and also with nonspecific stresses such as inflammation, pregnancy, and autoimmune diseases. Normal plasma concentration is 150–400 mg/dl.

Factor II is usually called *prothrombin,* and is a glycoprotein with a molecular weight of 70,000 daltons. It is closely related to factors VII, IX, and X, and together they are called the vitamin K-dependent factors. They are all manufactured in the liver and require fat-soluble vitamin K for synthesis. All four of these "liver factors" are heat-stable, retain their potency in stored blood or plasma and remain present in serum after the plasma has clotted. Prothrombin has a half-life of 0.5–3 days.

Factor III is more usually termed *tissue thromboplastin,* and the numerical designation is never used. The clot-promoting activity of tissue products is too poorly characterized to be described as a specific factor. The most active tissues are brain, lung, and placenta, but all tissues have this clot-promoting activity.

Factor IV, or *ionized calcium,* is necessary for activation of factor IX, factor X for conversion of prothrombin to thrombin by X_a and for polymerization of fibrin monomers. There must be at least 2.5 mg/dl of calcium before coagulation can occur *in vivo* or *in vitro.* Hypocalcemia never causes clinical bleeding difficulties, because more profound neurologic, hemodynamic, and cardiac arrhythmia occur well before clotting is disturbed. Anticoagulants such as citrate, oxalate, and ethylene diaminetetraacetic acid (EDTA) chelate calcium and anticoagulate blood by making calcium unavailable for participation in coagulation.

Factor V, also known as proaccelerin and *labile factor,* is a poorly characterized protein that is synthesized in the liver and may be low in patients with liver disease. Its activity disappears rapidly when anticoagulated blood or plasma is stored in the liquid state. It also disappears rapidly from the circulating blood and has a half-life of only 15–25 hours.

Factor VI: this term is not used.

Factor VII is variously called proconvertin, auto-prothrombin I, serum prothrombin conversion accelerator, and SPCA. The multiplicity of synonyms reflects uncertainty about its structure, origin, and function. Factor VII is usually referred to by number, has the shortest half-life of all coagulation factors (five hours), and is one of the vitamin K-dependent liver factors. It is the first clotting factor to decline after administration of vitamin K antagonists such as oral anticoagulants.

Factor VIII, also known as *anti-hemophilic factor (AHF)* is a large molecule that has several physiologic functions. *Procoagulant activity (VIII HF or VIIIC)* resides on a low-molecular-weight fragment determined by a gene on the X-chromosome. This factor is capable of normalizing the clotting time of Hemophilia A patients, and this activity is found on a 200,000-dalton molecular weight molecule in plasma. Males whose single X-chromosome carries a defective VIII;AHF gene suffer from Hemophilia A. Factor VIII refers to the procoagulant protein that corrects the coagulation abnormality in hemophilia A. This is sometimes referred to as VIII:C. Von Willebrand's factor (vWF) is the factor that corrects the bleeding time defect in von Willebrand's disease. vWF and factor VIII are two distinct proteins that circulate as a complex in plasma. The antigenic expression of the vWF is now called vWF:Ag but was previously referred to as VIIIR:Ag. Another property of vWF that promotes aggregation of platelets in the presence of the antibiotic ristocetin is called the ristocetin co-factor or vWF activity (previously referred to as VIIIR:RCo). Quantitative and qualitative abnormalities of vWF as seen in von Willebrand's disease are inherited in an autosomal manner. Factor VIII is one of the few clotting proteins not synthesized by the liver, and appears to be synthesized by endothelial cells in all tissue. Factor VIII has a short biologic half-life of approximately 12 hours, and disappears fairly rapidly from plasma stored at refrigerated temperatures. It is present in high concentrations in the cryoprecipitate fraction of plasma (see Transfusion Medicine section, Chapter 8).

Factor IX, also called *Christmas Factor,* plasma thromboplastin component, and PTC, is another vitamin K-dependent liver factor. Unlike factors II, VII, and X, factor IX deficiency exists as an isolated constitutional defect. The disease *Hemophilia B,* or *Christmas disease,* closely resembles Factor VIII deficiency (Hemophilia A) in clinical and laboratory aspects. The factor has a physiologic half-life of about 24 hours, but remains at high levels in stored liquid plasma. It is also present in serum. The molecular weight of the protein has been estimated at between 56,000–110,000 daltons.

Factor X, also called Stuart Factor or *Stuart-Prower Factor,* is another of the vitamin K-dependent liver factors and is the key protein in all activation pathways. Isolated congenital deficiency does occur, though rarely, causing moderately severe clinical bleeding. It also exists as an acquired deficiency in *amyloidosis.* This factor has a biologic half-life of about 40 hours.

Factor XI, also called *plasma thromboplastin antecedent* or *PTA,* is probably synthesized in the liver. This factor does not diminish in liver disease, however, and is not vitamin K-dependent. It is stable in stored blood or plasma, and is present in serum. Isolated deficiency occurs as an autosomal recessive trait. After factor VIII and factor IX deficiencies, it is the next most common congenital deficiency state, but the bleeding diathesis is rather mild. Biologic half-life is about two days.

Factor XII is commonly called *Hageman Factor* and has a molecular weight of between 20,000–100,000 daltons. It may, therefore, exist as subunits in human plasma. It appears to be one of the link coagulation factors between several physiologic pathways, including contact activation of clotting, activation of the kinin pathway, activation of complement, and activation of fibrinolysis. Its ability to activate factor XI is enhanced by two other factors, namely *Fletcher Factor* and *high molecular weight kininogen.* Deficiency of Hageman Factor is paradoxically not associated with substantial hemostatic problems, but more usually with a thromboembolic tendency. The half-life of Hageman Factor is 60–70 hours.

Factor XIII is also called *fibrin stabilizing factor,* or *FSF,* and stabilizes the conversion of fibrin monomer to polymerized fibrin and a stable clot. It appears to be synthesized in both the liver and the megakaryocytes, and more than half of blood factor XIII exists in platelets. Factor XIII has a long biologic half-life (5–10 days), but disappears when plasma is converted to serum.

Comparisons Between Plasma and Serum

Plasma is the liquid part of fluid blood. Outside the vascular system, blood can be kept fluid by either removing fibrinogen or by adding anticoagulants, most of which prevent coagulation by chelating or removing calcium ions. *Citrate, oxalate, and EDTA* are anticoagulants of the *chelating category. Heparin* prevents coagulation by directly *inhibiting thrombin;* it prevents the conversion of fibrinogen to fibrin by augmenting a natural anticoagulant molecule, *anti-thrombin III (ATIII)* to neutralize thrombin. Heparin fails to influence the calcium concentration in its anticoagulant effect. Freshly drawn plasma contains all the proteins present in circulating blood; as plasma is stored, however, factor V and factor VIII activity gradually declines.

Serum is the fluid remaining after blood coagulates. Coagulation converts all fibrinogen into solid fibrin and consumes factor VIII, factor V, and prothrombin in the process. The other coagulation proteins and proteins, not related to hemostasis, remain in serum at the same levels as plasma. Normal serum lacks fibrinogen, prothrombin, factor VIII, factor V, and factor XIII, but contains factors XII, XI, X, IX, and VII. If the coagulation process proceeds abnormally, serum may contain residual fibrinogen and fibrinogen cleavage products for unconverted prothrombin.

Absorbing plasma with barium sulfate or aluminum hydroxide removes the vitamin K-dependent "liver factors" (i.e., factors II, VII, IX and X). Barium-absorbed plasma contains fibrinogen, factor XIII, the labile factors VIII and V, and factors XI and XII. It does not coagulate because prothrombin and factor X are absent, as are factors VII (which is needed for extrinsic activation) and factor IX (which is needed for intrinsic activation). Factors XII and XI (contact factors) are stable in stored plasma, are not adsorbed by barium, and are not consumed in the coagulation process.

Antagonists of Hemostasis (Natural Anticoagulant Mechanisms)

Both platelet activation and coagulation are self-perpetuating processes. If coagulation proceeds unchecked, then massive intravascular coagulation would occur, producing massive impedance of blood flow. The circulatory system has natural mechanisms preventing disseminated coagulation and keeping local hemostasis in check. Local conditions of platelet activation and fibrin deposition dissipate if newly entering blood dilutes activated coagulation factors or disperses aggregated platelets. Partially activated coagulation factors are carried to the liver and reticuloendothelial system, where they are degraded. Briskly flowing blood also brings in antagonists to specific coagulation products and other mechanisms that facilitate the ultimate breakdown of a clot, once wound healing has occurred, and reestablish blood flow.

Fibrinolysis is the mechanism that dissolves unwanted clots, reestablishes blood flow, and keeps coagulation in check. It is one of the main natural anticoagulant systems. In addition, there are specific inhibitors to activated products of coagulation, and indeed inhibitors checking fibrinolysis that are important in keeping clot propagation and clot reduction in fine-tuned balance.

FIBRINOLYSIS

Concomitant with the activation of coagulation is activation of one of the natural anticoagulant defense mechanisms, namely the *fibrinolytic system.* This system is also a multi-component enzyme system that results in the generation of the active enzyme *plasmin.* Plasmin's function is to remove the fibrin clot by digesting fibrin into small fragments or degradation products (fibrin degradation products or FDP's). In this way, fibrinolysis enzymatically regulates the formation of fibrin as it is occurring in the site of fibrin deposition. It is, in this sense, an extremely integral part of normal hemostasis. Plasmin has a very high affinity for both fibrinogen and fibrin. Generation of plasmin occurs from the inactive plasma protein *plasminogen,* and this process is initiated by means of *plasminogen activators.* Stimulation of these activators can occur by activated Hageman Factor (factor XII_a) in the coagulation system, kallikrein and other plasminogen activators released by various tissues. A specific *tissue plasminogen activator (TPA)* released at the site of blood vessel damage is probably the most important activator, converting plasminogen to plasmin within the fibrin clot at the site of injury. This activator has an extremely high affinity for fibrin and not fibrinogen; therefore localizing the activation of fibrinolysis within the clot and not within the circulating fluid blood. Normal plasma contains 10–20 mg/dl of the precursor substance plasminogen. Plasminogen is converted to plasmin by other plasminogen activators, including *urokinase* and *streptokinase.* Urokinase is an activator that has full activity at the time it enters the circulation. It is an enzyme that is released from tissues of the genitourinary tract. Streptokinase is a streptococcal product that has plasminogen-activating capability. Urokinase and streptokinase have been used therapeutically to activate plasminogen to plasmin in an attempt to dissolve clots. The problem with these two compounds is that they are nonselective and their activity is widespread, producing fibrinolysis and breakdown of fibrinogen throughout the vascular system. There is much excitement on the therapeutic use of TPA in dissolving thrombi, since its affinity for the fibrin is more specific.

For normal hemostasis to be accomplished, a delicate and dynamic balance between the coagulation cascade and the fibrinolytic pathway needs to be maintained. Once generated, plasmin exerts rather indiscriminate proteolytic activity. Besides digesting fibrin, it also cleaves fibrinogen into peptide fragments that are incoagulable and prevent coagulation of normal fibrinogen. Plasmin also degrades factor VIII, factor V, and factor XIII. Normally, very little plasmin accumulates. Plasma contains two agents that neutralize plasmin: a rapidly acting *antiplasmin* and a slower-acting antagonist called *alpha-2 macroglobulin.* Under physiologic conditions, plasmin is protected from these antagonists because it is sheltered by its proximity to fibrin.

Plasminogen adsorbs to fibrin as fibrin deposits. Bound plasminogen is gradually activated by contact endothelial elements, a process that under normal conditions generates just the right amount of plasmin to prevent excessive fibrin accumulation. Excessive accumulation of activated plasmin can cause proteolysis directed locally at proteins other than fibrin. Systemic activation of plasmin may also occur, or plasmin antagonists may be exhausted. The section on disseminated intravascular coagulation discusses some of these consequences (see Chapter 6).

Three main *natural anticoagulant mechanisms* exist. Firstly, the *fibrinolytic system* that was discussed above is important in keeping the coagulation process localized and in dissolving clots that are formed. Two additional specific anticoagulant systems exist to keep blood in a fluid state. There are many checks and balances in the coagulation and fibrinolytic systems that prevent unnatural activation of either of these processes, and the specific inhibitors exist to limit the activated coagulation factors from proceeding in an unregulated manner. The most important specific anticoagulant inhibitor is *antithrombin III.*

Antithrombin III

Antithrombin III (ATIII) is a serine protease inhibitor that preferentially binds thrombin as well as some other serine proteases within the coagulation cascade, and neutralizes their activity. The ability of antithrombin III to neutralize thrombin's activity is rapidly enhanced by the presence of heparin. Antithrombin III inhibits serine proteases because it has an arginine that reacts preferentially with protease before it can act on other proteins. Antithrombin III abolishes activity not only of thrombin, but also of plasmin and activated factors X, XI, and XII. Another name for the antithrombin III is *heparin cofactor.* Heparin augments a hundredfold the affinity between ATIII and the serine protease enzymes. Patients whose blood lacks ATIII derive no therapeutic benefit from heparin. Naturally occurring heparinoid substances exist in the body that are probably released from the vascular endothelium. The heparin antithrombin III complex will rapidly neutralize any thrombin that is generated by activation of the coagulation cascade. Antithrombin III is formed in the liver and therefore can be depleted both as a result of *liver disease* and consumptive disorders such as *disseminated intravascular coagulation. Inherited deficiency of antithrombin III* can also occur, in which individuals are prone to intravenous thromboembolism (see Hypercoagulable States). Lysis of platelets releases platelet factor IV, which inhibits ATIII activity.

Protein C and Protein S

A third very recently discovered natural anticoagulant system is, strangely enough, dependent on vitamin K for its action. The action of vitamin K on these specific proteins, termed protein C and protein S, which work in unison, is different from vitamin K's activity on the vitamin K-dependent coagulation factors II, VII, IX, and X.

Protein C, like the vitamin K-dependent coagulation factors, is also a vitamin K-dependent polypeptide manufactured by the liver and circulates in its inactive form. Activation of coagulation, and specifically activation of prothrombin to form thrombin, facilitates protein C's conversion into its active form, protein C_a. This process is also modulated by an additional substance produced by the blood vessel termed *thrombomodulin,* which may help focus the neutralization at the site of vascular injury. Protein C's action as an anticoagulant is due to its rapid neutralizing activity of factors VIII_a and V_a. Protein S accelerates the inactivation of V_a and VIII_a by protein C. It is also possible that protein C may, through an interrelated pathway, activate fibrinolysis.

It therefore can be seen that there is a dynamic relationship between coagulation on the one hand and fibrinolysis on the other, with numerous interconnections both augmenting and neutralizing the respective pathways (see Fig. 5–5). This delicate balance can be altered by deficiencies of the various factors, and the clinical syndromes so produced may manifest either as hemostatic disorders or as thrombotic disorders. These will be discussed in the section dealing with disorders of hemostasis (Chapter 6).

Tests of the Coagulation System

Only the tests in common usage in the clinical laboratory will be discussed in this section. There are, however, multiple other tests of coagulation function using more sophisticated substrates that are available in reference laboratories. Table 5–3 shows the normal values for coagulation studies.

Lee-White Clotting Time

The oldest but least accurate test of coagulation is to measure how long it takes for blood to clot in a test tube. The Lee-White clotting time employs three tubes incubated at 37°C, each containing 1 ml of whole blood. These are gently tilted at 30-second intervals to enhance the contact between the blood and the glass surface to see when clotting occurs. Normal blood clots firmly within *4–8 minutes.*

Interpretation

This test is extremely insensitive. It was formerly a test to monitor heparin therapy, which prolongs the clotting time. When used as a test of heparin monitoring, the clotting time should be prolonged to double its baseline.

Activated Coagulation Time (ACT)

Some centers have found that adding *Celite,* a finely divided clay, shortens the whole blood clotting time, reduces test variability, and allows more precise correlations between heparin dosage and laboratory results. Normal blood clots in less than *100 seconds* when added to a tube containing *Celite.* With *heparin,* the goal is to achieve an *ACT of 300–600 seconds.* The ACT has found greatest use in monitoring

Table 5–3. NORMAL VALUES FOR COAGULATION STUDIES

Clotting time, Lee-White	4–8 min
Activated coagulation time (celite)	<100 sec
Prothrombin time (PT)	11–13 sec or within 2 sec of control
Partial thromboplastin time (PTT)	60–85 sec
Activated partial thromboplastin time (aPTT)	30–40 sec or within 5 sec of control
Thrombin clotting time (TCT)	10–15 sec or within 1.3 times as long as control
Fibrinogen	150–450 mg/dl
Clot dissolution (5-M urea)	Clot intact at 1 hr, 24 hr
Euglobulin lysis	Lysis in 2–6 hrs
Fibrinogen degradation products	
Latex particles	<20 μg/ml
Tanned red cells	<5 μg/ml
Antithrombin III	
Coagulation assay	≥50% of normal pool
Spectrophotometric	85–125% of normal pool

heparin therapy during extracorporeal circulation such as hemodialysis and hemapheresis. Repeated bedside determinations can be correlated with the patient's clinical status, and heparin or its antagonist (protamine) given to induce desired changes in direction. The ACT is less suitable for intermittent checks in heparin dosage, partly because it must be done immediately after the blood is drawn and therefore cannot be done on specimens submitted to a central laboratory. Many laboratories have found the activated partial thromboplastin time (see below) to be the most satisfactory test for hospital-wide monitoring of heparin therapy.

Partial Thromboplastin Time (PTT)

This test is performed on a specimen of *citrated blood.* The plasma is removed and placed in a sample tube, where it is recalcified, and a reagent containing surface-active *factors such as kaolin and phospholipid* is added. The kaolin enhances the speed of contact activation, the phospholipid provides a surface on which the coagulation enzyme substrate reactions can occur (see diagram), and the *calcium* replaces the calcium chelated by the citrate. The time taken for a clot to form represents the partial thromboplastin time (PTT). The *normal "activated" PTT varies from 28–40 seconds.* The test may be done manually; however, it is more usually evaluated using automated instruments that dispense the respective reagents. The PTT assesses the *intrinsic coagulation and common coagulation pathway.* If intrinsic coagulation is not enhanced by an activated compound, following the addition of the "partial thromboplastin" reagent and ionized calcium, the normal PTT is 60–85 seconds. This test measures the presence of factors VIII, IX, XI, and XII, which must all be present, at adequate levels, to have a normal partial thromboplastin time. In addition, factors X, V, prothrombin, and fibrinogen must also be present. Factor VII is not required for the PTT because the test bypasses the extrinsic system. The PTT is more sensitive in detecting minor deficiencies of the common pathway than is the prothrombin time (see below). As a general rule, factor levels below 30% of normal prolong the PTT. In general, the activated partial thromboplastin time is usually used, since it is more reproducible than the unmodified PTT and just as sensitive in detecting minimal deficiencies.

Prothrombin Time (PT)

Reagents for the prothrombin time (PT) are *tissue thromboplastin and ionized calcium.* When added to *citrated plasma,* these substitute for the extrinsic coagulation pathway to activate factor X directly without involving platelets or the procoagulants of the intrinsic pathway (see Fig. 5–5). To get a normal prothrombin time result, plasma must have at least 100 mg/dl of fibrinogen and adequate levels of factors VII, X, V, and prothrombin.

Brain extract is the tissue most often used as the tissue thromboplastin reagent that is standardized to elicit a firm fibrin clot in the *normal time of 11–13 seconds.* Test results are sometimes given as "percent" of normal activity, comparing the patient's result against a standardized curve that shows the prothrombin time occurring with plasma dilutions. Percent results have little clinical value, since dilution affects all the coagulation proteins and also changes the ionic composition. Sometimes a percentage activity is given where the patient result is expressed as a percentage activity of the normal result standardized to 100%. Prolongation of the PT occurs in patients whose plasma contains normal levels of most factors but lacks only a few specific factors. It is far preferable to report PT results as the actual time in seconds and also to give a normal or control value in seconds.

Thrombin Clotting Time (TCT)

This test measures the time taken for a citrated blood specimen to clot after calcium and a known amount of thrombin are added. The test consequently evaluates thrombin–fibrinogen interaction in that it bypasses both the extrinsic and intrinsic pathways and assesses the terminal steps of the common pathway. Consequently, the thrombin time may be prolonged if there is deficiency of fibrinogen or if there are circulating anticoagulants that are active and interfering with thrombin's action, such as heparin. Abnormal fibrinogen or abnormalities of the fibrinogen molecule may also be evaluated using this test.

Thrombin-induced clotting is very rapid, and the test result can be standardized to any desired normal, usually between 10–15 seconds. The TCT is prolonged if fibrinogen levels are below 100 mg/dl. In all the conditions that substantially prolong the TCT, the PT and PTT are prolonged as well. Fibrinogen deficiency can be distinguished from inhibitory conditions by adding small volumes of normal plasma to the patient's plasma and repeating the TCT.

Fibrinogen Titer

It is possible to estimate plasma fibrinogen levels by performing the TCT on serial dilutions of plasma. If the initial fibrinogen level is more than 100 mg/dl, thrombin produces a firm, visible clot after incubation with plasma diluted 1:32. With normal plasma, a good clot develops at dilutions of 1:64 or 1:128. Plasma that is significantly deficient in fibrinogen may clot after 15 seconds of incubation, but cannot clot following 1:2 or 1:4 dilution. This semiquantitative approach can be useful for quick estimation when quantitative tests are not available. More accurate and reasonably rapid tests for fibrinogen have superseded this procedure in most laboratories.

Fibrinogen Measurement

Fibrinogen is unique to plasma. After clotting has occurred, serum should contain no residual fibrinogen. To measure plasma fibrinogen, it is necessary to make one of several assumptions. *Classic procedures* depend on the assumption that adding thrombin will convert all the available fibrinogen to fibrin. What is actually measured is the amount of protein in the resulting clot; the quantity of precursor fibrinogen is extrapolated from this value. In *immunologic techniques,* the assumption is that the plasma constituent that reacts with anti-fibrinogen antibodies is indeed fibrinogen. Plasma levels are determined by comparing plasma reactivity against a curve derived from known fibrinogen concentrations. *Heat precipitation tests* proceed on the comparable assumption that all the material responsive to the precipitation technique really is fibrinogen.

Measuring protein in a precipitate or a clot gives an objective, quantitative result, but the techniques are time-consuming and require experienced, careful performance. Immunologic techniques in which anti-fibrinogen antibodies are adsorbed to inert indicator particles use visible agglutination or immunoprecipitation as the endpoint, and quantitation depends on the results observed with successively diluted samples. Reliability depends on the purity of the antibody and the accuracy of the original standardization done by the manufacturer of the kit. The test is quick and easy, but the user is entirely dependent on the quality of the kit.

Depletion of fibrinogen may occur in situations where there is decreased synthesis, as may occur in *liver disease;* however, this is uncommon. The other major reason for fibrinogen depletion is consumption of fibrinogen, which may occur in *intravascular coagulation or in the activation of fibrinolysis.*

Interpretation of PT and/or PTT Prolongations

It is possible to infer which factors are deficient by comparing the PT with the PTT result. A normal PT with a prolonged PTT points to factors VIII, IX, XI, and XII, or to von Willebrand's disease (abnormality of the intrinsic pathway). Fletcher Factor deficiency causes a prolonged PTT that reverts to normal if plasma is incubated with kaolin for ten minutes. A normal PTT with a prolonged PT occurs only with factor VII deficiency. Congenital isolated deficiency of factor VII is extremely rare, but the combination of a normal PTT and prolonged PT occurs fairly often in patients with liver disease or who are on vitamin K inhibitory anticoagulant factors such as warfarin. This is because factor VII has such a short half-life that it is the first of the liver factors to decline when hepatic synthesis falters. As warfarin dosage is changed or as hepatic disease is first developing, factor VII may be the only liver factor to decline significantly.

Both the PT and PTT are prolonged with severe liver disease or established warfarin therapy. Prolongation of both tests also occurs with disorders of factors V, X, or prothrombin; with acquired complex deficiencies, or inhibitors. With high heparin levels or with congenital or acquired fibrinogen defects and the resulting high levels of fibrin degradation products [(FDP) see also p 202], the PT and PTT are usually prolonged together. Neither test measures factor XIII activity. On a more practical level, the PTT is used to follow patients on heparin therapy and the PT is used to follow those taking warfarin treatment.

Mixing Studies

After a tentative diagnosis has been reached by observing abnormal screening results, presumptive confirmation is possible by adding different agents to the patient's plasma to see what corrects the abnormality. The usual diagnostic dilemma lies in separating factor VIII deficiency from factor IX deficiency. The clinical findings are indistinguishable: Both have prolonged PTT with normal PT, both occur in males with sex-linked inheritance pattern, and both are relatively common in the general population.

Normal serum contains levels of factors VII, IX, X, XI, and XII that are virtually equal to those of plasma, but lacks factors V, VIII, fibrinogen, and prothrombin. Fresh plasma containing all the clotting factors but factors II, VII, IX, and X can be prepared by adsorbing the plasma with barium sulfate or aluminum hydroxide. Absorbed plasma contains factors V, VIII, XI, and XII and fibrinogen. After the patient is known to have an abnormal PT or PTT, or both, the laboratory can repeat such tests on a mixture of the patient's plasma and added materials that contain clotting factors. In addition, the mixing studies can also determine whether there is a specific factor deficiency present, or whether there is a circulating inhibitor. When an inhibitor is present, mixing normal plasma with the patient's plasma fails to correct the apparent deficiency. In addition, patient's plasma may prolong the normal PT or PTT of normal plasma, indicating that inhibitor is present. Specific inhibitors can be determined by mixing studies—again using a specific plasma factor as the replacement and then mixing.

Factor Assays

Assays for specific factor levels require both a high degree of technical expertise and, often, a bank of frozen rare plasma. Factor assays are used to discriminate among mild, moderate, and severe deficiency patterns and to follow the course of a defined factor inhibitor. The factor assays are formed by evaluating the effects of dilutions of known specific factors to correct either the PT or the PTT on patients with prolonged tests. A specific percentage of the factor may be obtained from a standard curve.

Factor XIII

Deficiency of factor XIII is an uncommon cause of severe, lifelong hemorrhagic tendency. The diagnosis should be considered in a patient with a well-documented bleeding tendency, but without abnormalities of any of the tests previously described, including PT, PTT, TCT, fibrinogen quantitation, bleeding time, or platelet count. Factor XIII promotes stable cross-linkage between individual fibrin monomers. Without factor XIII, fibrin forms but the clot disintegrates easily. The screening test for factor XIII deficiency is very easy. A fibrin clot is generated by adding ionized calcium to the patient's citrated plasma. Once the clot is firm, 1 ml of 5M urea solution is added to the tube, which is incubated at 37°C for 12 hours or overnight. Normally, stabilized fibrin remains firm, but a factor XIII deficiency sample will completely reliquify. A 1% solution of monochloroacetic acid can be used instead of urea, or both can be used in parallel tubes. Normal control plasma should always be tested simultaneously. The test is not a quantitative test and reports the result as *presumptively normal or abnormal factor XIII.*

Tests of the Fibrinolytic Pathway

THROMBIN TIME

Thrombin time may also be used as a test to assess fibrinolytic pathway activation. Since fibrinolytic activation results in the release of plasmin, which cleaves fibrin and fibrinogen, fibrinogen may be decreased, or for that matter the fibrinogen degradation products so released may competitively inhibit thrombin/fibrinogen interaction. Consequently, if circulating fibrin degradation products are present, this competitive inhibition of thrombin/fibrinogen interaction may prolong the thrombin time.

FIBRINOGEN DEGRADATION PRODUCTS (FDP)

Plasmin degrades fibrin as its physiologic substrate, but it readily cleaves fibrinogen as well if disproportion develops between plasmin, fibrin, and fibrinogen. The fragments that remain after plasmin digestion not only fail to clot, they interfere with clotting of whatever fibrinogen has escaped proteolysis. High concentrations of fibrinogen degradation products (FDPs) also interfere with the formation of hemostatic platelet plugs. Whenever fibrin undergoes fibrinolysis, low levels of degradation products enter the circulation, but these are normally cleared by the liver and reticuloendothelial system. With excessive plasmin activity, *fibrin and fibrinogen degradation products (FDP)*—also called fibrin or fibrinogen split products—can circulate in levels high enough to cause serious hemostatic difficulty.

Tests for FDP are done on serum. Since FDPs do not coagulate, they remain in the serum after fibrinogen is removed through clotting. Their presence is documented immunologically so as not to require biologic activity from these functionally abnormal molecules. Anti-fibrinogen antibody is used, since it is neither desirable nor easy to generate antibodies against individual degradation fragments. One simple and widely used procedure employs antibodies adsorbed to inert indicator particles; such techniques as agglutination inhibition and immunodiffusion can also be used. These fragments may be immunologically quantitated by means of a latex test where latex particles coated with the specific antibodies are added to patients' serum. If agglutination occurs, this may be titrated and a value recorded.

Interpretation

Because normal serum contains neither fibrinogen nor FDP, there should be nothing present to react with anti-fibrinogen antibodies. In patients with widespread bleeding or brisk hemostatic activity, small quantities of FDP may circulate, enough to react at a low level with reagent antibody. Very high levels of FDP are seen if the fibrinolytic system is inappropriately active, or if there is widespread intravascular coagulation. Patients with these disorders have blood that clots poorly or not at all.

Euglobulin Lysis Time

Euglobulins are proteins that precipitate from acidified dilute plasma. The euglobulin fraction of plasma contains fibrinogen and all the plasminogen and plasminogen activators of plasma, but only traces of the antiplasmins. Thrombin added to a euglobulin solution converts fibrinogen to fibrin and activates plasminogen. In euglobulins prepared from normal blood, the initial clot undergoes dissolution in 2–6 hours. The main reason plasminogen or its active products, specifically plasmin, can dissolve fibrinogen is that it is now removed from its natural inhibitor in the euglobulin fraction, namely antiplasmin. Even with excessive fibrinolysis, there is usually sufficient fibrinogen to form a clot when thrombin is added, but its appearance is often abnormal from the start. Lysis may take place in minutes; if the process is less severe, complete dissolution may occur in 60–90 minutes. The euglobulin lysis time is abnormally short in blood with normal fibrinolytic activity but reduced fibrinogen, because less fibrin is present to be lysed. An alternative method in this case may be *fibrin plate lysis,* where euglobulin from a patient is applied to a standard fibrin plate and the degree of dissolution of the fibrin is determined.

Interpretation

These tests are generally not that practical, since it is difficult to differentiate whether the fibrinolysis has occurred through a primary mechanism specifically activating the fibrinolytic pathway, or through a secondary intravascular coagulation with secondary fibrinolytic activation. The tests are very rarely used, therefore, to differentiate between intravascular clotting or intravascular fibrinolysis.

Other tests are also available to assess fibrinolytic pathway activation, including quantitation of plasminogen or specific fragments. These, however, are not practical and are not readily available.

Table 5–4 summarizes the categories of hemostatic disorders and the effects on the screening coagulation tests. It must be emphasized that further work-up of the coagulation abnormalities may involve specific factor assays. The factors assayed will depend on which coagulation pathway (i.e., extrinsic, intrinsic, or fibrinolytic) is abnormal.

Laboratory Tests of Hypercoagulable States

A thrombus is an insoluble mass of particulate material in the bloodstream or in the cardiac chambers that is produced by the action of thrombin on fibrinogen to produce fibrin or the aggregation of platelets to form a platelet mass. Thrombosis may occur in either the venous or the arterial system, and the pathogenesis of each of these thrombotic events is somewhat different. Venous thrombosis involves venous stasis, vascular damage, and hypercoagulability. The hypercoagulability in this situation more generally occurs as a result of tissue thromboplastin, producing thrombin that subsequently acts with fibrinogen to produce fibrin. In arterial thrombosis, platelet interaction is much more evident. This may involve platelet–platelet

Table 5–4. LABORATORY EVALUATION OF DISORDERS OF HEMOSTASIS

Hemostatic Defect	Cause	Platelet Count	Bleeding Time	PT	PTT	TT
1. Vascular	Collagen disorder Vitamin C deficiency	N	Prolonged	N	N	N
2. Platelet disorders						
a. Thrombocytopenia	All causes except immune thrombocytopenic purpura	Low	Prolonged	N	N	N
b. Thrombocytopathy	Von Willebrand's disease	N	Prolonged	N	Prolonged	N
	Drugs: Aspirin Anti-inflammatory (non-steroidal)	N	Prolonged	N	N	N
	Renal failure	N	Prolonged	N	N	N
	Hematologic dyscrasias	Variable↓	Variable	N	N	N
3. Coagulopathies						
a. Inherited	Hemophilia (VIII deficiency)	N	N	N	Prolonged	N
	Hemophilia (IX deficiency)	N	N	N	Prolonged	N
b. Acquired	Vitamin K deficiency	N	N	Prolonged	Prolonged	N
	Disseminated intravascular coagulation	Low	Variable (N)	Prolonged	Prolonged	Prolonged
	Liver disease	Variable (N)	Usually normal	Prolonged	Prolonged	Prolonged
	Lupus anticoagulant	N	N	Variable (N)	Prolonged	N

interaction or platelet–vessel wall and thrombin interaction.

Laboratory assessment of those disorders associated with a propensity to thrombosis should involve analysis of deficiencies of the natural anticoagulant systems (Table 5–5). Their deficiency facilitates spontaneous thrombosis or thromboembolic disease. In addition, laboratory markers indicative of intravascular coagulation and increased platelet turnover may also represent markers of an increased propensity to thromboembolic disease. These conditions may broadly be classified as the hypercoagulable disorders.

The term hypercoagulability, therefore, refers to an unnatural tendency to pathologic thrombosis. Hypercoagulable states may be subclassified into those disorders where there are 1) laboratory abnormalities identifying a prethrombotic state, or 2) clinical conditions that are associated with an increased thromboembolic risk. Factors that favor thrombotic tendency are listed in Table 5–6.

Classification of the Hypercoagulable States

The hypercoagulable states may be classified as primary, where there is no underlying predisposing cause, or secondary, where thromboembolism is associated with some preexisting clincial condition or disease. These disorders include those conditions where there is an inherited predisposition to thrombosis, and may be associated with depleted levels of natural anticoagulants or increased or abnormal procoagulants. These categories are listed in Table 5–7.

Laboratory Tests of Hypercoagulability

The clinical laboratory has the potential for a considerable impact on the diagnosis of thromboembolic disease and defining the hypercoagulable state. Laboratory evaluation could be applied to 1) detection of prethrombotic changes—the truly hypercoagulable situation, 2) diagnostic enhancement (for example, in identifying subclinical or silent forms of thromboembolism), 3) monitoring high-risk patients (patients with known risk factors such as past history of thromboembolism, cardiac disease, cancer, genetic tendency, obesity, etc.), and 4) rational therapeutic intervention and monitoring with anticoagulant, anti-platelet, and fibrinolytic drugs.

An ideal screening test should be sensitive, specific, reproducible, easy to perform, and inexpensive. Unfortunately, in the evaluation of hypercoagulability, there are no ideal laboratory tests that can approach these standards.

Certain laboratory tests are, however, potentially useful and these will be discussed. Laboratory assessment of platelet turnover will not be presented, since its

Table 5–5. THE NATURAL ANTITHROMBOTIC MECHANISMS

1. Antiplatelet
    - Prostacyclin
2. Anticoagulant
    - Antithrombin III
    - Other serine protease inhibitors
    - Protein C
    - Protein S
3. Fibrinolytic mechanisms

Table 5–6. FACTORS FAVORING THROMBOTIC TENDENCY

1. Local factors
   - Blood stasis*
   - Vascular damage
2. Coagulation-fibrinolytic imbalance
   - Unimpeded activation of coagulation—DIC (intravascular thrombin generation)
   - Deficiency of natural anticoagulants
     - Antithrombin III
     - Protein C & S
   - Defective fibrinolysis and abnormal plasmin generation
     - Quantitative depletion
     - Qualitative abnormalities
3. Increased platelet turnover†
   - Prosthetic values
   - Valvular heart disease

*Usually venous thromboembolism.
†Usually arterial thromboembolism.

use in defining the hypercoagulable state existing in *arterial thromboembolism* is still controversial. The tests include *beta thromboglobulin, platelet factor IV release assays,* and *platelet survival studies.*

Since all of the recognizable primary hypercoagulable states are associated with defects of the coagulation system and/or the fibrinolytic system (see Table 5–7), and since hypercoagulability is manifested by pathologic hemostasis, study of the hemostatic and fibrinolytic system, as mentioned above, should always be performed. This would include screening tests for both extrinsic (PT), intrinsic (PTT), and thrombin–fibrinogen interaction (TCT) pathways. An appreciation of the disorders classified as primary hypercoagulable states is essential to the selection of laboratory tests for their evaluation. Most of the conditions listed in Table 5–7 are inherited, primary disorders; and in many instances, the patient may be entirely asymptomatic until some minor challenge predisposes them to thromboembolic phenomena. In other instances, the patients may be discovered as part of a routine evaluation for family studies and work-up of a relative with thrombosis.

Table 5–7. CLASSIFICATION OF THE HYPERCOAGULABLE STATES

Primary
- Antithrombin III deficiency
- Protein C & S deficiency
- Lupus anticoagulant
- Factor XII deficiency
- Dysfibrinogenemia
- Fibrinolytic deficiency

Secondary
- Acquired disorders of coagulation and fibrinolytic impairment
- Acquired platelet disorders

Antithrombin III Deficiency

Antithrombin III inhibits thrombin's ability to clot fibrinogen. An assay for antithrombin III deficiency is available in most large centers; however, it is generally unavailable in routine laboratories. The laboratory may determine immunologically the amount of antithrombin III, or else may use a functional assay of the ability of the protein to inhibit thrombin/fibrinogen interaction. Deficiency of this protein allows unimpeded thrombin-mediated conversion of fibrinogen to fibrin. Consequently, most patients with this disorder manifest clinically with spontaneous thromboembolic events. Furthermore, in most cases, the thrombotic events tend to be *venous thromboses.*

Depletion of ATIII may occur as an inherited disorder. The homozygous deficiency is probably incompatible with life, and most patients with heterozygous deficiency are asymptomatic. However, certain patients with heterozygous deficiency may present with spontaneous thrombosis. The incidence of this disorder is estimated to be approximately 1:2000, and patients who are heterozygotes may have ATIII levels ranging between 25–60% of normal. Other conditions that can be associated with a depletion of antithrombin III include pregnancy, liver disease, nephrotic syndrome, widespread thrombosis, and/or disseminated intravascular coagulation, and following L-asparaginase chemotherapy.

Protein C and Protein S Deficiency

It has recently been appreciated that two natural anticoagulants, protein C and protein S, which are vitamin K-dependent proteins, are important in the physiologic prevention of thrombosis. Again, these two proteins are synthesized by the liver, and their disorders are most frequently associated with congenital or hereditary deficiencies. The homozygous condition is incompatible with life, and heterozygosity is usually asymptomatic but can present with recurrent venous thromboses. *Protein C deficiency* may develop in patients who are on oral anticoagulant therapy because of the interference with vitamin K action. This is particularly evident in those rare patients who develop warfarin hypersensitivity, manifested by skin or digital necrosis. Unfortunately, these proteins cannot be assayed in most routine laboratories; but they will probably be available to predict those patients susceptible to thrombotic events in most clinical laboratories in the near future. Protein S deficiency is less recognized but may be equally as common.

The Lupus Anticoagulant

This circulating immunoglobulin factor is responsible for inhibition of the prothrombin time or partial thromboplastin time or both. It inhibits the phospholipid interaction with the coagulation proteins. The anticoagulant is most easily identified when citrated plasma from the patient is mixed with normal plasma in serial dilutions, and then a PTT is performed on the mixture. The anticoagulant prolongs the PTT, or less often the PT, of normal plasma. Stated another way, normal plasma does not correct the prolonged PTT of the patient's plasma as it would do if there was a coagulation factor deficiency. This signifies that an inhibitor is present (see Mixing Studies, p 201). Therefore, mixing studies would be very helpful in identifying the *lupus anticoagulant.* This substance is termed "lupus" because it has been identified in patients with systemic lupus erythematosus (SLE). However, this inhibitor is only found in approximately one third of patients with lupus, and also approximately only one third of patients with the anticoagulant have lupus erythematosus. Other conditions associated with the lupus anticoagulant include other autoimmune diseases and patients that are on chlorpromazine therapy. It is of interest that even though this is a "circulating anticoagulant," there is a greater propensity to thromboembolic phenomena than to bleeding problems. Again, venous thromboembolism is more commonly seen. The term anticoagulant really is a misnomer since it really only applies to the *in vitro* prolongation of the clotting times in the test tube, and is more often associated with clinical thromboembolic disease.

The 'lupus anticoagulant' has also been associated with habitual spontaneous abortions and is concomittantly associated with the presence of an anticardiolipin autoantibody in these cases.

Acquired Hypercoagulable States

A tendency for thromboembolic disease may be seen in a diverse group of conditions from their adverse effects on coagulation or fibrinolytic systems. Disturbance in platelet function or impairment of blood flow may occur in many disorders. Virchow, the eminent pathologist, proposed a triad of pathologic features that are associated with the development of venous thrombosis: hypercoagulability (which has already been discussed), vascular damage, and venous stasis. Diseases associated with impairment of venous blood flow such as pregnancy or abdominal tumors, varicose veins, conditions producing vascular damage such as inflammatory disorders of the vessels (vasculitis), or the hypercoagulable states listed above are included in this category. Laboratory evaluation should be directed toward excluding these secondary causes.

REFERENCES

1. Biggs, R and Rizza, CR: Human Blood Coagulation: Hemostasis and Thrombosis, ed 3. Blackwell Scientific Publications, Boston, 1984.
2. Brandt, JT and Triplett, DA: Laboratory monitoring of heparin. Effect of reagents and instruments on the APTT. Am J Clin Pathol 76:530, 1981.
3. Colman, R, et al: Hemostasis and Thrombosis, ed 2. WB Saunders, Philadelphia, 1987.
4. Comp, PC: Clinical implications of the protein C/S system. Ann NY Acad Sci 509:149, 1987.
5. Comp, PC: Hereditary disorders predisposing to thrombosis. Prog Hemostasis Thromb 8:71–102, 1986.
6. Dacie, JV and Lewis, SM: Practical Hematology, ed 6. Grune & Stratton, New York, 1984.
7. Glatzel, JW and Krause, SG: Laboratory methods in hematology and hemostasis. In Pittiglio, DH and Sacher, RA (eds): Fundamentals of Hematology and Hemostasis. FA Davis, Philadelphia, 1987, p 449.
8. Harker, L and Thompson, AR: Manual of Hemostasis and Thrombosis, ed 3. FA Davis, Philadelphia, 1983.
9. Kazniier, FJ: Thromboembolism, Coumadin, necrosis and protein C. Mayo Clin Proc 60:673, 1985.
10. Loeliger, EA: ICSH/ICTH recommendations for reporting prothrombin time in oral anticoagulant therapy. Thromb Haemost 53:155, 1985.
11. Lusher, JM, et al: Factor VIII/vWF and platelet formation and function in health and disease. Ann NY Acad Sci 509:53, 103, 118, 1987.
12. McGann, MA and Triplett, DA: Interpretation of antithrombin III activity. Laboratory Medicine 13:12, 1982.
13. Ogston, D: The Physiology of Hemostasis. Harvard University Press, Cambridge, 1983.
14. Shafer, E, et al: Monitoring activity of fibrinolytic agents. Am J Med 76:879, 1984.
15. Sirridge, MS and Shannon, R: Laboratory Evaluation of Hemostasis and Thrombosis, ed 3. Lea & Febiger, Philadelphia, 1983.
16. Zimmerman, TS and Ruggeri, MZM: von Willebrand's disease. Hum Pathol 18:140, 1987.

CHAPTER

6

DISORDERS OF HEMOSTASIS

OUTLINE

CHAPTER

6

DISORDERS OF HEMOSTASIS

Patients with hemostatic disorders may present a spectrum of conditions ranging from no symptoms to severe hemorrhage. Patients may seek medical attention 1) because the patient has noticed abnormal bleeding manifestations, 2) because a responsible clinician notices abnormal physical signs or elicits a suspicious history, or 3) because the clinician specifically tests for hemostatic abnormalities before undertaking a surgical, obstetric, or dental procedure. Medical history, physical examination, and laboratory tests are all important in evaluating the significance and nature of bleeding problems.

COAGULATION FACTOR DISORDERS

Medical History

Specific information obtained from the patient can be very helpful in directing the nature of laboratory tests. The medical history should include:

PRESENTATION OF SYMPTOMS

It is important to find out whether the bleeding tendency is a new problem, or whether the individual has noticed easy bruising since childhood. The presentation of hemostatic abnormalities in a male infant at the time of circumcision may suggest a congenital or hereditary bleeding problem. Certainly a lifelong history of bleeding will suggest a congenital coagulation or platelet disorder.

ONSET OF BLEEDING

Is the bleeding provoked by injury, or does it occur spontaneously? *Spontaneous* bleeding is more commonly seen in the hemophilia syndromes and von Willebrand's disease. Hemostatic abnormalities only manifesting with *trauma* or *surgery* may suggest a mild coagulation factor deficiency or factor XI or XIII deficiency. Factor XIII deficiency more commonly presents 24–48 hours after surgery.

Location of the Bleeding

Coagulation factor abnormalities such as hemophilia rarely present with mucous membrane bleeding, and more commonly present with spontaneous hemorrhages into the joints, in particular the knees and elbows. Platelet disorders more commonly present with mucous membrane bleeding or cutaneous bruising and bleeding, and are indicated by the presence of petechiae (see later).

Family History

Family history is important since a sex-linked preponderance may suggest hemophilia (Factor VIII deficiency) or Christmas disease (Factor IX deficiency). Obviously, in this situation male members, and in particular male members on the maternal side, are affected. An autosomal dominant inheritance is more commonly seen with von Willebrand's disease.

Drugs and Medications

Certain drugs may be associated with impairment of platelet function, in particular aspirin and the nonsteroidal anti-inflammatory agents. Some drugs and medications, such as quinidine or quinine, are associated with rapid reduction of platelet count on an allergic basis; other drugs, such as thiazide diuretics, are notorious for suppression of bone marrow production of platelets. Many drugs may cause idiosyncratic reactions that may affect platelet function or production.

Other Systemic Diseases

Patients should always be questioned regarding the possibility of other systemic diseases that can be associated with bleeding abnormalities, such as recent infections, the presence of other hematologic diseases, nutritional deficiencies, autoimmune disease, and liver disease.

Bruising is difficult to evaluate by history since it occurs so commonly, particularly on the thighs and upper arms, and especially in postmenopausal women. Duration of symptoms may determine whether the condition is congenital or acquired, and the anatomic site of hemorrhage is important in determining the nature of the hemostatic abnormality.

Physical Examination

General physical examination may reveal evidence of a bleeding abnormality. Notable categories of bleeding episodes include bleeding into joints *(hemarthroses)* and into soft tissues *(hematomas)*, especially muscles, diffuse oozing from mucosal surfaces, blood in the urine *(hematuria)*, and pinpoint or spreading hemorrhages into skin *(petechiae, ecchymoses,* or *purpura)*. Poorly healed scars may be seen in patients with connective tissue diseases and coagulation factor deficiencies or with factor XIII deficiency. Chronic bleeding into the joints may produce, in addition, joint deformities or impaired joint mobility. Acquired disorders such as lymphomas or leukemias may present with anemia or enlargement of the liver, spleen, or lymph nodes. Rapid bone marrow expansion due to infiltrative marrow disease such as leukemia may be associated with bone marrow tenderness.

Laboratory Screening Tests

For an apparently normal patient about to undergo an operation, the prothrombin time (PT), partial thromboplastin time (PTT), and platelet count probably constitute an adequate screening profile. If the history is suggestive, the bleeding time and thrombin time should also be performed. In this manner, the extrinsic coagulation pathway (PT), intrinsic coagulation pathway (PTT), thrombin/fibrinogen interaction (TCT), and platelet count, as well as platelet function screen (bleeding time), may elucidate whether a bleeding problem exists, and its nature. If these screening tests are all normal despite a suggestive clinical history, it is highly unlikely that the patient has a significant bleeding problem. If an abnormality of one or the other of these tests is identified, then further characterization can be performed to elucidate the specific nature of the problem and to define a preventive measure or specific treatment. The laboratory work-up of many of the disorders of coagulation has been presented in Chapter 5. Specific disorders are discussed in this chapter and the confirmatory laboratory tests are explained.

Clinical and Laboratory Observations

Although acquired bleeding problems are far more common than congenital disorders, characterization and treatment of congenital syndromes is far easier. Congenital deficiency syndromes attract investigators who use these isolated defects as experiments of nature that elucidate fundamental physiologic and pathologic events. Acquired disorders often accompany other diseases. Aside from treating the underlying disease, the clinician may have few options other than to treat the hemorrhagic diathesis empirically with platelets and plasma for factor replacement. Coagulation problems are probably less common than platelet disorders, but the coagulation mechanisms can be studied and manipulated more readily than can functional disorders of platelets.

Laboratory tests that are useful in evaluating hypercoagulability are generally not easy to perform and not reproducible except in some rare inherited deficiencies or in association with the lupus anticoagulant. These are discussed in Chapter 5 and mentioned briefly in this chapter.

Congenital Disorders of Coagulation

Deficiencies of Factor VIII and Factor IX (Hemophilias)

Hemophilia, in general terms, refers to a severe, lifelong tendency toward excessive bleeding, occurring almost exclusively in men and following an X-linked inheritance pattern. Defects of *factor VIII* or *factor IX* produce this syndrome. Hemophilia has been recognized for thousands of years. The Talmud states that a male infant should not be circumcised if two or more of his brothers died from postcircumcision bleeding. In the United States, approximately 1 out of 10,000 boys has hemophilia of greater or lesser severity; four out of five cases are factor VIII deficiencies, and thus factor IX problems are less common. *Factor VIII (Hemophilia A* or *classical hemophilia)* and *factor IX* deficiency *(hemophilia B* or *Christmas disease)* were not differentiated until 1952. Clinical findings and genetic transmission are identical. The conditions can be distinguished by cross-correctional studies (mixing studies) or specific factor assays (see Chapter 5).

Clinical Findings. Depending on the level of available circulating factor, clinical severity of both hemophilia A and B can range from severe to mild or almost asymptomatic. As a rule, affected males in any one family tend to have comparable factor levels and comparably severe clinical disease. *Severely* affected patients have *less than 1%* activity, *moderately* affected patients have between *1 and 5%*, and *mildly* affected patients have between *6 and 30%* activity (Table 6–1).

Excessive bleeding after obvious trauma is only part of the problem, an aspect that usually can be treated successfully. Of more serious, long-term consequence is bleeding into joints, which often occurs without any apparent incitement and is extremely painful. The sequelae of progressive joint deformity produce severe crippling. This more often affects the lower extremities. Before the advent of effective therapy, hemophiliac patients who survived early bleeding episodes almost invariably became severely crippled by adolescence and young adulthood. Even though present day therapy controls most lethal and many disabling symptoms, hemarthroses have not been eliminated; however, their frequency, magnitude, and crippling effects have been markedly reduced.

Soft tissue bleeding, especially subcutaneous and intramuscular hemorrhage, can cause compressive damage to muscles and nerves. Hematomas into soft tissues of the head and neck may compress respiratory passages and cause death by asphyxiation. Bleeding into the urinary or alimentary tract is common, but usually causes no long-term complications. Intracranial hemorrhage, on the other hand, sometimes occurs without apparent predisposing trauma and can be extremely dangerous.

Persons with hemophilia suffer not only from hemorrhage, but also from delayed wound repair. Before adequate therapy was available, dental or surgical procedures were extremely hazardous. Bleeding after an operation or tooth extraction often can be the first sign of the disease in mildly affected persons with previously unsuspected hemophilia.

Laboratory Findings. Initial diagnostic procedures have been discussed in Chapter 5. After a presumptive diagnosis has been made, it is important to determine the *level of factor activity* and to *test* whether an *inhibitor* exists. *Anti-factor VIII antibodies* develop in as many as 5–10% of treated classical hemophiliacs; it is rare to find antibodies at initial diagnosis. Factor IX antibodies are less common. When adequate replacement fails to have therapeutic effect, or if the PTT remains severely abnormal after treatment, an antibody should be suspected. The presence of inhibitor is demonstrated by incubating the patient's plasma with a known concentration of factor VIII or factor IX, and measuring the coagulant activity of the resulting mixture. This can be done either by determining the PTT or by performing a specific inhibitor assay that determines how much factor VIII or IX is neutralized by the inhibitor.

Treatment. *Factor VIII* is available as a highly potent *concentrate* prepared from large pools of cryoprecipitated plasma, and as a moderately rich factor VIII

Table 6–1. CLINICAL/LABORATORY CLASSIFICATION OF HEMOPHILIA

Degree of Severity	Level of Factor
Mild	5–30%
Moderate	1–5%
Severe	<1%

cold precipitated plasma or *cryoprecipitate* prepared from single donor plasma. Pooled cryoprecipitate can be freeze-dried from thousands of donors, and dispensed as a factor VIII concentrate of predetermined activity (see Chapter 8). It can be reconstituted by adding a diluent solution. Cryoprecipitate gives good results in treating minor or uncomplicated problems. Concentrates are ideal for treating severe hemorrhagic episodes and for elevating factor VIII levels prior to surgical procedures (Table 6–2). In these circumstances, the therapeutic benefits of concentrates outweigh the moderate risk of hepatitis. These issues are also discussed in Chapter 8. Mild factor VIII deficiency is now effectively treated by the administration of desmopressin (DDAVP).

Factor IX is not available as a product separate from other liver factors (prothrombin, factor VII, and factor X). The concentrate of these four ''vitamin K-dependent factors'' carries a very high risk of hepatitis transmission. Single donor plasma, either freshly frozen or salvaged from stored liquid blood, contains substantial factor IX and should be used for treatment of minor difficulties; for major episodes the concentrate is preferred.

Carrier State. Women, who have two X chromosomes, almost always have one normal gene to balance the hemophilia gene. Theoretically, a woman who received an abnormal gene from her carrier mother, and another from her hemophiliac father, would have true hemophilia. Such a case is extremely rare in humans. When there is one normal and one abnormal gene, the woman often has less than the normal level of factor activity. This deficiency is highly variable and usually too mild to be detected in routine PTT. The presence of the normal gene supplies an adequate amount of activity to normalize the PTT in most cases. The carrier state, therefore, cannot be diagnosed reliably by quantitative assays of factor activity. Sufficient variation occurs that a woman can have normal or near normal assays and still be a carrier. The diagnosis of the carrier state can be determined by comparing the percentage level of coagulant factor with the percentage level of factor VIII antigen. As was mentioned in Chapter 5, the von Willebrand factor antigen (vWF: Ag—also called VIII:RAg) is invariably normal or even high in hemophiliacs and the basic defect is a defect or deficiency of the procoagulant activity. Therefore in hemophilia carrier states the ratio of von Willebrand factor antigen to factor VIII coagulant is greater than unity. This assay system is also useful in differentiating mild classical hemophilia from mild von Willebrand's Factor. In the latter disorder, procoagulant (VIII:C) is equally decreased, as is vWF:Ag. These assay systems were discussed in Chapter 5.

Factor IX carriers have not been as substantially characterized as factor VIII carriers, and the carrier status may be difficult to diagnose.

FIBRINOGEN

Plasma may contain no fibrinogen or severely abnormal fibrinogen. Patients with *afibrinogenemia* are paradoxic in having totally incoagulable blood, but nevertheless bleed less often and less dangerously than patients with procoagulant deficiencies. Bleeding episodes, bruising, and poor wound healing characterize this disorder, which is usually inherited as an autosomal recessive trait. In rare autosomal dominant conditions, the fibrinogen molecule is structurally or functionally defective. These *dysfibrinogenemias* cause relatively mild hemorrhagic symptoms; a few patients, indeed, have a thrombotic tendency.

Laboratory Findings. Blood that lacks fibrinogen fails to clot in the PT, the PTT, or the TCT, but the addition of afibrinogenemic plasma to normal plasma does not inhibit fibrinogen formation. All the tests that measure fibrinogen measure zero.

Table 6–2. TREATMENT SCHEDULE FOR SEVERE HEMOPHILIA (1% OF FACTOR PRESENT) WITHOUT AN INHIBITOR

Disorders	Degree of Hemorrhage	Initial Dose of Concentrate in Units	Subsequent Doses	
Hemophilia A Classic hemophilia (factor VIII deficiency)	Minor Hemoarthrosis Muscle hematoma Mild hematuria	18 units/kg*	10 units/kg every 8–12 hr	Until objective bleeding and pain resolves; single dose may be sufficient.
	Moderate	26 units/kg*	14 units/kg every 8–12 hr	7–10 days to permit adequate healing
	Severe Life-threatening surgical procedure Major trauma Head injury	35 units/kg*	18 units/kg every 8–12 hr	7–10 days to permit adequate healing
Hemophilia B Christmas disease (factor IX deficiency)	Minor Hemarthrosis Muscle hematoma Mild hematuria	25 units/kg†	5 units/kg every 12–24 hr	Until objective bleeding and pain resolves; single dose may be sufficient.
	Moderate	35 units/kg†	8 units/kg every 12–24 hr	7–10 days to permit adequate healing
	Severe Life-threatening surgical procedure Major trauma Head injury	45 units/kg†	10 units/kg every 12–24 hr	7–10 days to permit adequate healing

*Factor VIII concentrates.

†Factor IX concentrates.

From Sacher, RA. Hemophilia. In Tintinalli, UE, Rothstein, RJ, and Krome, RL (eds): Emergency Medicine: A Comprehensive Study Guide. American College of Emergency Physicians, McGraw-Hill, New York, 1988, p 530, with permission.

There is no precipitate to analyze and nothing reacts with anti-fibrin/fibrinogen antibodies.

The *dysfibrinogenemias,* on the other hand, show qualitative as well as quantitative abnormalities. When incubated with normal plasma, this dysfibrinogenemic plasma inhibits clotting. Discrepancy exists, often strikingly, between the amount of coagulable fibrinogen and the quantity of immunoreactive or precipitable protein. Therefore, the functional tests show discrepant values with the protein assays. Another test that is useful in diagnosing dysfibrinogenemia, which empirically gives a prolonged thrombin clotting time, is the *Reptilase Time.* This is a test that is very similar to the thrombin clotting time; however, it uses the snake venom reptilase to produce cleavage of the fibrinopeptide molecules from fibrinogen. Therefore, following this direct cleavage, which bypasses the clotting pathway, fibrinogen can form an insoluble fibrin monomer and a fibrin clot. If an individual has an abnormal fibrinogen molecule, the reptilase time is substantially prolonged. As was mentioned in Chapter 5, most of the tests of fibrinogen utilize a functional assay that requires the addition of thrombin to clot an unknown amount of fibrinogen. Heparin is a powerful antithrombin, and is used as an anticoagulant because of this property. Reptilase can be used to assay fibrinogen in the presence of heparin.

OTHER FACTORS

Except for the hemophilias and the dysfibrinogenemias, inherited deficiencies of coagulation factors follow an autosomal recessive inheritance pattern. All are rare (less than 1:500,000) except for *factor XI deficiency,* which occurs in up to 1:10,000 in certain Jewish populations. Most cause a lifelong tendency toward severe bleeding episodes, but hemarthroses are rare. Factor XI deficiency causes much milder symptoms, often menorrhagia, epistaxis (nosebleeds), or bleeding after dental or surgical procedures. *Factor XII* and *Fletcher factor deficiencies* do not cause any symptoms at all, and indeed, as was previously mentioned in Chapter 5, deficiency of factor XII (Hageman factor) may, paradoxically, be associated with a thrombotic tendency. Table 6–3 lists the clinical features of congenital deficiency syndromes for all the coagulation factors.

VON WILLEBRAND'S DISEASE

Von Willebrand's disease (vWD) is a hemostatic disorder that is transmitted as an autosomal dominant trait with variable penetrance. It occurs with equal frequency in both sexes. The condition and the clinical manifestations may vary, despite the inheritance patterns. Since factor VIII levels are low, von Willebrand's disease earned the name *pseudohemophilia* or *Hemophilia C,* and created much confusion for early workers studying hemophilia. Besides the low factor VIII:C levels, there is a *prolongation of the bleeding time,* a phenomenon inspiring the alternate name *"vascular hemophilia"* for this disease.

Pathophysiology. Factor VIII has at least *three* different molecular properties: the *procoagulant activity* (VIII:C), the *antigenic activity* (vWF:Ag formally called VIII:RAg), and the *von Willebrand factor activity* ((vWF:activity formally called VIII:vWF). This third function is important in the interaction between the vascular endothelium and the platelets, and prevents excessive capillary bleeding by enhancing platelet plug formation. The name von Willebrand factor has been applied to the protein properties with these complex results. In *classical hemophilia,* the procoagulant activity of factor VIII is low, but von Willebrand factor and cross-reactive antigenic factor (vWF:Ag) are normally active. In vWD, all three aspects are variably abnormal, and the degree to which these abnormalities may manifest produces

Table 6–3. INHERITED FACTOR DEFICIENCIES

Factor	Deficiency	Minimum for Hemostasis	Half-life	Laboratory	Clinical
I	Afibrinogenemia Autosomal recessive-homozygous Rare	50–100 mg	3.2–4.5 days	No clot formation <5 mg fibrinogen	Umbilical stump bleeding, easy bruising, ecchymosis, epistaxis, gingival oozing, hematuria, poor wound healing.
	Hypofibrinogenemia Autosomal recessive-heterozygous Rare			Abn: PT APTT TCT Low fibrinogen	Mild bleeding, thrombotic episodes.
	Dysfibrinogenemia Variable inheritance Uncommon—variants			Fibrinogen— Qualitative abnormal Quantitative normal	Possible hemorrhage, possible thrombosis, possibly asymptomatic.
II	Hypoprothrombinemia Autosomal recessive Extremely rare	30–40%	2.8–4.4 days	Abn: PT APTT	Postoperative bleeding, epistaxis, menorrhagia, easy bruising.
V	Parahemophilia Autosomal recessive 1/1,000,000–homozygote	10–25%	20 hr	Abn: PT APTT BT	Epistaxis, easy bruising, menorrhagia.
VII	Hypoproconvertinemia Incomplete autosomal recessive—variable expression 1/500,000	10–20%	100–300 min	Abn: PT Norm: APTT	Epistaxis, menorrhagia, cerebral hemorrhage.
VIII	Hemophilia A (Classic hemophilia) Sex-linked recessive 1/100,000	10–40%	9–18 hr	ABN: APTT Norm: PT BT	May be severe, moderate or mild—spontaneous hemorrhage, hemarthroses, crippling, ecchymoses,

					muscle hemorrhage, post-traumatic and postsurgical bleeding.
	von Willebrand's syndrome Variable inheritance—variants—autosomal dominant, variable penetrance; 1/80,000	20–40%	16–24 hr	Variable results: Platelet studies BT APTT	Mucous membrane bleeding, superficial wound bleeding—variable depending on VIII:C levels.
IX	Hemophilia B (Christmas disease) Sex-linked recessive 1/100,000	20–50%	18–30 hr	Abn: APTT Norm: PT	May be severe, moderate or mild—spontaneous hemorrhage, hemarthroses, crippling, ecchymoses, muscle hemorrhage, posttraumatic and postsurgical bleeding.
X	Stuart-Prower defect Autosomal recessive < 1/500,000–homozygous 1/500–heterozygous	15–20%	32–48 hr	Abn: PT APTT	Menorrhagia, ecchymoses, CNS bleeding, excessive bleeding after childbirth.
XI	Incomplete autosomal recessive—pseudo—dominant Rare	15–25%	40–84 hr	Abn: APTT Norm: PT	Mild bleeding, bruising, epistaxis, retinal hemorrhage, menorrhagia.
XII	Hageman trait Autosomal recessive Rare	?	48–52 hr	Abn: APTT Norm: PT	Asymptomatic—rarely bleed, may thrombose.
XIII	Factor XIII deficiency Autosomal recessive Rare	1%	12 days	Norm: PT APTT Clot soluble in 5 M urea	Umbilical cord bleeding, delayed wound healing, minor injuries cause prolonged bleeding, fetal wastage, excessive fibrinolysis, male sterility, intracranial hemorrhage.

Table 6–3. INHERITED FACTOR DEFICIENCIES *(Continued)*

Factor	Deficiency	Minimum for Hemostasis	Half-life	Laboratory	Clinical
PK	Fletcher trait Autosomal recessive Rare	?	?	Abn: APTT (normal after prolonged activation)	Asymptomatic.
HMWK	Fitzgerald deficiency Autosomal recessive Rare	?	?	Abn: APTT	Asymptomatic.
Plasminogen	Abnormal functional Plasminogen Autosomal Rare	?	2–2.5 days	Abnormal plasminogen function—normal clotting tests	Thrombosis.
Protein C	Protein C deficiency Autosomal dominant	?	6–8 hr	Normal clotting tests	Thrombosis—thrombophlebitis, recurring pulmonary emboli.

From Pittiglio, DH, et al: Treating hemostatic disorders. A problem-oriented approach. In Pittiglio, DH (ed): Hemostasis Overview. American Association of Blood Banks, Arlington, VA, 1984, p 28, with permission.

Key: PK=prekallikrein. HMWK=high molecular weight kininogen.

the several different types of von Willebrand's disease syndromes, which are classified according to their relative abnormalities. Most patients have mild clinical symptoms. Small vessel bleeding (such as mucocutaneous bruising), nosebleeds, and menorrhagia are the most common events. Aspirin enhances the bleeding tendency and exaggerates the defective interaction between the platelets, plasma Factor VIII, and vessel wall that characterizes vWD.

Laboratory Findings. Routine tests of hemostatic functions are somewhat unpredictable. The classical findings are a prolonged bleeding time and an abnormally long PTT due to the low factor VIII levels. Bleeding time varies only moderately in most patients, but there may be a marked fluctuation in factor VIII levels. The platelet count and clot retraction are normal, but there exists a characteristic abnormality of platelet activity that provides the best single diagnostic test for vWD. When exposed to *ristocetin,* platelets from vWD patients fail to exhibit aggregation (see Chapter 5). In addition, when passed through a column of glass beads, they fail to adhere. Infusion of plasma or factor VIII-rich cryoprecipitate causes temporary improvement of ristocetin aggregation and glass bead retention tests, as well as an increase in procoagulant activity that lasts much longer than the survival of passively administered factor VIII.

In most vWD patients, there are comparably low levels of antigenic and procoagulant activity. A minority of patients have a normal quantity of protein with aberrant immunologic activity. There seem to be several different fundamental mechanisms involved. Most patients have quantitatively normal synthesis of the entire factor VIII complex, whereas others have a qualitative defect of synthesis. Not surprisingly, laboratory observations vary more widely among patients with qualitative or structural variants than among those with quantitative deficiency.

PLATELET DISORDERS

Disorders of platelet number or function cause prolonged bleeding time and poor clot retraction. The platelet count allows quantitation of circulating platelets. To evaluate how many platelets are being produced, it is necessary to examine the bone marrow megakaryocytes. If platelet counts are normal but clinical symptoms and screening laboratory tests suggest platelet failure, qualitative tests of platelet function are indicated, as was outlined in *Chapter 5.*

Quantitative Platelet Abnormalities

Platelets may be either *decreased (thrombocytopenia)* or *increased* (*thrombocytosis* or *thrombocythemia).*

THROMBOCYTOPENIA

The major causes of thrombocytopenia may be classified into two categories: 1) the failure of the bone marrow to produce an adequate number of platelets and 2) increased peripheral destruction or sequestration of platelets.

The diagnosis of thrombocytopenia is usually made using *automated platelet counters.* It is essential, however, that these counts be verified by examination of the *peripheral blood smear.* Corroboration with the peripheral smear may also reveal other possible causes of the apparently low platelet count such as *artifactual thrombocytopenia (pseudothrombocytopenia).* In this condition, platelet clumping occurs after collection of the blood sample, particularly in blood collected in the anticoagulant EDTA. The automated platelet counter interprets this as an apparent decrease in the platelet count due to the multiple platelets adherent in one aggregant mass. These clumps may readily be seen on a peripheral smear examination. Furthermore, the peripheral smear may also reveal clues as to the cause of the disorder. For example, fragmented red cells (schistocytes) would suggest a *microangiopathic hemolytic anemia* in association with thrombocytopenia, as may occur in *disseminated intravascular coagulation, hemolytic uremic syndrome,* and *thrombotic thrombocytopenic purpura.* The presence of altered red cell and white cell morphology may suggest a *megaloblastic anemia,* a *marrow failure syndrome,* or *leukemia.* In most cases, however, evaluation of a bone marrow is essential for categorizing the cause of the thrombocytopenia.

If bone marrow examination reveals abundant megakaryocytes with normal maturation of all the other cell lines, this strongly suggests a peripheral destructive process causing reduction in the platelet count. This may occur in *autoimmune thrombocytopenia* or *splenic platelet sequestration.* The bone marrow may also reveal *abnormal hematopoiesis, marrow fibrosis,* the presence of *foreign cells, leukemia,* or marked reduction in hemopoietic tissue, as may occur in *aplastic anemia.* It is also extremely important that any patient presenting with thrombocytopenia be thoroughly examined and have a detailed medical history, particularly with emphasis on recent viral syndromes, family history, and a drug history.

Thrombocytopenia Due To Decreased Platelet Production. Conditions that generally affect bone marrow cellular maturation often cause thrombocytopenia as one of several hematologic manifestations; therefore, anemia and leukopenia often coexist. Table 6–4 lists causes of thrombocytopenia associated with decreased platelet production.

Aplastic anemia is discussed in Chapter 3, and usually occurs as a result of some undefined insult to the pleuripotent or multipotent stem cell in the bone marrow. Consequently there is failure of one or all of the major hemopoietic cell lines, producing variable degrees of anemia, leukopenia, and thrombocytopenia. Disorders in which there is abnormal growth or maturation of the pleuripotent or multipotent stem cell occur in the *clonal hematologic diseases* that are discussed in Chap-

Table 6–4. ACQUIRED THROMBOCYTOPENIA SECONDARY TO DECREASED PLATELET PRODUCTION

Aplastic anemia
Paroxysmal nocturnal hemoglobinuria
Leukemia (acute, chronic, hairy cell)
Preleukemia syndromes (myelodysplasia)
Metastatic lymphoma or carcinoma
Myelofibrosis (primary or secondary)
Folate and vitamin B_{12} deficiencies
Cytotoxic and immunosuppressive chemotherapy
Viral infections*
Drugs*
Idiopathic*

*Conditions in which thrombocytopenia is often the predominant hematologic finding.

ter 4, and include *leukemia,* the *myelodysplastic syndromes,* and *paroxysmal nocturnal hemoglobinuria. Metastatic malignancies* and *lymphomatous involvement* of the bone marrow may produce a gross disturbance of the bone marrow architecture with the production of a *leukoerythroblastic (myelophthisic)* peripheral blood picture (see Color Plate 39). In *megaloblastic anemia,* folate and vitamin B_{12} are necessary for maturation and normal development of all rapidly dividing cells; and although these conditions usually produce a more profound anemia, more often pancytopenia occurs. Cancer chemotherapeutic *drugs* usually produce suppression of all marrow elements; however, in some situations, more profound thrombocytopenia may exist, such as the agents mitomycin C and the nitrosoureas.

These disorders are often associated with specific findings on history and physical examination as well as laboratory examination. In most cases, examination of a bone marrow aspirate and biopsy is necessary to confirm the correct diagnosis. Some *viral infections* are associated with thrombocytopenia (HIV, Epstein-Barr virus, cytomegalovirus, and hepatitis B). These conditions can also be associated with immune destruction of platelets.

Relatively few drugs affect platelet production selectively. *Chlorothiazide* causes mild thrombocytopenia in some patients, but this rarely causes bleeding. *Alcohol* depresses platelet production; low platelet counts are found in most alcoholics examined during or immediately after acute or continued ingestion. Alcohol may have varied effects on the bone marrow and may produce thrombocytopenia by direct suppression of platelet production, hypersplenism secondary to cirrhosis of the liver, and folate and other nutritional deficiencies. Thrombocytopenia from direct alcoholic suppression is usually associated with recovery of the platelet count in a few days after alcohol withdrawal.

Rarely, thrombocytopenia may occur as a result of selective *deficiency of megakaryocytes.* This may be as a result of a primary or constitutional defect, or may be acquired in association with myelodysplastic syndromes. Occasionally this disorder may be seen in *collagen–vascular diseases* and may occur as a result of autoimmune destruction of platelet precursors.

Thrombocytopenia as a Result of Platelet Sequestration. Thrombocytopenia associated with normal megakaryocytes in a bone marrow aspirate indicates that the lifespan of the platelets is significantly shortened. The presence of abundant megakaryocytes in association with a peripheral thrombocytopenia is the hallmark of these conditions. These disorders associated with shortened platelet survival are classified according to the mechanisms of platelet destruction. In addition to alloantibodies and immune complexes, antibodies can be directed specifically against the platelet membrane, producing an autoimmune thrombocytopenic syndrome.

The spleen, under normal conditions, contains up to one third of all circulating platelets, although relatively few platelets undergo destruction in any one passage through the spleen. *Massive splenic enlargement* increases the number of platelets removed from active circulation by splenic sequestration, and reduces the survival time of all circulating platelets. *Liver disease, portal hypertension,* and *the lymphomas* are common causes of splenomegaly great enough to affect platelet numbers (see also Table 3–19).

Since platelets adhere to damaged endothelial surfaces, platelet counts often drop dramatically in conditions characterized by widespread endothelial damage. *Rocky mountain spotted fever* and the hemorrhagic rash of *meningococcemia* are outstanding examples. In these cases, the infection and the localized capillary damage cause hemorrhage and thrombocytopenia; it is not the thrombocytopenia that causes the hemorrhagic rash. Other causes of *vascular inflammation (vasculitis)* can be associated with thrombocytopenia (due to platelet destruction or adherence to vessel walls) and similar hemorrhagic rash.

Thrombocytopenia Due to Immune Destruction of Platelets. *Alloantibodies.* Platelets may be destroyed by *autoantibodies,* by *alloantibodies,* and by the action of antibodies directed against *drugs.* Alloantibodies cause problems relatively rarely, except in thrombocytopenic patients who receive multiple platelet transfusions and develop antibodies to human leukocyte antigens (HLA). Such patients are refractory to platelet transfusions from random donors, and require platelets from donors of compatible HLA phenotype (see Chapter 8).

Much rarer are antibodies to specific platelet antigens; anti-PL^{A1} is the usual offender and pregnancy is the usual immunizing event. Occasionally, maternal anti-PL^{A1} crosses the placenta and destroys fetal platelets. The newborn suffers from *neonatal alloimmune thrombocytopenia,* a disorder that is pathogenetically similar to hemolytic disease of the newborn, except in this situation thrombocytopenia is the end result (see Chapter 8). If purpura or the threat of hemorrhage makes it necessary to transfuse PL^{A1}-negative platelets, the mother is usually the best donor if her clinical condition permits. Very rarely, PL^{A1}-negative women become profoundly and symptomatically thrombocytopenic six or seven days after receiving whole blood or red cells. In this *posttransfusion purpura* (see Chapter 8), the patient's own platelets are destroyed, but the inciting event is exposure to PL^{A1}-positive material in the transfusion. Immune complex formation (see Chapter 7) may be at fault. Later transfusions exacerbate the problem, which can be treated by plasma exchange.

Drugs and Immune Complex Formation. Many drugs have been implicated in acute thrombocytopenic episodes; most cases are isolated *idiosyncratic* reactions. Frequent offenders are *quinine* and its optical isomer *quinidine. Digitoxin, heparin,* and the *thiazides* occasionally cause problems.

Characteristically, the antibody is directed against the drug (such as quinidine), not against the platelets. If platelets adsorb the drug from the plasma, the antibody damages the platelet while attaching to the drug. High blood levels are often necessary before platelets become coated with the drug.

High drug doses are not necessary for the quinine antibodies and others with comparable activity. These antibodies unite with free drug to form *immune complexes,* insoluble macromolecules that settle onto the receptive surface of circulating platelets. The immune complex activates complement; because the immune complex attaches to the platelets, the activated complement sequence acts on the platelets and actively destroys them. Although neither the antibody nor the complement has specific affinity for the platelet, it is the platelet that suffers as an "innocent bystander."

Autoimmune Thrombocytopenia. This condition, formerly called *idiopathic thrombocytopenic purpura* (ITP), results from the effects of an IgG antibody that coats circulating platelets and causes them to be rapidly destroyed in the reticuloendothelial system. Idiopathic thrombocytopenic purpura is a disorder in which the individual develops an autoantibody against undefined antigens on the platelet membrane. As a consequence of this attack, platelet survival is markedly shortened and thrombocytopenia occurs. Idiopathic thrombocytopenic purpura is a *diagnosis of exclusion* and may occur as a *primary or idiopathic* condition, or as *a secondary disorder* in association with other diseases such as collagen vascular disorders, lymphomas, carcinomas, and drugs. The clinical manifestations of this disorder may be *acute* (less than 6 months) or *chronic* (persisting for longer than one year). The *acute type* occurs more commonly in children and is usually transient and self-limiting in more than 80% of cases, irrespective of whether treatment is administered or not. The *chronic type* is more commonly seen in adults and is usually exacerbating. The IgG antibody coats both the patient's own platelets and also transfused donor platelets if they are administered. In general, platelet transfusions are not recommended and usually are unsuccessful in elevating the platelet count. The transfused platelets would also be destroyed by the underlying disease process at the same rate as the patient's platelets, which are being produced in vastly greater quantities.

Many elegant studies have demonstrated the pathogenesis of this condition, but in the individual patient the diagnosis of ITP is not easy to make because there is no simple, reliable *in vitro* test for plasma antibody. Procedures to demonstrate IgG on circulating platelets are not available in most clinical laboratories; reference laboratories use antiglobulin consumption tests, radiolabeled antiglobulin tests, tests using radiolabeled staphylococcal protein A, or enzyme-linked immunosorbent antiplatelet antibody tests. All these tests are designed to detect, using different mechanisms, the presence of IgG on the platelet surface. It is important to remember that ITP is a diagnosis of exclusion, and all the secondary causes listed in Table 6–5 must be excluded. Laboratory studies, therefore, are also addressed at excluding some of the secondary causes. The spleen, although the site of major platelet destruction, is not enlarged in ITP. Splenomegaly, if present, requires investigation for other causes of thrombocytopenia.

The usual *treatment* is corticosteroid therapy (completely successful in only one third of chronic cases), which if unsuccessful is often followed by splenectomy. Splenectomy not only removes the site of platelet destruction, but also a significant site of platelet sequestration (see above). Table 6–5 gives a list of the causes of thrombocytopenia producing increased platelet destruction. As can be seen, a systematic approach to this cytopenia is similar to that discussed in Chapter 3, that is, the exclusion and diagnosis of autoimmune hemolytic anemia. Occasionally, autoimmune hemolytic anemia and immune thrombocytopenia may coexist. This condition is called *Evan's syndrome.*

Table 6–5. THROMBOCYTOPENIA SECONDARY TO INCREASED PERIPHERAL DESTRUCTION OF PLATELETS

Immune-mediated thrombocytopenia
- Idiopathic thrombocytopenic purpura (ITP)
  - Acute ITP
  - Chronic ITP
  - Intermittent/recurrent ITP
- Secondary immune thrombocytopenias
  - Viral infections
  - Collagen vascular diseases
  - Lymphoproliferative malignancies
  - Carcinomas
  - Drugs
  - After blood transfusions

Non-immune-mediated thrombocytopenias
- Thrombotic thrombotcytopenic purpura
- Hemolytic uremic syndrome
- Disseminated intravascular coagulation
- Complications of pregnancy
- Infections

Secondary Immune Thrombocytopenia. As with autoimmune hemolytic anemia (see Table 3–17), immune destruction of platelets may also occur in association with *viral syndromes.* In about 50% of cases of idiopathic or primary-type, an antecedent viral infection may have predated ITP. Virus disorders such as *EBV* infections, *CMV,* and *hepatitis B* may also be associated with ITP. Recently, the association with HIV infections has been recognized. In any patient presenting with ITP, serologic work-up for exposure to the HIV must be performed. *Lupus erythematosus* and other *collagen–vascular disorders* may produce immune destruction of platelets or may be associated with sequestration of platelets in conjunction with vasculitis, as was described previously. Thrombocytopenia may be a presenting feature of a collagen–vascular disease such as *systemic lupus erythematosus.* Immune thrombocytopenic purpura may also occur secondary to hematologic malignancies such as *chronic lymphocytic leukemia, Hodgkin's and non-Hodgkin's lymphomas,* and other solid tumors such as *adenocarcinoma of the large bowel.* These conditions should also be excluded before the diagnosis of primary or idiopathic ITP is made.

Nonimmune Thrombocytopenia with Destruction of Platelets. Destruction and consumption of platelets may occur in the bloodstream in clinical syndromes not associated with immune (antibody) destruction of platelets. Two main clinical syndromes in which this occurs are themselves associated with complex hematologic problems. These are 1) *disseminated intravascular coagulation* and 2) syndromes of *thrombotic thrombocytopenic purpura (TTP)* and *hemolytic–uremic syndrome (HUS).* The syndrome of DIC is discussed fully under Acquired Complex Bleeding Disorders later in this chapter.

Thrombotic Thrombocytopenic Purpura and the Hemolytic–Uremic Syndrome. These conditions may be part of a similar spectrum of diseases that represent the sequelae of different stimuli. *Thrombotic thrombocytopenic purpura (TTP)* is a disorder in which there is disseminated *intravascular platelet aggregation* occurring for unknown reasons associated with deposition of mainly platelet thrombi in the microcirculation. Many vessels in different organs are affected, and the consequence is organ circulatory insufficiency (particularly of the brain and kidneys), and microangiopathic hemolytic anemia as well as thrombocytopenia. Thrombotic thrombocytopenic purpura classically presents as a pentad of clinical features that include: 1) thrombocytopenia, 2) microangiopathic hemolytic anemia, 3) renal disorders, 4) neurologic impairment, and 5) fever.

Disseminated intravascular coagulation is generally *not a feature of TTP* since the syndrome rarely reflects localized fibrin deposition, but is more an intravascular platelet consumption and aggregation. The peripheral blood smear shows a striking *schistocytosis* of erythrocytes and profound thrombocytopenia. The *reticulocyte count* is invariably *elevated,* and chemical analyses on the serum show variable *impairment of renal function,* usually including an elevated blood urea nitrogen and creatinine. A urine sediment is usually active. Since the microvasculature of many organs can be involved, including the liver and the heart, variable enzyme changes or other test parameters reflecting insufficiency of these organs may be seen.

Thrombotic thrombocytopenic purpura is a serious disorder that formerly was associated with a greater than 80% mortality. In recent times the mortality has decreased; however, it still carries approximately a 40–50% mortality. It is usually a disease of young adults who have a viral-like prodrome in many instances. The clinical features are typically those of the predominant organ failure, thrombocytopenia, and anemia. Other laboratory studies reflecting hemolysis may also be evident, including an *elevated indirect bilirubin, reticulocytosis, elevated lactate dehydrogenase (LDH),* and often an *elevated leukocyte count* reflecting panhyperplasia of the bone marrow.

The pathophysiology of this disorder is unclear, and it may be associated with collagen–vascular diseases, infections, drugs, or a postpartum state. Treatment is directed toward removing a presumed plasma/platelet aggregating factor, replacement of a deficient anti-aggregant (prostacycline) by means of plasmapheresis and fresh frozen plasma infusion, and interference with abnormal platelet aggregation by means of drugs or medications known to inhibit platelet aggregation such as the antiplatelet drug dipyridamole and aspirin. Corticosteroids are also generally used.

Hemolytic–Uremic Syndrome. The hemolytic–uremic syndrome may represent a focal manifestation of TTP involving, predominantly, the kidneys. The main features are a severe microangiopathic hemolytic anemia with schistocytes in the peripheral blood and a *reticulocytosis,* as well as all the other clinical and laboratory features of *hemolysis.* However, in this condition, a major feature is the presence of *renal failure.* Hemolytic anemia and thrombocytopenia appear to be secondary to local renal abnormalities. Fever and neurologic impairment, which may occur in TTP, are generally absent. This condition more usually occurs in children who present with profound reduction of urine output and hematuria. Platelet consumption occurs in the microcirculation of the kidney.

Hemolytic–uremic syndrome can also occur following pregnancy (postpartum hemolytic–uremic syndrome), and has been reported following chemotherapy with the agent mitomycin C.

Quantitative Platelet Abnormalities: Thrombocytosis

Thrombocytosis is the term that refers to an *elevated platelet count,* usually as a result of secondary stimulation. The term *thrombocythemia* is used for *unregulated, uncontrolled production of platelets,* as occurs in the *myeloproliferative syndromes* (see Chapter 4). Elevated platelet counts are commonly encountered in the hospitalized population, and may be seen in conditions such as inflammatory disorders, infections, malignancy, and following acute bleeding. Platelets may be elevated as part of an acute phase response to inflammation or infection. Table 6–6 is a list of the causes of thrombocytosis.

The laboratory determination of the platelet count by electronic counters will document the presence of an elevated platelet count. Sustained platelet count *elevations above a million* are generally not encountered in reactive thrombocytosis and are more commonly seen in *primary thrombocythemia;* however, occasionally more marked platelet counts may be seen in the reactive disorders. The peripheral smear may also show the appearance of giant or large platelets, which are usually more indicative of either abnormal production or increased platelet turnover (see Fig. 6–1). Sample testing, particularly serum samples, may give *spurious elevation of potassium levels* (spurious hyperkalemia) since platelets contain intracellular potassium and as the blood clots, potassium is released. This produces a *spurious hyperkalemia.* A more accurate determination of blood potassium is achieved by a plasma potassium, which is the determination of choice in patients with elevated platelet counts. In *reactive thrombocytosis, platelet function* studies are usually *normal* and patients are not at increased risk for thrombotic events. In *thrombocythemia, platelet function* studies may be quite *abnormal,* including abnormal aggregation studies, and patients may be at risk for both bleeding or thrombotic events.

Thrombocytosis may also occur in patients who have had a splenectomy, since the normal splenic pool consitutes one third of the total platelet mass. Splenectomy will result in an immediate increase in platelet count and the platelet count may return to a normal or high normal value within 1–2 months.

Table 6–6. CAUSES OF THROMBOCYTOSIS

Myeloproliferative syndromes
Essential thrombocythemia
Polycythemia vera
Myelofibrosis with agnogenic myeloid metaplasia
Chronic myelogenous leukemia
Secondary (reactive) thrombocytosis
Mobilization of pooled platelets
Postsplenectomy
After epinephrine administration
Rebound thrombocytosis
After blood loss (including surgery)
Accompanying bone marrow recovery
After cytotoxic chemotherapy
After treatment of vitamin B_{12} or folate deficiency
Iron deficiency
Malignancy
Chronic inflammatory conditions
Collagen vascular diseases
Inflammatory bowel diseases
Chronic infections
Tuberculosis
Osteomyelitis

Qualitative Platelet Disorders

Abnormal platelet function in the presence of a *normal platelet count* suggests a *qualitative platelet abnormality.* These defects in platelet function may be *inherited* (von Willebrand's disease) or *acquired* (drugs, infections, renal disease, or dysproteinemias). The *commonest* qualitative platelet abnormality is that occurring in association with *drugs,* and in particular *aspirin* and the *nonsteroidal antiinflammatory agents. Alcohol* may also produce qualitative platelet malfunction. Patients with qualitative platelet abnormalities usually have an abnormally *prolonged bleeding time* and variable disturbances of *platelet aggregation.* These are discussed in Chapter 5. Table 6–7 is a list of the qualitative platelet abnormalities that may occur. One of the most common inherited disorders of platelet function is *von Willebrand's disease,* and this is discussed earlier in this chapter. Reduction of platelet numbers is far commoner than disorders of function. Most dysfunctional syndromes do occur as part of other diseases. Note: Constitutional defects of platelet function are very rare. Of these, von Willebrand's disease is the commonest but, as already mentioned, it is not primarily a platelet disorder.

Platelet Disorders Secondary to Other Diseases

Severe uremia impairs the platelet release reaction (see Chapter 5); the patient's own platelets behave abnormally, and transfused normal platelets acquire this abnormality. Oozing and mucocutaneous bleeding often complicate *advanced uremia.*

Table 6–7. QUALITATIVE PLATELET ABNORMALITIES

Inherited platelet abnormalities
Intrinsic platelet defects
Bernard-Soulier syndrome
Glanzmann's thrombasthenia
Storage pool disorders
Extrinsic platelet abnormalities
von Willebrand's disease
Congenital afibrinogenemia
Acquired platelet abnormalities
Intrinsic platelet abnormalities
Preleukemic and acute nonlymphocytic leukemia
Myeloproliferative syndromes*
Paroxysmal nocturnal hemoglobinemia*
Drug-related platelet abnormalities
Aspirin and other nonsteroidal anti-inflammatory agents
Sulfinpyrazone
Dipyridamole
Dextran
Heparin*
Penicillins
Extrinsic platelet abnormalities
Uremia
Paraproteins (multiple myeloma, Waldenstrom's macroglobulinemia)

*Associated with increased risk of thromboembolic events.

Although dialysis often restores platelet function to normal, the bleeding problem may remain difficult to control.

Platelets also experience difficulty in functioning normally when there are high levels of *abnormal serum proteins,* as seen in *multiple myeloma* and other *dysproteinemias.* High molecular weight dextrans produce the same effect.

The presence of *fibrin–fibrinogen split products* seems to inhibit both aggregation and release. The normal liver clears from the circulation the low levels of degradation products that occur with everyday trauma and repair. Platelet function is diffusely abnormal in *severe liver disease* and failure to clear fibrin split products may contribute to this situation.

The high platelet counts that accompany *myeloproliferative syndromes* often predispose, paradoxically, to both bleeding problems and a thrombotic tendency.

Effect of Drugs

Many drugs impair platelet function; aspirin is undoubtedly the leading offender. Once exposed to aspirin, platelets have impaired release reactions for their entire lifespan. Other anti-inflammatory drugs have comparable effects, but may not irreversibly impair platelet function. Alcohol inhibits ADP-related aggregation; this probably does have clinical significance, at least in patients whose liver functions also have been damaged by alcohol.

ACQUIRED COMPLEX BLEEDING DISORDERS

Disseminated Intravascular Coagulation (DIC)

The complex disorder variously called *disseminated intravascular coagulation (DIC), consumption coagulopathy,* and *defibrination syndrome* is a common, acquired cause of bleeding tendency. It is a complex disorder that is due to pathologic generation of thrombin in the vascular compartment. As a consequence, there is *intravascular coagulation* with *consumption of coagulation factors, thrombin generation,* and secondarily, *consumption of platelets.* Disseminated intravascular coagulation usually occurs as a complication of some other life-threatening illness; the superimposed bleeding problem is often the last event in a rapidly deteriorating situation.

Pathophysiology

The mechanisms that lead to DIC are exaggerated physiologic processes, in which the coagulation cascade is activated, leading to fibrin deposition in the small blood vessels of many tissues and organs. Several stimuli activate the coagulation cascade (Table 6–8). The result of this process is impaired oxygenation of multiple organs, consumption of coagulation proteins, consumption of platelets, and secondary activation of the fibrinolytic system in an attempt to remove the fibrin. Without the checks and balances that normally regulate thrombin and plasmin, both these powerful proteolytic enzymes meet little resistance to their lytic attack on whatever factor VIII, factor V, fibrinogen, and platelets survive the coagulation process. The severity, chronicity, and natural history of DIC is extremely variable, and prognosis often depends on the primary disease causing the DIC rather than the syndrome itself.

Clinical Findings

A complex clinical syndrome with thrombotic and hemostatic–hemorrhagic features occurs. In the full-blown state of DIC, there is severe depletion of all coagulation proteins, especially of factors V and VIII, platelets are markedly decreased, little or no clottable fibrinogen exists, and high levels of fibrin–fibrinogen degradation products circulate and inhibit fibrin formation. The reticuloendothelial system and the liver attempt to clear these abnormal proteins and restore a semblance of normal coagulation protein synthesis. Unfortunately, DIC usually occurs in a setting of circulatory stasis, shock, hypovolemia, or increased vascular permeability. These conditions impair circulation and make it very difficult to initiate compensatory activity.

Inciting Events

The classic stimuli to DIC are infectious, surgical, obstetric, or traumatic events that allow thromboplastic material to enter the circulation. These events include *amniotic fluid embolism,* trauma, or large-scale *operations,* especially those involving the brain, lungs, or the genitourinary system, *severe burns,* and conditions in which blood cells undergo intravascular destruction such as *hemolytic transfusion reactions, bacterial toxemia,* and *acute promyelocytic leukemia. Generalized sepsis*

Table 6–8. PROFILE OF DIC

Synonyms	Condition Associated with DIC	Suggested Triggering Mechanisms	Clinical Manifestations	Clinical Laboratory Findings	Sequential Therapy
1. "Consumptive coagulopathy" 2. Defibrination syndrome	Obstetric accidents Intravascular hemolysis Septicemia Viremia (varicella) Leukemias: Acute Promyelocytic Other Solid malignancy Acidosis/alkalosis Burns Crush injury and tissue necrosis Vascular disorders	Amniotic fluid Retained fetus Byproduct of red cell hemolysis Antigen/antibody complexes Endotoxin release Chronic stasis Complement activation	1. *General signs:* hemorrhaging (usually from 3 unrelated sites), fever, hypotension, acidosis, hypoxia, proteinuria, hematuria 2. *Specific signs:* petechiae, purpura, gangrene 3. *Microthrombi* 4. *End organ dysfunction*	Hypofibrinogenemia Abnormal PT Abnormal PTT Abnormal thrombin time Abnormal platelet count Abnormal factors V and VIII Positive fibrin(ogen)-split products Leukocytosis Schistocytosis Thrombocytopenia Reticulocytosis	1. Remove or treat triggering process 2. Stop or slow coagulation process a. Heparin b. Antiplatelet drugs c. AT-III concentrates 3. Blood component replacement a. Platelets b. Fibrinogen c. Prothrombin complex d. AHF (b–d: Cryoprecipitate) 4. Antifibrinolytic therapy* a. Epsilon amino caproic acid (EACA)

*Sequential therapy used only after clotting is stopped. (3% of patients may require this therapy.) Generally used in conjunction with heparin.
From Pittiglio, DH and Sacher, RA: Clinical Hematology and Fundamentals of Hemostasis. FA Davis, Philadelphia, 1987, p 389, with permission.

Table 6–9. CLINICAL CONDITIONS ASSOCIATED WITH DIC

Thromboplastin release—factor VII activation
Placental abruption
Trauma
Fat emboli syndrome
Sepsis*
Promyelocytic leukemia
Retained dead fetus syndrome
Acute intravascular hemolysis*
Amniotic fluid embolus*
Cardiopulmonary bypass surgery
Endothelial cell damage—factor XII activation
Immune complex disease
Intravascular hemolysis*
Liver disease*
Heat stroke
Sepsis*
Burns
Vasculitis
Anoxia
Acidosis
Factor X and II activation
Snake venoms
Acute pancreatitis
Liver disease*
Fat emboli syndrome*

*More than one mechanism may be involved.

and severe liver disease can cause acute or gradually developing DIC. Other conditions that can be associated with DIC are listed in Table 6–9.

Laboratory Diagnosis of DIC

Laboratory assessment of DIC must take into consideration that:

1. There is activation of coagulation with thrombin generation and fibrin formation,
2. There may be consumption of coagulation factors, particularly factors VIII and V,
3. There is consumption of platelets,
4. There is secondary activation of the fibrinolytic pathway with parts of fibrin and fibrinogen digestion increasing in the bloodstream, and
5. The clinical syndromes inciting the DIC may have their own inherent clinical and laboratory manifestations. Table 6–8 is an outline of the laboratory tests reflecting these manifestations.

Activation of the coagulation cascade and *thrombin* generation can be assayed in the clinical laboratory. Simple screening tests of thrombin/fibrinogen interaction make use of the property that thrombin cleaves two fibrinopeptides from fibrinogen called *fibrinopeptide A* and *fibrinopeptide B*. These may be assayed by radioimmunoassay techniques. In addition, following cleavage of these fibrinopeptides, *fibrin monomer complexes* with fibrinogen may be determined in the laboratory by the *paracoagulation tests*. Two tests, namely *protamine sulfate precipitation* and *ethanol gelation* tests, will detect the presence of fibrin monomer. These tests have all been used as an index of intravascular thrombin generation. The fibrinopeptide assays are more specific than the paracoagulation tests, since a positive paracoagulation test can also occur following fibrinolytic activity and plasmin cleavage of fibrin and fibrinogen.

Consumption of the coagulation factors V, VIII, and fibrinogen will obviously, by necessity, prolong the PTT and the PT to a variable degree, depending on the degree of consumption.

Platelet determination can easily be performed by electronic counters and may be verified by examination of the peripheral blood smear. In addition, *large platelets* may be seen reflecting increased platelet turnover (see Fig. 6–1). Furthermore, *microangiopathic hemolytic anemia* and *schistocytes* may be seen, and are indicative of mechanical damage to the erythrocytes (see Color Plate 14).

Fibrinolysis causes liberation of the active enzyme *plasmin,* which cleaves fibrinogen and fibrin into degradation products. These are consequently increased in DIC, as fibrinogen is decreased.

The *primary condition* inciting the DIC may, in addition, be evident on laboratory testing, for example positive blood cultures in association with sepsis, abnormal leukocytes in association with promyelocytic leukemia, evidence of liver cell decompensation with liver disease, clinical evidence of trauma, or the postpartum state.

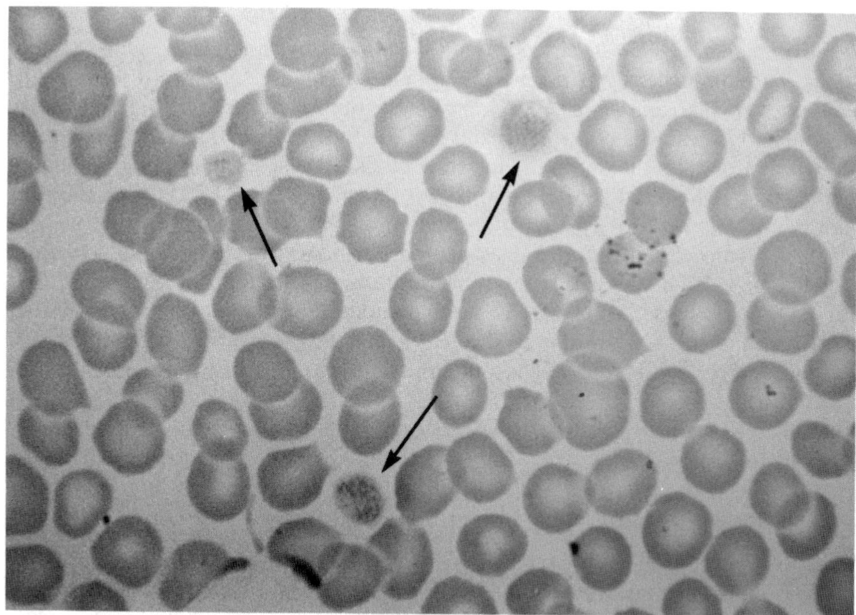

Figure 6–1. Peripheral blood smear showing giant platelets (arrows).

MANAGEMENT

The best therapy is to correct or reverse the initial inciting events. With massive trauma, sepsis, cardiogenic shock, and other clinical catastrophes, this tends to be difficult. The second major therapeutic thrust is to maintain blood volume and hemostatic function by means of replacement of the coagulation factors that have been consumed and attention to cardiovascular hemodynamics. Usual blood component replacement includes red cells for the anemia, platelet transfusions to correct the thrombocytopenia, and cryoprecipitate to correct factor VIII and fibrinogen deficiencies. Fresh frozen plasma is also used in an attempt to correct a complex coagulopathy. There is very little role for heparin in the treatment of DIC unless complicated by profound thrombotic events.

Liver Disease

Patients with severe liver disease nearly always have abnormal results in laboratory tests of hemostatic function, and may bleed significantly after liver biopsy or other surgical procedures. Spontaneous bleeding, however, is surprisingly uncommon unless there is an obvious hemorrhagic lesion such as esophageal varices or hemorrhagic gastritis. The liver manufactures so many coagulation proteins that factor *deficiencies* are to be expected when hepatic function fails. *Platelet problems,* excessive *fibrinolysis,* and low-grade *intravascular coagulation* are additional complicating events.

LIVER FACTORS

Deficiency of the *Vitamin K–dependent factors* (II, VII, IX, and X) is the most frequent coagulation abnormality. This deficiency affects both PT and PTT. Early in the disease, factor VII may be the only depressed factor; this leads to a *prolonged PT* with a *normal PTT.*

If liver cells are badly diseased, giving vitamin K does nothing to increase factor levels, but administering parenteral vitamin K can help to *distinguish obstructive from nonobstructive jaundice.* In biliary obstruction, factor levels are low because fat-soluble vitamin K is not being absorbed. The liver is capable of synthesizing the proteins but no bile salts reach the intestine to facilitate absorption of fat, including the fat-soluble vitamin K. After vitamin K is injected, PT and PTT should improve within 48 hours in cases of biliary obstruction.

When hepatocellular failure has caused coagulation factor deficiencies, albumin production is also depressed. In addition, antithrombin III and factor protein C and protein S are decreased. It is rare to have hypoprothrombinemia without pre-existing hypoalbuminemia. A *prothrombin time more than 1.5 times normal* correlates with *poor clinical prognosis,* but it is hepatic insufficiency rather than hemorrhagic complications that causes clinical deterioration. When hemorrhage occurs, large volumes of fresh or fresh frozen plasma may correct the coagulation defect temporarily.

OTHER ABNORMALITIES

Factor V levels decline unpredictably in liver disease, but it is not clear whether this contributes to clinical bleeding. Factor VIII, by contrast, may give higher than normal results. Recall that *factor VIII* is synthesized by *endothelial cells* and is probably the only major factor *not* synthesized by the liver. Fibrinogen levels are variable, depending on whether or not fibrinolysis occurs. Even when fibrinogen levels appear normal, coagulation may be qualitatively abnormal. There is a defect in polymerization, but it is not clear whether the abnormality lies in the fibrinogen molecules or in factor XIII.

Activated products of both coagulation and fibrinolysis normally circulate in small quantities and are cleared by the liver. With hepatic failure, *activated coagulation and fibrinolytic factors* may persist and accumulate. These factors affect laboratory tests for *disseminated intravascular coagulation* and for the occurrence of fibrin–fibrinogen degradation products.

Severe liver disease impairs both platelet production and platelet function; this is especially marked in alcoholics. The transfusion of platelet concentrates gives disappointing clinical results, although it may be necessary if active bleeding is present.

Inhibitors to Coagulation Factors

In addition to the inhibitory antibodies that develop in repeatedly transfused factor-deficient patients, antibodies have been observed to develop *spontaneously*. Antibodies to factor VIII, or rarely to factors V and VIII, occur in previously normal individuals of either sex. Usually IgG, these antibodies resemble autoimmune red cell or platelet antibodies. They occur without discernible stimulus, they react with tissue or protein from other humans as well as from the patient, and they can cause clinically significant disease.

Spontaneous anti–factor VIII usually occurs in older people, although it has been reported in young patients with chronic *immuno-inflammatory diseases* such as rheumatoid arthritis, lupus erythematosus, and ulcerative colitis. There is also a puzzling association with *pregnancy*. Pregnancy-associated anti–factor VIII usually develops after delivery rather than during the pregnancy itself. Its management may be quite complicated.

A patient with antibody to factor VIII has bleeding symptoms very like those of constitutional hemophilia, including hemarthroses, soft tissue hematomas without apparent trauma, and excessive bleeding after minor injuries. The patient's plasma has low or absent levels of procoagulant activity and, after incubation, inhibits the coagulation of previously normal plasma (''mixing study''). Treatment is extremely difficult; non–human Factor VIII concentrates can be used for one-time correction of a crisis, but these products are immunogenic under the best of circumstances. Coagulation factor replacement usually consists of replenishing activated products of coagulation or excessive amounts of factor VIII concentrate. Immunosuppression has been tried with variable success. Another approach has been to administer concentrates of the ''liver factors,'' including factors IX and X, thereby bypassing the step that involves factor VIII.

REFERENCES

1. Colman, RW, et al (eds): Hemostasis and Thrombosis: Basic Principles and Clinical Practice, ed 2. JB Lippincott, Philadelphia, 1987.
2. Gill, FM: Congenital bleeding disorders: Hemophilia and von Willebrand's disease. Med Clin North Am 68:601, 1984.

3. Hirsch, J: Therapeutic range for the control of oral anticoagulant therapy. Arch Intern Med 145:1187, 1985.
4. McKee, PA: Disorders of blood coagulation. In Wyngaarden, JB and Smith, LH (eds): Textbook of Medicine, ed 17. WB Saunders, Philadelphia, 1987, p 1040.
5. Ogston, D: The Physiology of Hemostasis. Harvard University Press, Cambridge, MA, 1983.
6. Rock, G: Defects of plasma clotting factors. In Pittiglio, DH and Sacher, RA (eds): Fundamentals of Hematology and Hemostasis. FA Davis, Philadelphia, 1987, p 365.
7. Shattil, S: Diagnosis and treatment of recurrent venous thromboembolism. Med Clin North Am 68:577, 1984.
8. Silgals, RM and Sacher, RA: Quantitative and qualitative vascular and platelet disorders, both congenital and acquired. In Pittiglio, DH and Sacher, RA (eds): Fundamentals of Hematology and Hemostasis. FA Davis, Philadelphia, 1987, p 346.
9. Suchman, AL: Diagnostic uses of the activated partial thromboplastin time and prothrombin time. Ann Intern Med 104:810, 1986.
10. Thompson, AR and Harker, LA: Manual of Hemostasis and Thrombosis, ed 3. FA Davis, Philadelphia, 1983.
11. Weiss, HJ: Von Willebrand's disease. In Williams, WJ, et al (eds): Hematology, ed 3. McGraw-Hill, New York, 1983, p 1413.

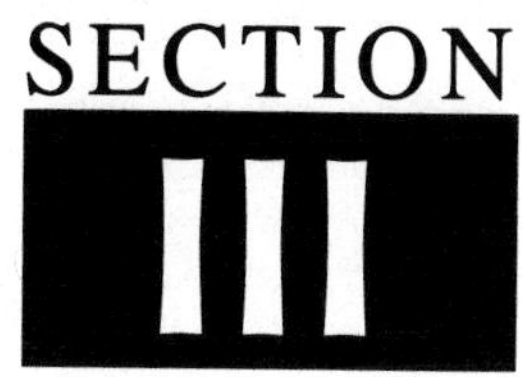

IMMUNOLOGY

OUTLINE

TESTS

CHAPTER

7

Principles of Immunology and Immunologic Testing

The fields of immunology and microbiology have grown hand-in-hand with discoveries of infectious agents and the body's host defenses against them. Further knowledge of the specifics of antigens and antibodies has also come from developments in blood banking and the practice of crossmatching transfusion products from donor to recipient.

Different immune responses to challenges from bacteria, fungi, viruses, and parasites or from other foreign antigens such as transfused blood cells result from various degrees of involvement of the three major divisions of the immune system:

1. humoral immunity (immunoglobulins or antibodies),
2. complement and its cascade of activation, and
3. cell-mediated immunity.

Although these three divisions do have distinct components, they frequently, if not usually, work in concert when confronted with a foreign material such as a microorganism.

Beyond this role in infectious diseases, principles of immunology have major significance in autoimmune diseases, in allergy and hypersensitivity, in immunodeficiency states, and in modalities of therapy involving immunosuppression for organ transplantation and immuno-enhancement for rejection of malignancies.

This chapter details elements of the immune system, laboratory procedures that measure the activity of the immune system, and how such laboratory tests can be used effectively for diagnosis and monitoring of immune disorders.

HUMORAL IMMUNITY

This portion of the immune system refers to the *immunoglobulins* or *antibodies* that circulate in the plasma phase of blood and that are also secreted at mucosal surfaces of the body. Immunoglobulin molecules are proteins composed of heavy chains (50,000 daltons in molecular weight) and light chains (25,000 daltons). The basic structure of an immunoglobulin molecule consists of two *light chains* plus two *heavy chains.* The light chains are attached to the heavy chains by way of disulfide (S–S) bonds between cysteine residues in the amino acid backbone of each chain. The heavy chains are also linked to one another through disulfide bonds (Fig. 7–1). This basic monomeric structure has a molecular size of approximately 150,000 daltons. Spatially, it points in three directions: two arms with identical *Fab regions* that can combine with a specific antigen and a third *Fc portion* that is constant in structure between different antibodies. The Fab region varies considerably in amino acid composition between different antibodies. This difference in Fab structure is what accounts for the extremely diverse range of different antigens to which specific antibodies can be synthesized by the immune system.

Both heavy and light chains have what are called *variable regions* near their amino ends in the Fab segments and also *constant regions* toward their carboxy ends in the Fc segment. It has recently been discovered that the variable nature of immunoglobulin chains derives from reorganization of the DNA in genes that encode both heavy and light chains. This process works by selecting a few short DNA segments from many tandemly aligned segments and then recombining them in such a way as to yield a unique gene that has a specific variable region and is linked with a constant region. If other DNA segments are recombined, antibodies with totally different antigenic combining powers will result.

The particular cells that make immunoglobulins for release into the circulation are called *plasma cells* (see also Chapter 4). They reside in the bone marrow along with precursors of the blood cells. An individual plasma cell produces only a single type of immunoglobulin molecule, which recognizes its specific antigen. As that plasma cell divides and produces a line of descendent cells (also termed a clone or clonal line), those resultant cells continue to synthesize the same antibody specific for that single antigenic site. Monoclonal antibodies are used extensively as diagnostic reagents for measurement of such substances as drugs and hormones and are also now finding therapeutic applications (e.g., to facilitate removal of digoxin from the circulation of digoxin-overdose cases by intravenous administration of a monoclonal anti-digoxin antibody).

The *class* of an immunoglobulin is determined by the type of its heavy chain. Immunoglobulin G *(IgG)* has gamma-heavy chains, *IgM* has mu-heavy chains, *IgA* has alpha-heavy chains, *IgE* has epsilon-heavy chains, and *IgD* has delta-heavy chains. The antibody molecules made by a single clone of plasma cells have exactly the same heavy chains and also contain only a single type of light chain. There are two general types of light chains, designated *kappa* and *lambda.* Both kappa and lambda light chains occur in all classes of antibodies. Overall, there is a slight predominance of kappa versus lambda by a ratio of roughly 3:2 in the serum of normal individuals. The major clinical use of measuring light chain type is in distinguishing whether proliferations of plasma cells or lymphoid cells are *monoclonal* (in which case there is almost complete predominance of only kappa or only lambda) or *polyclonal* (both kappa and lambda are present in major amounts [see Chapter 4]).

Subclasses of immunoglobulins exist due to minor differences between heavy chains that occur in the constant regions of some classes. There are four subclasses

CHAIN	WEIGHT
Light	22,500
Heavy	55,000
Heavy	55,000
Light	22,500

S S S S S S S S

A

NH_2 COOH

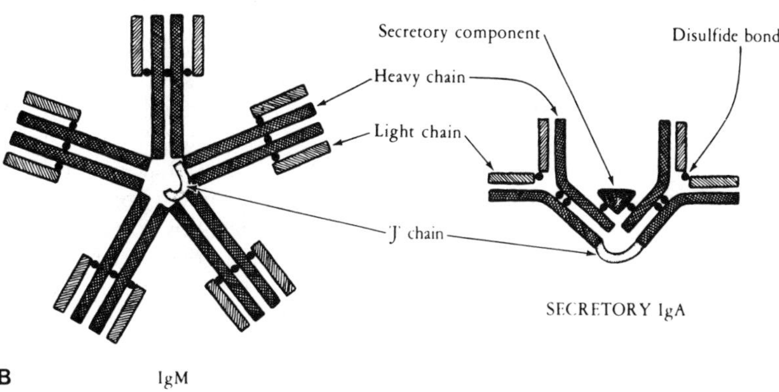

B IgM

Figure 7–1. (*A*) Schematic diagram of human IgG1 showing the location of interchain disulfide bonds. The molecule consists of two light chains and two heavy chains. The amino-terminal end is at the left and the carboxyl-terminal end is at the right. The structure depicted here is also applicable to other immunoglobulins with varying heavy-chain composition and polymerization. (*B*) Models of IgM and secretory IgA. The former is shown in its usual pentameric form with a J chain involved in the pentamer formation. Secretory IgA is shown as a dimer attached to a secretory component. Note the absence of the light–heavy interchain bonds in the IgA. The IgA predominant in secretions is of the IgA2 subclass, which lacks such bonds. (From Bernier, GM: Antibody and immunoglobulins: Structure and function. In Bellanti,[1] p 92, 93, with permission.)

of IgG (IgG1, IgG2, IgG3, and IgG4), two of IgA (IgA1 and IgA2), and two of IgD. Some of these subclass differences result in altered function of an immunoglobulin. For example, IgG1, IgG2, and IgG3 molecules generally can fix complement (see below), while IgG4 cannot. IgG3 has a structure that allows it to remain in the circulation for a much shorter period than the other IgG subclasses before it is cleared. Maternal IgG2 does not cross the placenta to the fetal circulation, although the other IgG subclasses can. IgA1 can be cleaved and thereby inactivated by some bacterial (streptococcal and gonococcal) enzymes, whereas IgA2 is not susceptible to those proteases.

In addition to the basic monomeric immunoglobulin structure mentioned above as two heavy chains plus two light chains (H_2L_2), there are polymeric linkages in which IgM and IgA participate. Normally, IgM in the serum is a pentameter of five monomeric units as $(H_2L_2)_5$ with interconnection through the mu-heavy chains in their Fc regions. There is another small fragment designated the *J chain,* which is involved in joining these IgM monomers together (see Fig. 7–1). In the case of IgA, the J chain allows for dimerization of two IgA molecules linked similarly through their alpha chains at the Fc location. One further modification of IgA occurs as it passes across epithelial cells and enters body secretions such as saliva where IgA is the major immunoglobulin. This modification entails the attachment to IgA of another protein segment designated *secretory piece.*

A typical *immune response* consists initially of a rise in IgM antibody directed against the stimulating antigen (immunogen). This phase is followed by production of IgG antibody against the antigen. Repeated stimulation with the antigen leads to greater production of the IgG antibody, but with shorter time lag after each succeeding antigenic stimulus. This ability of the immune system to remember and respond more efficiently to an antigen is called an *anamnestic response.* The time sequence of IgM followed by IgG is used extensively in the diagnosis of infectious diseases (see Fig. 15–1). In general, significant levels of IgM antibody against a virus, bacterium, or other infectious agents is interpreted as evidence for acute infection, whereas a high level of specific IgG is consistent with persistence of immunity in the convalescent phase after a previous infection. A common application of this principle is the measurement of IgM antibody against hepatitis A virus to diagnose acute or recent infection with that virus. Antibody of the IgG class against hepatitis A virus merely indicates infection in the (distant) past and is not very useful clinically for the evaluation of current hepatitis (see also Chapter 15).

ANTIGENS

The chemical nature of materials that can be recognized by antibodies is extremely wide and includes proteins, lipids, nucleic acids, and small molecules such as drugs and steroid hormones. This is due in part to the fact that any particular antibody reacts with only a small region of an antigen. This antigenic site is designated an *epitope. Monoclonal antibodies* by their very nature are very specific for a single epitope. This degree of specificity has allowed the development of different antibodies that can distinguish between such closely related antigens as thyroxine (T_4) versus triiodothyronine (T_3), hemoglobin A versus hemoglobin S, and procainamide (parent drug) versus N-acetyl procainamide (drug metabolite).

Polyclonal antibodies are typical of the immune response in a normal animal on stimulation with foreign antigens, such as by immunization or by infection. Polyclonal antibodies consist of many different clones, each with potentially different specificities for a large number of epitopes on the surface of the foreign antigen. A distinct advantage for having many different antibody clones recognize an array of epitopes on an invading microorganism is that mutation by the infectious agent will likely alter only one epitope. The microbe may then escape one clone of antibody, but the other clones can still recognize the remaining epitopes. Polyclonal immune responses to infectious agents can therefore be seen to confer significant survival advantage to an animal.

Whether or not an antigen elicits an antibody response depends on the ability of the immune system to recognize that antigen as foreign and not as a *self antigen.* The vast number of self antigens present on our own tissues, cells, and proteins do not trigger immune responses except in cases of autoimmune disorders.

A foreign antigen is essentially one that has not been present in the body during development nor afterwards until it is introduced by infection, by trauma, or injection, as with immunization, by blood transfusion with erythrocytes, or by pregnancy with fetal cells that cross the placenta to the mother (e.g., Rh incompatibility). Even some small molecules normally present in the circulation can be made immunogenic (i.e., capable of stimulating an immune response) by coupling them to large foreign proteins. Examples of this strategy include coupling of thyroxine or steroid hormones to an enhancer called keyhole limpet hemocyanin that induces an intense immune response when injected into animals. Some of those antibody clones will react with the small hormone molecule even though it was previously tolerated as a self antigen. In other instances, drugs such as penicillin or heparin on rare occasion can cause autoimmune responses when those drugs become bound to cell surfaces, thereby converting a self antigen to a foreign-appearing one.

Antigens of similar chemical structure may be able to cross-react with the same antibody. There is very likely a measurable difference in affinity or binding strength between an antibody and those different antigens, but when the antibody is present in high concentration, the reaction may be clinically significant. An example of this may be similar epitopes on the surface of a virus or bacterium and also on some protein in the body. Infection with such a microorganism could then trigger an antibody response, which has the undesired side effect of attaching to the common epitope on tissues and causing damage to the body. Examples of this type are streptococcal antigens and rheumatic fever or acute glomerulonephritis.

IMMUNE COMPLEXES

When antibodies interact with antigens, the two Fab arms of the immunoglobulin monomer can bind to separate antigen molecules, each containing the same epitope. If the antigen is large enough for another antibody to combine with another epitope on its surface, there can result a large *matrix* of alternating antigen and antibody molecules. This meshwork is referred to as an *immune complex.* It can be so large as to be physically insoluble and may actually form a visible precipitate, thereby removing both antigen and antibody from solution.

If the concentration of either antigen or antibody greatly exceeds that of the other, a matrix cannot form. When the antigen is in excess, the Fab regions are saturated with individual antigens. When the antibody is in excess, available antigen is coated with antibody. The point where concentration of antigen and antibody form an interlocking matrix is termed *equivalence.*

These different states of immune complexes have importance for laboratory test procedures that use the point of equivalence to detect assay end points by immunodiffusion or by nephelometry. They also can have enormous clinical significance because large immune complexes that form at equivalence in the circulation are filtered by the kidney, potentially giving rise to glomerulonephritis. In addition, any infectious disease can be separated into a stage in which there is excess antigen (early in the disease before an immune response is mounted) and another in which the antibody is in excess (convalescence). For example, human immunodeficiency virus (HIV) and its antigens are present in an infectious form in the body and blood of individuals for several weeks after initial infection before there is sufficient time to develop a detectable antibody response to that virus.

COMPLEMENT

Once an antibody has lodged on the surface of an invading microorganism, an orderly sequence of plasma proteins called *complement* may be activated (Fig. 7–2). These complement proteins are capable of delivering a fatal blow to the invader. This process is initiated by a conformational change in the Fc region of an antibody on combining with an antigen. If that antigen were floating freely in the circulation as an individual molecule, the immune complex that formed may bind complement components to it. Complement in the complex could then help to attract phagocytic cells, which will engulf and remove the inactivated antigen from the circulation.

If the antigen is part of a bacterial cell wall, complement can fix onto the bound antibody, ultimately weakening the bacterium and killing it. The same process can occur with transfused red blood cells if they are incompatible with the recipient, thereby leading to hemolysis.

By the so-called *classical pathway of complement activation,* the first component C1q attached to Fc regions of two adjacent IgG molecules that have been brought into proximity by binding onto a foreign surface. Alternatively, a single IgM molecule can attract C1q since each IgM has five Fc regions. Next, the subunits C1r and C1s bind to C1q. These subunits have enzymatic activities that cleave two other components (C4 into C4a and C4b and C2 into C2a and C2b). C4b binds directly to the surface near where it was generated, and C2a binds to the C4b. The C4b–C2a complex then cleaves C3 into C3a and C3b, which in turn binds nearby on the surface. The interaction of C2a and C3b cleaves C5, which then binds C6 and C7 and also attaches to the surface. C8 and C9 are attracted to form the final additions to this complex. At this point, the surface of the cell or bacterium is seriously damaged, leading ultimately to lysis. This sequence of complement activation is the same regardless of the specific antigens involved in the immune complex. It is the specificity of the antibody that directs and initiates the whole process (see Fig. 7–2).

There is another means by which complement can be activated, the *alternative pathway.* This pathway is independent of antibody. It occurs when C3 combines with *factor B* and binds to a substance such as bacterial cell wall. This complex further activates more C3, which then continues the activation and attachment of C5 through C9.

Complement activation is *down-regulated* by individual plasma proteins that selectively inhibit C1, C4b, or C3b. Congenital deficiency of one such protein, *C1 esterase inhibitor,* results in a clinical syndrome called *hereditary angioedema.* In this disorder, edema occurs in the gastrointestinal and respiratory tracts when complement is activated by trauma or for frequently unrecognized reasons.

Congenital deficiencies of individual complement components may manifest themselves as increased susceptibility to infections with pyogenic bacteria (deficiency of C1, C4, C2, or C3) or *Neisseria* (C3, C5, C6, C7, C8, or C9). In addition, there is a greater frequency of rheumatic diseases (in particular systemic lupus erythematosus) with deficiencies of C1, C2, or C4, perhaps due to impaired clearance of immune complexes.

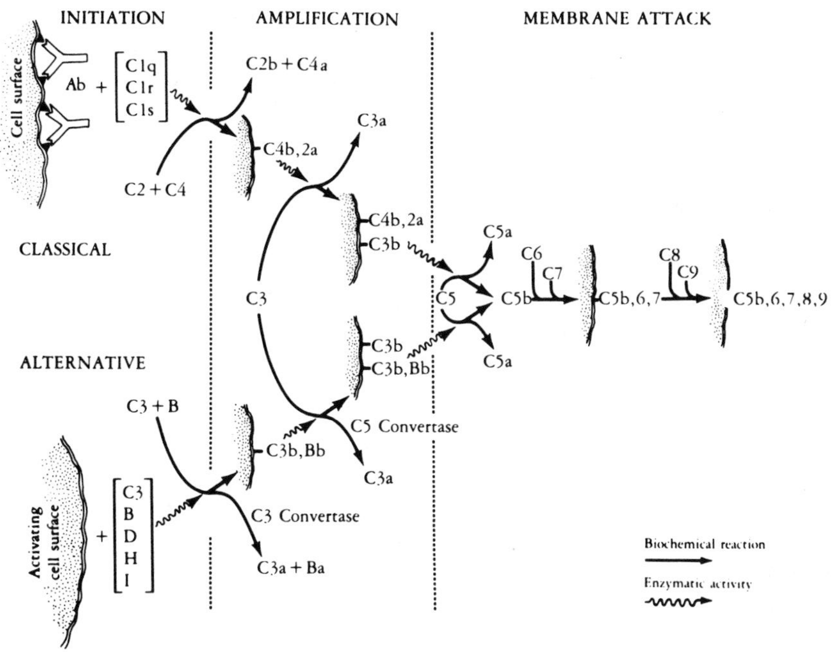

Figure 7–2. Schematic representation of the 2 pathways of complement activation. (From Kunkel, SL, et al: The complement system. In Bellanti,[1] with permission.)

CELL-MEDIATED IMMUNITY

The recognition, uptake, and processing of foreign antigens is performed by cellular elements of the immune system. These include *macrophages,* which initially ingest foreign materials and then present them to *T-lymphocytes* in a process that relies on complex cell-to-cell and antigen recognition signals supplied by surface markers on cell membranes. With all these control signals acting properly, a subset of the T-lymphocytes called *T-helper cells* then stimulates *B-lymphocytes* to produce antibody against the processed antigen. These B-lymphocytes are also stimulated to divide as a further means to amplify antibody production. This sequence is slowed down by other types of T-lymphocytes called *T-suppressor cells,* which limit the antibody response. This on–off feature of the immune response permits a multitude of different antibodies to be made and subsequently to be turned off when the need for those particular antibodies is over. Discovery of unique antigenic markers on the surfaces of lymphocytes has led to the classification of helper T cells as T_4 (also called CD4; CD = cellular determinant) cells and suppressor T cells as T_8 cells (also called CD8 cells [Table 7–1]).

One other type of lymphocyte is *cytotoxic killer T cells,* which have the capacity to lyse target cells. An example is interaction of cytotoxic T cells with virally infected cells. If the infected cells have both viral antigens and major histocompatibility antigens on their membranes, they constitute targets that the cytotoxic T cells

Table 7–1. WORLD HEALTH ORGANIZATION RECOMMENDED NOMENCLATURE FOR HUMAN LEUKOCYTE DIFFERENTIATION ANTIGENS*

Antigen	Monoclonal Antibodies	Positive Leukocytes
CD1	Leu 6, T6, OKT6	Thymocytes
CD2	Leu 5B, T11, OKT11	T and NK cells (E-rosette receptor)
CD3	Leu 4, T3, OKT3	Mature T cells
CD4	Leu 3, T4, OKT4	Helper-inducer T cells, monocytes
CD5	Leu 1, T1, T101	T cells, B-cell subset, CLL cells, PLL cells
CD6	T12	T cells
CD7	Leu 9, 3A1	T, T-ALL, and NK cells
CD8	Leu 2, T8, OKT8	Suppressor-cytotoxic T cells, NK subset
CD9	BA-2	Lymphoid leukemia-associated antigen
CD10	CALLA, J5	Granulocytes, pre-B leukemia cells
CD11	CR3/Leu 15, OKM1, MO-1	(C3bi receptor) Monocytes, granulocytes, NK cells
CDw13	MY7	Neutrophils and monocytes
CDw14	MY4, MO-2	Monocytes
CD15	Leu M1	Monocytes, granulocytes
CD16	Leu 11	(lgG Fc receptor) NK cells, PMNS
CD19	Leu 12, B4	B cells, Pre-B-ALL cells
CD20	Lau 16, B1	B cells
CD21	CR2, B2	(C3d receptor) Mature B cells
CD22	Leu 14	B cells
CD23	Blast-2	
CD24	BA-1	B cells, pre-B-ALL cells
CD25	IL-2 receptor (Tac)	HTLV-I and HTLV-II infected T cells, subset of B cells, activated T cells

*CLL = chronic lymphocytic leukemia; PLL, prolymphocytic leukemia; ALL, acute lymphocytic leukemia; CALLA, common ALL antigen; NK, natural killer.

Note: Newer antigens have been discovered since this list was formed and more than 50 have now been described.

From James, K: Immunophenotyping of lymphomas and leukemias. Lab Med 19:225, 1988, with permission.

recognize and kill, thereby protecting the body from further virus production and release.

HISTOCOMPATIBILITY ANTIGENS

The immunologic identity of human cells is determined by histocompatibility antigens on the surface membranes of all cells except for erythrocytes and trophoblasts. These tissue antigens are what account for rejection of transplanted organs. *Class I antigens* consist of two protein components: heavy chains from one of the three different genetic loci designated HLA-A, HLA-B, and HLA-C and a common light chain called beta-2-microglobulin. The large number of alleles for the heavy chain genes accounts for an almost unlimited number of different antigen combinations. For this reason, a perfect cross-match between organ transplant donor and recipient is virtually impossible to achieve except in the case of identical twins.

Another set of antigens is restricted primarily to monocytes and lymphocytes. These are the *class II antigens,* which consist of two protein chains. Class II antigens include HLA-D, HLA-DP, HLA-DQ, and HLA-DR, which also has multiple alleles. The function of all these antigens appears to be at the level of cell-to-cell communication regulating the immune response.

Human leukocyte antigen typing is used clinically for cross-matching solid organ and bone marrow transplants and also for better typing of platelet transfusion products in patients who have become HLA sensitized after multiple transfusions. Human leukocyte antigen typing is also used medico-legally for paternity testing because of the relatively high degree of certainty in tracing lineages through familial inheritance of the HLA alleles or *haplotypes* (see Chapter 8).

The genes for both class I and class II, antigens are located on chromosome 6 along with genes for some complement components. Some HLA types have been associated with diseases that have an autoimmune etiology, perhaps because of faulty immune regulation related to antigen type. In particular, HLA-B27 has an association with the rheumatic diseases, ankylosing spondylitis and Reiter's syndrome and other HLA types with multiple sclerosis, diabetes mellitus, and Grave's disease (thyroid) (see Chapter 8).

DISORDERS OF THE IMMUNE SYSTEM

Immune Deficiencies

Deficiencies of selective parts of the immune system usually result in increased susceptibility to infection with different microorganisms. These immune deficiencies can be *inherited* or *acquired* (Table 7–2; see Table 4–3).

Congenital deficiency typically presents early in the life of a newborn as recurrent infections, sometime after maternally transferred immunity has waned (IgG immunoglobulins that cross the placenta; IgA swallowed in breast milk). There are distinct hereditary deficiencies of immunoglobulins, of lymphocyte functions, and of complement (discussed above). In general, absence of antibodies (agammaglobulinemia) or severely reduced levels of antibodies (hypogammaglobulinemia) are manifested by increased susceptibility to bacterial infections. Immunoglobulins that normally bind to bacterial cell walls (opsonization) promote phagocytosis and removal by leukocytes.

However, impaired cellular immunity typically shows infections with viruses or fungi. This is because it requires lymphocytes to recognize and kill other cells infected with viruses and to kill the large cellular forms of the fungi.

Combined immunodeficiencies involving both immunoglobulins and cell-mediated immunity are severe disorders that show multiple infections and usually result in early death unless treated with heroic measures such as immune system reconstitution by bone marrow transplantation (e.g., severe combined immunodeficiency disease).

Acquired immunodeficiency may be due to replacement of normal plasma cells in the bone marrow by leukemia or to loss of cells with aplastic anemia. The resulting

Table 7–2. CONDITIONS ASSOCIATED WITH IMMUNOGLOBULIN DEFICIENCIES*

Condition	Population Affected	Immunoglobulin Abnormality	Other Findings
Acquired hypogamma-globulinemia	Malignancy of lymphoreticular system Autoimmune diseases Protein loss or malnutrition Immunosuppressive drugs	Unpredictable	T cell function also depressed Findings of primary disease
Selective IgA deficiency	1 in 500–1000 persons	↓↓ IgA Other Ig normal	Sinopulmonary infections frequent Often asymptomatic May have anaphylactoid response to transfused IgA
X-linked hypogammaglobulinemia	Males, from birth	All Ig classes very low	No B-lymphocytes or plasma cells T cell function intact
Wiskott-Aldrich syndrome	X-linked	IgG, IgA normal or ↑ IgE ↑, IgM ↓	Eczema, thrombocytopenia, recurrent infections T cell function decreased; may have ↓ number of T cells
IgG and IgA deficiency	X-linked or acquired	↓ IgG; ↓ IgA; ↑ IgM, to 10 × normal	Frequent infections Plasma cells numerous
Ataxia telangiectasia	Rare; both sexes	↓ IgA in 70%	Neurologic symptoms prominent Cutaneous vessels abnormal Lymphoid malignancies often develop
Severe combined immunodeficiency (SCID)	Very rare	All Ig classes ↓↓, except sometimes IgM present	Deficiency of progenitor lymphocyte Absent T cell functions Lymphoreticular malignancies develop in those who do not succumb to infection

*Listed in approximate order of decreasing incidence.
Adapted from Roitt,[15] Reinherz and Schlossman,[13] and Tomar.[17]

hypogammaglobulinemia can leave a patient susceptible to pneumococcal pneumonia or other bacterial infections. Malignancy involving the immune system, such as lymphoma, can also impair cellular immunity, resulting in such infections as herpesvirus and candida.

During the last decade, there has emerged a previously unrecognized disorder known as acquired immune deficiency syndrome (AIDS). This disorder is due to a new virus, human immunodeficiency virus (HIV), that infects and destroys the helper T-lymphocytes. Loss of these helper cells affects the body's ability to produce antibodies and to induce cellular immune responses. Patients with this syndrome therefore become infected with a wide array of microorganisms, many of which are not normally pathogenic except in such severe disorders. These include *Pneumocystis carinii,* candida, *Mycobacterium avium-intracellulare,* and many species of parasitic organisms (see also Chapters 13 and 14).

Immunosuppression/Enhancement

Chemotherapy with antimetabolites such as methotrexate is designed to kill rapidly dividing cancer or leukemia cells. One of the undesired side effects of chemotherapy is suppression of bone marrow and also of the immune system, which limits the extent to which cancer treatment can be tolerated.

Organ and bone marrow transplantation recipients must be treated with immunosuppressive agents and/or irradiation in order to prevent rejection of the grafted organ or cells as foreign antigens. These strategies are directed primarily at cellular immunity. In addition to using antimetabolites, physicians employ steroids, cyclosporine, antithymocyte globulin, and leukapheresis to control the immune response.

Exciting new developments in cancer therapy are based on the idea that tumor cells have escaped destruction by the immune system due to a breakdown in normal immune surveillance for antigens that are present on the tumor cells. The new strategies of therapy are based on enhancing or reconstituting the body's own immune response by activating lymphocytes with one or more of the chemicals that normally modulate immune function. These substances are the *lymphokines* such as interleukin-2 (IL-2). By injecting IL-2 into the body or by treating lymphocytes outside the body and then returning those cells to a cancer patient, the hope is that lymphokine-activated killer (LAK) cells will target the tumor for destruction. Other *biologic response modifiers* that affect the immune system and are undergoing clinical trials include alpha and gamma interferons.

Autoimmunity

When the immune system produces antibodies against (self) antigens of the body, there can be serious damage to many organ systems. A classic example of autoimmunity is *systemic lupus erythematosus* (SLE), in which extensive damage occurs in the kidneys due to deposition of circulating immune complexes in the glomeruli followed by activation of complement that indiscriminately injures the glomeruli. A target antigen for these autoantibodies is frequently DNA as well as other nuclear antigens such as ribonuclear protein (RNP) and also many cytoplasmic antigens. Other forms of autoimmune diseases include mixed connective tissue disorder (MCTD), rheumatoid arthritis, and many organ-specific diseases (e.g., thyroid-Graves disease, adrenal, skin).

Allergy/Hypersensitivity

Inappropriate excess activity of the immune system is sometimes an undesirable reaction on exposure to allergens such as pollens, dust, animal hairs, or foodstuffs. These reactions are mediated by IgE, which is the only immunoglobulin class to bind onto mast cells or basophils (see Chapter 2, p. 61). These cells contain granules of histamine and similar substances that are the direct chemical mediators of allergy. When an allergen such as ragweed pollen comes in contact with antiragweed IgE bound onto mast cells in the respiratory tract, the mast cells release their contents, causing constriction of smooth muscle around bronchioles. This action results in limited air movement, mucus secretion, and wheezing—a condition known as asthma. Other manifestations of this IgE-mediated reaction can occur in other parts of the body. These reactions can be relatively mild, in the form of hayfever and nasal congestion, or they can be extremely severe and result in sudden death from anaphylactic shock which produces circulatory collapse (Table 7–3).

DIAGNOSTIC TEST PROCEDURES IN IMMUNOLOGY

Serum Immunoglobulins

There are several methods commonly available to evaluate the level of immunoglobulins present in serum and other body fluids. Major elevations or reductions of immunoglobulins are broadly indicated by measurement of *total proteins* and *albumin* in serum. The difference between these two values yields a quantity called *globulins,* of which immunoglobulins form a major component in the *gamma globulin* fraction (see Chapter 9, Proteins). Since other globulin fractions can also vary, a better appreciation of the immunoglobulin quantity can be obtained from *serum protein electrophoresis,* which gives a direct measure of total gamma globulins. The gamma globulins can be qualitatively identified as having a monoclonal (narrow) versus polyclonal (wide) distribution by visual examination of the electrophoresis strip or of the densitometric scan (see Chapter 4 and Fig. 4–4).

Table 7–3. IMMUNOLOGIC MECHANISMS OF TISSUE INJURY

Type	Manifestations	Mechanism
I.	Immediate hypersensitivity reactions	IgE and other immunoglobulins
II.	Antibody directed against cells	IgG and IgM
III.	Antigen–antibody complexes	IgG mainly
IV.	Delayed hypersensitivity (cell-mediated)	Sensitized T-lymphocytes
V.	Mixed reactions	

From Henson, PM: Mechanisms of tissue injury produced by immunologic reactions. In Bellanti, JA (ed): Immunology III. WB Saunders, Philadelphia, 1985, p 219, with permission.

The next step in qualitative evaluation of elevated gamma globulins is *immunoelectrophoresis* (IEP), using as reagents (animal) antibodies directed against the heavy and light chains of human immunoglobulins. This technique gives information on whether there is a predominance of IgG, IgA, or IgM versus elevation of all three. In rare cases an otherwise unidentified protein band in the gamma region may be IgD or IgE, both of which can be detected by IEP using anti-IgD and anti-IgE antibodies. With predominance of a single immunoglobulin class, it is essential to establish whether that protein component is monoclonal or polyclonal. This determination is based on the presence of only one light chain type by IEP (i.e., kappa or lambda) indicating *monoclonal gammopathy.* This finding is typical of multiple myeloma and other plasma cell dyscrasias and lymphoreticular disorders (see Chapter 4 and Fig. 4–4). If, on the other hand, both kappa and lambda light chains are present in large amounts, the elevation of immunoglobulins is polyclonal. This type of response is frequently seen in states of chronic inflammation or chronic infection.

Quantitation of immunoglobulin types is useful for monitoring progress in diseases such as myeloma, where the amount of monoclonal protein in serum is related to disease activity. Serial measurements should be separated by at least a few weeks to allow for natural clearance from the circulation even after successful treatment of myeloma. In cases where the patient's plasma is replaced by plasmapheresis to reduce high levels of a monoclonal immunoglobulin causing hyperviscosity and circulatory problems (usually an IgM), success of the removal can be ascertained by *quantitative immunoglobulin levels* soon after the procedure is completed. The methods for quantitation usually employ diffusion through agarose to form precipitin rings (one- to two-day procedure) or precipitation in solution with nephelometry on automated equipment (a few minutes for assay time)—both making use of class-specific antihuman immunoglobulin antibodies.

The diagnosis of immunodeficiency states also relies heavily on quantitative immunoglobulin levels. Very low levels of IgG, IgA, and IgM near zero are characteristic of *agammaglobulinemia.* Selective deficiency of one immunoglobulin class is also established by quantitation. An extremely important example is *IgA deficiency.* In this condition there is a unique risk of anaphylactic reactions from blood transfusion containing IgA into deficient individuals, due to immune anti-IgA antibodies (see Chapter 8).

In addition to clear-cut deficiency states and high-level gammopathies, immunoglobulins are measured to define and to monitor moderate elevations as an index of disease progression in autoimmune conditions such as systemic lupus erythematosus and rheumatoid arthritis. Documentation of below-normal levels may also be useful for explaining mild immunodeficiencies, particularly in children. In that light, it should be well noted that immunoglobulin levels normally increase throughout childhood till maturity. Thus, interpretation of quantitative immunoglobulin levels in children requires age-specific reference ranges.

Some patients develop a high concentration of an immunoglobulin that precipitates in the cold. These precipitates can cause blockage of small capillaries in regions of the body (e.g., fingertips, ears) exposed to cold in winter weather. These *cryoglobulins* are measured by collecting a blood sample, keeping it warm while centrifuging, and then cooling the serum in a refrigerator to observe the formation of a precipitate in one to two days. This procedure is performed in a special graduated tube. The volume of sedimented precipitate is then read as a percentage of the whole serum sample to yield a numerical value of the *cryocrit* analogous to hematocrit. The cryoglobulin can be further washed, redissolved at warm temperature, and specifically identified as to immunoglobulin class by IEP or other immunologic analysis.

When immunoglobulins are produced in a disordered manner by myeloma and similar cells, there is opportunity for light chains to be synthesized in excess and released into the circulation. These free kappa or lambda light chains enter the urine because of their small molecular size. Such a finding in urine is termed *Bence-Jones protein.* It can be detected by traditional heating methods that cause a precipitate that redissolves at higher temperatures. Modern methods for Bence-Jones protein are based on immunologic detection (i.e., IEP). This protein can be toxic to the tubule cells of the kidney that become overloaded with intracellular protein while attempting to reabsorb it from the renal filtrate. Further modification of light chains by proteolytic enzymes in the body can in some patients lead to deposition of insoluble protein complexes termed *amyloidosis.* In this condition, the extracellular deposition of the protein causes pressure on normal cells (e.g., of spleen, liver, heart, gastrointestinal tract, etc.). The normal functioning cells of those organs are gradually replaced with the acellular amyloid. Diagnosis of this disorder is established by tissue biopsy (rectal or gingival usually). Amorphous deposits that demonstrate optical birefringence of polarized light when stained with Congo red dye are characteristic of amyloidosis.

Tissue biopsies are sometimes stained by immunofluorescent techniques to demonstrate the deposition of immunoglobulins as part of a pathologic process. Kidney biopsies are commonly evaluated for deposition of IgG, IgA, and IgM in the glomeruli to help make the diagnosis of glomerulonephritis. Circulating immune complexes of antigens and antibodies are normally filtered out of the circulation by the glomeruli. The presence of those complexes in glomeruli activates complement, leading to localized tissue destruction. This filtration of immune complexes performed in the circulation (e.g., in systemic lupus erythematosus) leads to an irregular or lumpy-bumpy staining pattern for immunoglobulin in the glomerulus. When the antibody is directed against the glomerulus itself (e.g., post-streptococcal glomerulonephritis), the immunoglobulin staining pattern is smooth and more homogeneous within the glomerulus. Deposition of immunoglobulin is also of diagnostic significance in other autoimmune disorders (e.g., in the skin), although assessment of autoimmunity rests largely on the demonstration of autoantibodies in the serum.

Serum Complement

The integrity of the entire complement system and all its components is conveniently screened for by a *hemolytic assay* designated the CH_{50}. In this assay, dilutions of human serum to be tested for complement activity are mixed with a standardized suspension of sheep erythrocytes presensitized by the adsorption of specific antibody. The complement present in the test serum leads to hemolysis, which is quantitated spectrophotometrically as the amount of hemoglobin released from lysis of the sheep erythrocytes. The CH_{50} should be used to screen for complement function in such conditions as suspected congenital deficiency of one component. The CH_{50} has been used in the past to provide quantitative information of complement activation as part of a disease process. However, modern immunoassays for individual components (see below) has largely supplanted the role of CH_{50} in disease monitoring. One reason that even excellent immunochemistry laboratories may show marked variation in the CH_{50} levels is that the sheep cells demonstrate a seasonal fluctuation in stability. Thus, the functional CH_{50} assay should be deferred in most instances in favor of more specific component assays that are rigorously standardized over indefinite periods of time.

CH_{50} has a normal range of approximately 50–200 units. Levels just below normal range can indicate increased consumption (and hence active disease process) or decreased synthesis. The hemolytic assay has particular sensitivity to levels of the components C2, C4, and C5. A zero value of hemolytic activity indicates deficiency of one or more components and should be followed up by detailed investigation to delineate the abnormality. An elevated level of CH_{50} has no significance except that of other acute phase reactants.

The components of complement most frequently measured in serum are C3 (75–175 mg/dl) and C4 (15–45 mg/dl). They are normally the most abundant of the complement factors in serum and so are naturally most easily quantitated by immunologic methods (usually immunodiffusion or nephelometry). Reductions in their levels can be related to one another serially with time to provide a reasonable monitor of autoimmune disease activity. Low levels indicate depletion due to activation secondary to disease progression. Normal or high levels indicate the opposite: disease regression or response to therapy. Other more sophisticated component assays are available from specialized reference laboratories. These include determinations of C1q, C2, C3, C4, C4d, C5, C6, factor B (properdin), and C1 esterase inhibitor. These assays can be used to distinguish immunologic disorders from other inflammatory states and also to diagnose specific deficiencies.

Immune Complexes

The combination of antigen and antibody leads to the formation of immune complexes. When there is continuous release of antigen into the circulation plus release of antibody to that antigen, immune complexes can form in the blood. Circulating immune complexes (CIC) are significant in many diseases such as acute glomerulonephritis, systemic lupus erythematosus, chronic viral hepatitis, and vasculitis. Immune complexes probably mediate and direct the pathologic response involving chemotaxis, infiltration of cells, and release of proteolytic enzymes at sites in the kidney, heart, lung, synovium, etc.

Immune complexes can be grossly screened for as cryoprecipitable substance from serum held in the cold (1–4°C). This approach is sensitive only to very large amounts of CIC. There are two major methods commonly used to detect and quantitate CIC down to very low levels. The first is *C1q binding* in which radiolabeled C1q is added to a serum sample. If there are CIC present, some of the C1q will preferentially bind to the Fc portion of immunoglobulins engaged in that complex. Addition of polyethylene glycol differentially precipitates the CIC, which have now become labeled with radioactivity proportional to the number of Fc sites on the CIC. Radioactivity trapped in the precipitate is counted. The C1q binding is expressed as a percentage of total C1q added, which should be less than 15% roughly (see the laboratory report form for specific ranges).

The second method for evaluating CIC is the *Raji cell assay.* This is a lymphoblastoid B cell line that came originally from a patient with Burkitt's lymphoma. Raji cells have receptors for complement components (e.g., C3) that are participating in the CIC. They do not specifically bind immunoglobulins, but bind complement, thus their specificity is for CIC that activate complement. In the assay, Raji cells are mixed with test serum samples and incubated. Any CIC present bind to the Raji cells through the complement attachment. The cells are then washed and incubated with radiolabeled antihuman immunoglobulin, which binds in turn to CIC on the surface of the Raji cells. The cells are finally washed and counted for radioactivity as a measure of CIC. This assay is conveniently standardized with known amounts of aggregated human globulin to simulate various concentrations of actual CIC.

Cellular Immunity

This branch of the immune system can be assessed both by provocative tests performed on the body and with procedures done on lymphocytes collected outside of the body. *Skin tests* utilize extracts of various infectious microorganisms such as mycobacteria, yeasts (candida), and bacteria (streptococcus) that are injected intradermally. If the individual has functioning cellular immunity, there will develop a region of redness and induration around each injection site that contains antigen to which the individual has immunologic experience. If an individual shows no such positive reaction to any common antigen to which all humans are exposed, that person has a defective cellular immune response and is said to be *anergic*. This is a severe disorder that can leave a patient susceptible to infections from many opportunistic viruses, fungi, bacteria, protozoa, and parasites.

Lymphocytes can be separated from the other cells of heparinized whole blood by centrifugation in a special density-adjusted medium (e.g., Ficoll-Hypaque). Those lymphocytes can then be stimulated with materials such as phytohemagglutinin (PHA) that act as foreign antigens and cause normal lymphocytes to undergo blastic transformation. Such *lymphocyte stimulation* and transformation are measured by adding radiolabeled thymidine, which becomes incorporated into the DNA of the lymphoblasts that are stimulated to divide. Low level incorporation indicates a poor capacity to mount an immune response.

A variation of this procedure is used for cross-matching organ donors and recipients, particularly for bone marrow transplantation. In this procedure, lymphocytes are isolated from the blood of both recipient and the potential donors and then mixed in various combinations to test the reactivity of antigens on the donor's lymphocytes with the recipient's lymphocytes and vice versa. This assay is termed the *mixed lymphocyte culture* (MLC). It is based also on lymphoblastic transformation and incorporation of radiolabeled thymidine after ten days of co-culturing the lymphocytes. Incompatibility of cross-match is indicated by greater counts of radioactivity incorporated into the lymphocyte DNA. Very low counts indicate probability of a good match. The MLC is used as a more definitive test of compatibility after screening for HLA typing has been done to establish candidate donors.

Surface Markers

Lymphocytes carry antigens on their surfaces that are related to specific functions and subgroups of those cells. These antigens have been defined by the use of antibodies against each one. Early methods employed to delineate these markers included immunoflourescent staining of cells fixed on a glass slide. Modern methods for surface marker analysis are based on *flow cytometry,* which uses antibodies to stain the cells but also classifies them according to size and light scattering. Flow cytometry requires sophisticated instrumentation, but has the advantages of excellent quantitation and fast analysis time. The markers commonly used include ones for total B cells, total T cells, and subsets of the T cells (see Table 7–1). Subset analysis has a particularly lengthy (sometimes confusing) list of markers with different systems of nomenclature. The monoclonal antibodies specific for each cell type have given rise to designations such as OKT3 or T3 or Leu-4 for total T cells; OKT4, T4, or Leu-3 for helper T cells; and OKT8, T8, or Leu-2 for suppressor

T cells. Those markers for total T cell, helper T cell, and suppressor T cell have been assigned the cluster of differentiation (CD) categories of CD3, CD4, and CD8, respectively. Other markers are specific for thymocytes (CD1), early T cells (CD5), and several other antigens (see Table 7–1).

This spectrum of markers is used for clinical classification of immunodeficiency states, lymphoid leukemias, autoimmune diseases, and for monitoring their response to therapy. The T4 and T8 cell measurements have gained great popularity for assisting in the diagnosis of AIDS. In this disorder, the T4 cells are depleted by infection with HIV, whereas the T8 cells persist. The result is a characteristic reduction in the ratio of T4/T8 cells from a normal value of roughly 2.0 to far below 1.0. The absolute number of T4 (CD4) cells is also a marker of progression of HIV infection to more overt AIDS. This ratio is also useful for assessing success of immunosuppressive therapy with cyclosporin A in transplant patients.

Tissue Typing

The histocompatibility antigens are so named because of the role they play in the rejection of allogeneic tissue grafts and organ transplants. They are encoded by genes on the short arm of the sixth pair of chromosomes in humans in a group called the major histocompatibility complex (MHC). These antigens are present on most cell surfaces, but because they were initially discovered on human lymphocytes, they are termed *human leukocyte antigens (HLA)*. The class I antigens are HLA-A, HLA-B, and HLA-C, each of which consists of a unique heavy chain plus a common light chain called beta-2-microglobulin. Class II antigens are related to the HLA-D locus and consist of two peptide chains without beta-2-microglobulin. Human leukocyte antigen typing is performed with defined antisera that are specific for the individual antigens. The binding of an antibody to lymphocytes leads to cell death on addition of complement. This microcytotoxicity assay is a common means for identifying the corresponding antigen on the lymphocyte surface membrane.

Human leukocyte antigen typing is used for histocompatibility typing as in organ transplantation and in paternity testing and also for disease association or risk assessment (e.g., specific linkages of disease with HLA types: hemochromatosis, ankylosing spondylitis [see Chapter 8, p. 315]).

Autoantibodies

The diagnosis, classification, prognosis, treatment, and monitoring of the progression of autoimmune diseases depend on the detection and quantitation of various autoantibodies (Table 7–4). These autoantibodies have reactivities with specific antigens frequently characteristic of distinct diseases. In general, autoantibodies are screened for by a few common methods. The first of these is *indirect immunofluorescent antibody (IFA)* staining of fixed cells or tissues prepared and mounted on glass slides in a standardized manner. These substrate slides contain multiple antigens (both protein and nucleic acid) for detection of whichever autoantibodies may be present in a patient's serum. The test procedure consists of incubating a dilution of the patient's serum in contact with the cells or tissue on the slide. Unbound serum immunoglobulins are then washed off along with the rest of the serum sample. A second incubation is performed with fluorescein-labeled antihuman immunoglobulin to detect the autoantibodies bound to their respective antigens. Microscopic examination is done with ultraviolet illumination to excite the fluorescein, which gives

Table 7–4. AUTOANTIBODIES FREQUENTLY ANALYZED IN SERUM

	Disease
Antinuclear Antibodies	
Nuclear staining	
Homogeneous (diffuse) and peripheral (rim)	SLE, MCTD, RA, PSS, SS
Speckled	SLE, MCTD, SS, PSS, RA
Nucleolar	PSS, SS
Centromere	CREST syndrome
Cytoplasmic staining	
Mitochondria	Primary biliary cirrhosis
Smooth muscle	Chronic active hepatitis
Extractable Nuclear Antigens (ENA)	
Sm*	SLE
RNP	MCTD, SLE, RA, PSS
SS-A (Ro) and SS-B (La)	SS, SLE
Scl-70*	PSS
Histones	Drug-induced SLE
Anti-immunoglobulin	
Rheumatoid factor	RA, SS

SLE = systemic lupus erythematosus; MCTD = mixed connective tissue disease; RA = rheumatoid arthritis; PSS = progressive systemic sclerosis, scleroderma; SS = Sjogren's syndrome; CREST = calcinosis, Raynaud's phenomenon, esophageal dysfunction, sclerodactyly, telangiectasia.

*Highly specific disease marker.

off the visible light from the cellular and subcellular locations where the autoantibodies are bound (see Color Plates 48 and 49). A titer is reported as the highest dilution of patient serum that yields a strong fluorescent response under the microscope. This procedure is referred to as *antinuclear antibody (ANA)* testing because of its ability to detect antibodies against many different nuclear antigens. As detailed below, the ANA can identify antibodies to cytoplasmic antigens as well.

Another method for detecting autoantibodies utilizes a soluble extract of tissue such as spleen or thymus, which is particularly rich in a variety of nuclear antigens. The preparation of *extractable nuclear antigens (ENA)* is tested for reactivity with patient samples by double diffusion in agarose gels or by counterimmunoelectrophoresis in agarose. Since the ENA is performed with a mixture of antigens, identification of any particular reactivity depends on lines of identity between the patient's serum and positive prototype serum samples containing known autoantibodies. Other tests currently under development make use of purified antigens to detect autoantibodies instead of relying on prototype antibodies as the standard for reactivity.

A combination of ANA and ENA is typically used to screen patients suspected of having autoimmune diseases. The ANA and ENA identify autoantibodies directed against antigens present in virtually all cells of the body. For those patients suspected of having autoantibodies that react with only selective organs (e.g., thyroid, adrenal, heart, etc.), their serum is tested by IFA using as substrate fixed and mounted tissue slices of those organs from animals or autopsy material. By this means, *organ-specific autoantibodies* can be detected and quantitated in serum to assist in diagnosis and to mark disease progress.

ANTINUCLEAR ANTIBODY

This procedure can identify autoantibodies against DNA, histones, or soluble nuclear antigens. The microscopic fluorescent staining distributions within cell nuclei assume characteristic distributions. A *homogeneous* pattern may be due to antibodies directed against either DNA or histones or a combination of both. A homogenous stain indicates uniform staining throughout each nucleus with all nuclei staining to the same extent (see Color Plate 48A). Mitotic cells show positive staining corresponding to daughter chromosomes along the metaphase plate and in the newly formed nuclei just before final cell division. This finding is frequently associated with systemic lupus erythematosus (SLE). The titer of a homogeneous ANA is also a useful index for monitoring the progress of SLE. If the staining pattern is distributed more toward the nuclear membrane where native DNA is concentrated, it is referred to as a *peripheral* or *rim* staining pattern and is usually a reliable index of activity of SLE.

Further discrimination of whether these above types of positive ANAs are due to *anti-DNA antibodies* versus *antihistone antibodies* is conveniently accomplished by specific assay for the anti-DNA antibody by staining of the microorganism crithidia (which has an organelle called the kinetoplast that contains DNA but is devoid of histone) or by an assay using purified DNA as antigen (e.g., enzyme-linked solid phase assay). This distinction has clinical significance since SLE associated with antihistone predominant antibodies has been associated with a drug-induced etiology that can be reversible with discontinuation of that drug (e.g., procainamide) whereas anti-DNA antibodies are more associated with idiopathic SLE. Antibodies against DNA can also be classified into those specific for the native or double-stranded molecule (n-DNA or ds-DNA), those specific for the denatured or single-stranded molecule (ss-DNA), and those that react with both ds-DNA and ss-DNA. SLE frequently demonstrates high levels of ds-DNA antibodies; those levels are frequently correlated with a degree of glomerulonephritis most likely due to immune complex formation with DNA released from tissue destruction. Other autoimmune diseases besides SLE may sometimes have positive homogeneous ANAs that can be used as markers of those diseases' progression as well.

A staining pattern that is localized to the nucleus but consists of multiple small intersecting globules is designated as the *speckled* pattern (see Color Plate 48B). It typically shows negatively staining regions within the nucleus corresponding to the position of nucleoli. In addition, in contrast to a homogenous pattern that stains the DNA within chromosomes of dividing cells, speckled staining shows negative regions corresponding to chromosomes in mitotic cells. Thus, speckled pattern antibodies are directed against antibodies other than DNA and histones. These antigens are called the soluble or extractable nuclear antigens (ENA), which include Sm (initially designated for a patient named Smith who had SLE) and RNP (for ribonucleoprotein). High titers of anti-Sm antibody are suggestive of SLE, whereas high levels of anti-RNP antibody are characteristic of *mixed connective tissue disorder (MCTD)* as well as SLE and some other rheumatic disorders. Because of varying sensitivities and specificities of the test procedures, it is reasonable to perform both ANA and ENA assays in order to establish the precise autoantibody present and also its titer.

Another striking finding of the ANA is a positive *antinucleolar* pattern (see Color Plate 49A). This pattern is complementary to a true speckled pattern in that it shows stain deposition in the precise regions that are negative in the speckled pattern. The antigen in this case is nucleolar RNA. While this autoantibody may occur in SLE (often in association with other ANAs), it is more specific for *scleroderma,* also called *progressive systemic sclerosis* (PSS), a progressive disorder involving fibrosis and degeneration of skin, blood vessels, muscles, joints, and other organs (viscera). In addition to reacting with nucleolar antigens, autoantibodies characteristic of PSS can also react with the centromeres on each of the chromosomes. The anticentromeric pattern consists of multiple small positive dots distributed uniformly throughout the nucleus of interphase cells, but aligned with the chromosomes in metaphase cells. Results of ENA testing in PSS frequently show reactivity with an antigen designated Scl-70, although this autoantibody may also occur in other rheumatic diseases.

Two other commonly noted soluble antigens are *SS-A* and *SS-B,* which have a particular association with *Sjogren's syndrome,* a disorder of keratoconjunctivitis sicca and xerostomia with other connective tissue disease. These ENA reactivities can be of great clinical help in the diagnosis of Sjogren's syndrome, which can have no positive immunofluorescent findings. In another terminology, the SS-A antigen is the same as the Ro antigen and the SS-B is the same as the La antigen.

There are several other ENA autoantibodies identified by routine testing of large numbers of patients with rheumatic diseases. Some of these antibodies also have disease correlation (rheumatoid arthritis-associated nuclear antigen, RANA; proliferating cell nuclear antigen, PCNA; PM-1, Jo-1, and Ku antigens in polymyositis, dermatomyositis, and overlapping syndromes).

Since there is considerable overlap between antigenic reactivity and rheumatic disease classification, a practical clinical approach is simply to identify those autoantibodies present in a particular patient early in the stage of the disease and then to monitor the titer of those antibodies with time. Occasionally there will be detected autoantibodies that have almost amazing specificities for antigens without any recognized disease correlation. Among these findings are antibodies against the spindle apparatus, centrioles, Golgi apparatus, ribosomes, and other nondescript subcellular antigens. It is important that the laboratory performing the ANA recognize these autoantibodies as well and correctly classify them so as to avoid confusion with autoantibodies of true clinical significance and so that they will be reflected as an accurate baseline against which to gauge any change in the patient's status in later years.

Two very important anticytoplasmic autoantibodies are *anti-smooth muscle (SMA)* and *anti-mitochrondial (AMA),* both of which can usually be detected by ANA test procedures using fixed cells grown in monolayers (see Color Plate 49B). However, for accurate identification and for determination of antibody titer, it is necessary to test patient serum against fixed slices of tissues rich in those antigens, usually mouse stomach and kidney. The finding of a high titer SMA is strongly suggestive of *chronic active hepatitis,* whereas low titers may be found in other liver pathology, other rheumatic disease, malignancies, or healthy persons. The AMA is a useful marker for *primary biliary cirrhosis* and also for other obstructive hepatic disorders.

A final procedure that has gained wide usage in rheumatic diseases is that for *rheumatoid factor (RF),* an autoantibody (usually IgM) that reacts with other immunoglobulins (usually IgG) to form immune complexes. As indicated by its name, the RF has particular application to diagnosis and monitoring of *rheumatoid arthritis.* There are numerous methods for quantitating the RF based on its ability to induce flocculation visible to the eye. Unfortunately for purposes of diagnosis, RF is *not usually positive* in cases of *juvenile rhuematoid arthritis.*

A frequently employed marker for degree of disease activity in addition to specific autoantibody titer is the quantitation of *C-reactive protein (CRP),* which shows a very good correlation with amount of tissue necrosis, as may occur with inflammatory destruction (see Table 7–3; also Chapter 10, serum proteins).

ORGAN-SPECIFIC AUTOANTIBODIES

Many patients with disease of a particular organ have antibodies directed against antigens unique to that organ (Table 7–5). It is often difficult to untangle cause and effect, to know whether the antibody has caused the tissue problem, or whether organ damage provoked the antibody response. Patients with autoantibodies reactive against the diseased organ often have additional antibodies that react with other tissues. Thyroid and stomach are often linked in this way: many patients with *immune thyroiditis* (Hashimoto's disease) have antibodies to gastric parietal cells, and many patients with *pernicious anemia* have antithyroid antibodies in addition to antibodies against intrinsic factor and gastric parietal cells. Another confounding observation is that first-degree relatives of patients with autoantibody-related diseases often have the same circulating antibodies but no evidence of disease.

The role of cell-mediated immunity in diseases characterized by autoantibodies is another field of inquiry. Insulin-dependent *diabetes mellitus* is especially challenging; antibodies to pancreatic islet cells are moderately common, but seem to have minimal diagnostic significance. It may be that cell-mediated autoimmunity plays a significant etiologic role in the disease after some primary insult to the pancreas

Table 7–5. ORGAN-SPECIFIC AUTOANTIBODIES IN HUMAN DISEASE

Antibody Directed Against	Disease Produced	Antibody Detected By
Thyroglobulin; other thyroid antigens	Thyroiditis	Hemagglutination for thyroglobulin, IIF for others
Thyroid-stimulating hormone receptors	Graves' disease	Radioassay, bioassay
Erythrocyte membrane	Autoimmune hemolytic anemia	Coombs antiglobulin test
Platelet membrane	Immune thrombocytopenic purpura	Refinements of antiglobulin test, platelet survival studies
Glomerular basement membrane	Glomerulonephritis; Goodpasture's syndrome	IIF; direct immunofluorescent study of kidney biopsy
Acetylcholine receptor; striated muscle	Myasthenia gravis	Radioassay, IIF
Intrinsic factor; gastric parietal cells	Pernicious anemia	Neutralization in blocking tests; IIF

IIF = indirect immunofluorescence.

such as acute viral infection. In fact, recent immunosuppressive therapies have been successful in modifying the course of juvenile diabetes if begun soon after the onset of the disease.

Kidney Diseases. Several types of renal disease result from autoimmune activity. In glomerulonephritis of lupus erythematosus and of poststreptococcal states, immune complexes deposit on the glomerular membranes and induce complement-mediated damage. A different form of glomerulonephritis occurs in patients with antibodies directed specifically against glomerular basement membrane (anti-GBM). These antibodies damage not only the patient's kidneys but may, if persistent, damage transplanted kidneys also. The anti-GBM also reacts with alveolar basement membranes in the lungs. The clinical condition of antibody-mediated hemorrhagic damage in lungs and kidneys is called *Goodpasture's syndrome.*

Other Organs. Indirect immunofluorescence is used to demonstrate most organ-specific antibodies, but other procedures are used in special cases when the antigens can be solubilized or purified. *Antithyroid antibodies* are measured by an agglutination procedure in which antigen is adsorbed to red cells. Intrinsic factor antibodies are measured by radioimmunoassay. Other radioassays are used to detect antibodies against the *acetylcholine receptor* in *myasthenia gravis* and against cell surface receptors in *Grave's disease* (THS receptor) and also in some forms of diabetes mellitus. Many other organs can be seen to have autoantibodies directed against them. These include adrenal (Addison's disease), myocardium, skeletal muscle, various endocrine cells, skin components, colonic mucosa, salivary gland ducts, and more. While most of these antibodies may simply reflect existing tissue damage rather than the cause of it, there is the possibility of extending the damage or of stimulating cell-mediated immunity to those tissues that could cause the primary insult or contribute to it.

Allergy Testing

Persons suffering from asthma can be tested for sensitivities to a wide variety of potential allergens by *skin tests* in which each allergen is applied separately through a scratch in the skin. The development of redness and swelling around a scratch application site indicates that the patient is allergic to that particular antigen. Because of the discomfort involved and a limited number of sites that can be used at any one sitting, other procedures involving detection of IgE have been introduced. Diagnosis of allergic disorder can be further substantiated by quantitation of *total IgE levels* in the blood. Allergic individuals tend to have higher than expected concentrations of total IgE. Solid phase immunoassays are also available to detect the presence of IgE antibodies against a battery of individual allergens. These include different food groups, pollens, animal hairs, and other common environmental exposures. These allergens are linked to a solid bead that is incubated with the patient's serum in the test procedure to allow any IgE against that antigen to attach to it. The bead is then washed and further incubated with a labeled anti-IgE antibody. The bead is then washed one more time and the amount of bound label is quantitated (either radioactive or enzymatic label) as a direct measure of the specific IgE in the patient's serum directed against that particular antigen. These allergen-specific IgE assays are called RAST or RIST assays. Before embarking on a blind survey of these allergens (most of which will likely show no reaction), it is extremely useful to determine by careful history what classes of allergens may be within the exposure experience of the patient.

Within allergy and allergic reaction testing, it is frequently useful to determine the absolute count of eosinophils in the blood and also to look for eosinophils in nasal secretions to confirm an allergic origin.

REFERENCES

1. Bellanti, JA: Immunology III. WB Saunders, Philadelphia, 1985.
2. Bigazzi, PE and Rose, NR: Tests for antibodies to tissue-specific antigens. In Rose, NR and Friedman, H (eds): Manual of Clinical Immunology, ed 2. American Society for Microbiology, Washington, DC, 1980, p 874.
3. Burek, CL and Rose, NR: Detection of autoantibodies. In Sonnenwirth, AC and Jarett, L (eds): Gradwohl's Clinical Laboratory Methods and Diagnosis. CV Mosby, St. Louis, 1980, p 1257.
4. Editorial: Identifying T cells in man. Lancet 2:781, 1980.
5. Fritzler, MJ: Fluorescent antinuclear anatibody test. In Rose, NR and Friedman, H (eds): Manual of Clinical Immunology, ed 2. American Society for Microbiology, Washington, DC, 1980, p 852.
6. Froelich, CJ and Williams, RC, Jr: Tests for detection of rheumatoid factors. In Rose, NR and Friedman, H (eds): Manual of Clinical Immunology, ed 2. American Society for Microbiology, Washington, DC, 1980, p 871.
7. Gaither, TA and Frank, MM: Complement. In Henry, JB (ed): Clinical Diagnosis and Management by Laboratory Methods, ed 17. WB Saunders, Philadelphia, 1984, p 879.
8. Ishizaka, K: Structure and biologic activity of immunoglobulin E. Hosp Pract 12(1):57, 1977.
9. Krane, SM: Rheumatoid arthritis. In Rubenstein, E and Federman, DD (eds): Scientific American Medicine. Scientific American, New York, 1981, pp 15–II:1–23.
10. Muller-Eberhard, HJ: Chemistry and function of the complement system. Hosp Prac 12(8):33, 1977.
11. Nathan, CF, Murray, HW, and Cohn, ZA: The macrophage as an effector cell. N Engl J Med 303:622, 1981.
12. Primer on Allergic and Immunologic Diseases. JAMA 248 (20:00, 1982.
13. Reinherz, EL and Schlossman, SF: The characterization and function of human immunoregulatory T-lymphocyte subsets. Immunology Today 2:69, 1981.
14. Robinson, DR: Systemic lupus erythematosus. In Rubenstein, E and Federman, DD (eds): Scientific American Medicine. Scientific American, New York, 1981, pp 15–IV: 1–16.
15. Roitt, IM: Essential Immunology, ed 4. Blackwell Scientific Publications, Oxford, 1980.
16. Stobo, JD: Autoimmune antireceptor diseases. Hosp Pract 16(3):49, 1981.
17. Tomar, RH: Gammopathies, hypersensitivity, immunologic deficiency. In Henry, JB (ed): Clinical Diagnosis and Management by Laboratory Methods, ed 16. WB Saunders, Philadelphia, 1979, p 1381.
18. Wells, JV and Nelson, DS: Clinical Immunology Illustrated. Williams and Wilkins, Baltimore, 1986.
19. Wiggins, RC and Cochrane, CG: Immune-complex-mediated biologic effects. N Engl J Med 304:518, 1981.
20. Zweiman, B and Lisak, RP: Autoantibodies: Autoimmunity and immune complexes. In Henry, JB (ed): Clinical Diagnosis and Management by Laboratory Methods, ed 17. WB Saunders, Philadelphia, 1984, p 924.

OUTLINE

CHAPTER

8

TRANSFUSION MEDICINE

IMMUNOHEMATOLOGY OF ERYTHROCYTES

The red cell membrane contains many different proteins and carbohydrates capable of evoking antibody formation. More than 300 antigenic configurations have been discovered and classified. For a few, the molecule's biologic role has been inferred; for a few others, the chemical composition has been characterized; for the most, the structure, function, and reasons for their immunogenicity all remain mysterious. However, the genes that determine red cell antigens seem to follow the mendelian laws of inheritance. If the individual possesses a specific genetic pattern (genotype), these antigens usually express themselves on the red cell (phenotype). This inheritance pattern is called codominant. Chemically, red cell antigens may be proteins such as Rh, M, and N blood group substances, or glycolipids such as the ABH, Lewis, Ii, and P blood group substances. The antigenicity of these various compounds is influenced by biologic and chemical properties, molecular size, and three-dimensional configuration. Some blood group substances, such as the HLA antigens, are distributed widely throughout the body tissues. Others are more restricted to red cells such as the Rh antigens and the Kell blood group substances.

The most practical aspect of these antigens on red cells is their ability to evoke antibody formation when transfused into recipients. Some of the more important antigen systems will be discussed in this chapter.

BLOOD GROUPS

The ABO Blood Group System

Discovered in 1900 by the Austrian-born pathologist Karl Landsteiner, the ABO system is of paramount importance in blood banking and transfusion medicine. The major antigens are called A and B; the major antibodies are anti-A and anti-B. The genes that determine the presence or absence of A or B activity reside on chromosome 9. Normal persons older than 6 months of age almost always have naturally occurring antibodies that react with A or B antigens that are absent from their own cells. The occurrence of these antibodies and their specificity are not genetically determined. Instead, antibodies develop after exposure to apparently ubiquitous environmental antigens that share structure and specificity with red cell antigens. Although exposed to both A and B activity in the environment, individuals will not produce antibodies that react with their own red cell antigens.

Genes and Antigens

The ABO system is not as simple as it first appears. Antigenic activity depends on specific sugar linkages located at the end of a short sugar chain that is attached to a large, complex molecule with either protein or lipid structure. Most of the red cell antigens reside in membrane lipids called *glycosphingolipids,* but glycoproteins also possess ABO activity. The nature of the short sugar chain attached to the complex molecule is well characterized. The A antigen results when N-acetylgalactosamine links to a D-galactose moiety. B activity occurs if a D-galactose is present on that terminal D-galactose moiety. The A gene characterizes the presence of a *transferase enzyme* that is responsible for attaching N-acetylgalactosamine to galactose; the B gene produces a galactose transferase. These transferase enzymes encoded by the genes are capable of adding sugars to the basic precursor substance.

Figure 8–1 shows the schematic structure of the A, B, and H antigens. Before the D-galactose can accept the sugars that determine A or B activity, it must have a fucose sugar already attached. A D-galactose moiety with fucose already attached, but without A-active N-acetylgalactosamine or B-active D-galactose, has antigenic activity described as H. Cells with only the H-active sugar configuration have neither A nor B activity and are called *Group O.*

The transferases determined by the A and B genes depend on the presence of precursor H substance for their activity to become apparent. Attachment of fucose to D-galactose provides this precursor. Fucose attachment is mediated by another enzyme, fucose-transferase, the presence of which is determined by the *H gene.* The H gene is independent of the ABO locus; its chromosomal location is unknown. The H gene is extremely common and nearly everyone has H substance on the red cells. A few people are homozygous for an inactive gene at that site, called h. Since persons with two h genes cannot generate the enzyme needed to attach fucose, their red cells have no H activity. In the absence of H substance, A- or B-active transferases have no substrate on which to work; therefore the red cells of these persons lack A or B activity as well. Individuals whose red cells lack A, B, or H activity consistently have strong anti-A, anti-B, and anti-H in their serum. This constitution is called a *Bombay phenotype* because it was first discovered in that city and the very rare, inactive h gene seems to have its greatest concentration there (Fig. 8–2).

Many alleles exist at the ABO locus. The three commonest are A, B, and O. A and B produce sugar transferases that alter H activity. The O gene has no detectable product; it is called an *amorph.* Persons with two O genes produce no enzymes capable of transforming the H substance into A or B. Their cells possess only H activity, and their serum contains anti-A and anti-B. A single A or B gene can generate enough enzyme to fully convert the H substance to A or B, respectively. The red cells of a person with the genotype A-O do not differ from those with the genotype A-A. Persons with both A and B genes attach N-acetylgalactosamine to some of their H, and D-galactose to the rest of it. These group AB individuals have both A and B activity on their cells, with very little residual H, and their serum contains neither anti-A nor anti-B. Table 8–1 shows the blood findings and the frequency of the common ABO groups.

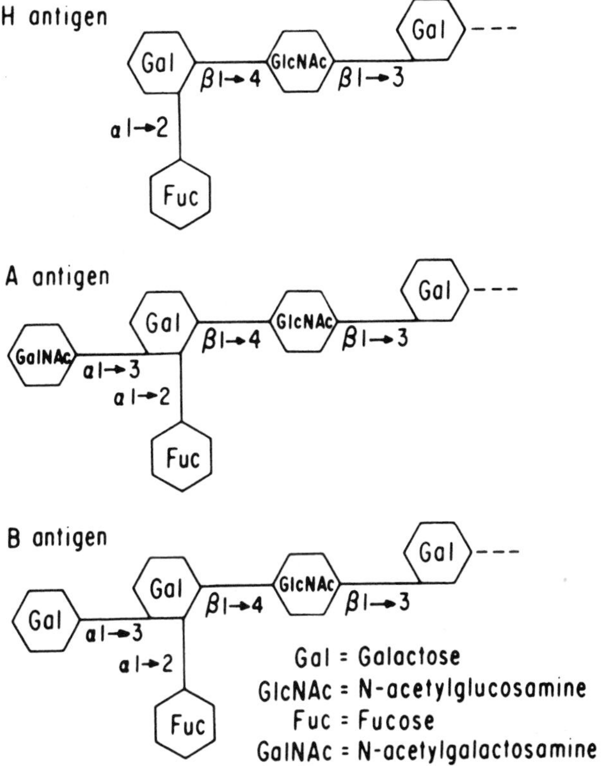

Figure 8–1. The sugar attached to the 3 carbon of galactose determines antigenic activity. N-acetyl-galactosamine confers A activity; galactose confers B activity. Unless the fucose moiety that determines H activity is attached to the 2 carbon, galactose does not accept either sugar on the 3 carbon. (From AABB Technical Manual,[18] p 119, with permission.)

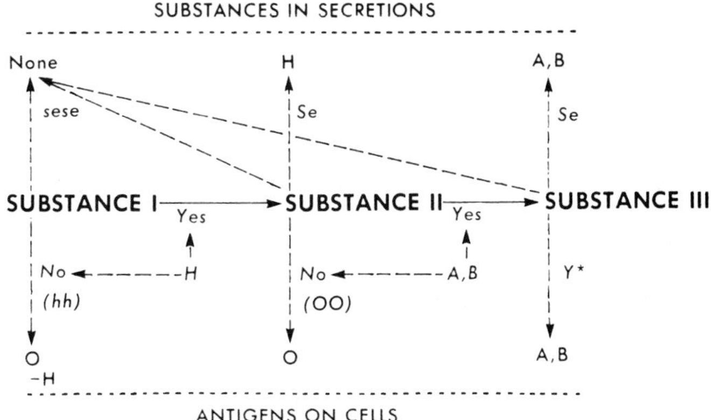

Figure 8–2. Possible genetic pathways in the biosynthesis of ABO antigens and ABH substances. *In the absence of a Y gene, one may have A substance in secretions but no A antigens on erythrocytes. (From Henry, JB: Clinical and Diagnosis and Management by Laboratory Methods, ed 17. WB Saunders, Philadelphia, p 988, with permission.)

Table 8–1. ANTIGENS AND ANTIBODIES IN ABO BLOOD GROUPS

Blood Group	Antigens on Red Cells	Antibodies in Serum	Frequency (%) in US Population			
			Whites	Blacks	American Indians	Orientals
A	A	Anti-B	40	27	16	28
B	B	Anti-A	11	20	4	27
O	Neither	Anti-A Anti-B	45	49	79	40
AB	A and B	Neither	4	4	<1	5

Adapted from Widmann, FK (ed): Technical Manual, ed 8. American Association of Blood Banks, Washington, DC, 1981.

Subgroups of A

Two different A genes are common in the general population: A_1 and A_2. The A_2 transferase is less efficient than the A_1 transferase in converting H to A. A single A_1 gene produces a transferase that converts nearly all the available H to A, but A_2 produces red cells with weaker A antigenic activity and more residual H antigen. Persons with genotypes A_2-A_2 or A_2-O have red cells of the A_2 phenotype. Persons with one A_1 gene and one A_2 gene have A_1 red cells. A coexisting B gene does not alter A_1 or A_2 activity. About 20% of AB are A_2B, whereas the majority are A_1B, just as 20% of group A persons are A_2.

Still other variant A genes exist, producing progressively less active transferases. These are uncommon, but occur sufficiently often that the number of weak A subgroups has been identified and classified. Inheritance of these weak variants follows normal mendelian distribution. The reason for their ''deficient'' activity is unknown. Also unexplained is the fact that variant A transferases exist so often, whereas B variants are uncommon. Only a few ''weak B'' genes have been found.

The presence of the A_2 antigen cannot be determined in the presence of A_1 antigen. It is felt that this may merely represent a simple quantitative deficiency; however, certain qualitative change in the A antigen may also be present in A_2 individuals. Certain A_2 and A_2B individuals can have anti-A_1 in their serum. Subgroups of A can, in this instance, give discrepant ABO grouping characteristics, as may occur when an individual's red cells type as AB, yet the serum contains anti-A. This is, in fact, an anti-A_1, and the correct blood groups are A_2 or A_2B, respectively.

Antibodies in the ABO System

Although anti-A and anti-B react strongly and specifically with the corresponding red cell antigens, the stimulus to anti-A and anti-B production is not exposure to red cells. The same linkages of galactose with N-acetylgalactosamine or galactose that characterize red cell glycosphingolipids also exist in bacterial cell walls. Continuous environmental exposure to these widely distributed antigens elicits continuous antibody production in immunocompetent persons, provided the antigen is not a ''self constituent'' of the individual's own red cells. Group A subjects form only anti-B, and those in Group B have only anti-A. Persons of Group O have both anti-A and anti-B, whereas Group AB individuals have neither antibody (see Table 8–1).

Infants are too young to form antibodies and patients with defective humoral immunity will not have these antibodies.

Environmental bacteria also possess the galactose–fucose linkage that confers H activity. Anti-H, however, occurs very rarely because nearly all red cells possess H antigen in quantities ranging from slight to substantial. A_1 or A_1B persons occasionally develop weak anti-H, but the only people who form strong anti-H are those of the Bombay phenotype, whose red cells are devoid of H activity.

Anti-A and Anti-B are strong agglutinins, easily demonstrated in the laboratory. In the circulation they cause rapid, complement-mediated destruction of any incompatible cells that chance to enter the bloodstream. Except for the few fetal cells that enter the mother's bloodstream during pregnancy and delivery, the only way that ABO-incompatible cells get into the circulation is by incorrectly identified transfusions. Incorrect identification of patients, blood samples, or donor blood, or incorrect clerical notations, cause the vast majority of hemolytic, ABO-incompatible transfusion reactions.

Most anti-A and anti-B activity resides in the IgM class of immunoglobulins, which produce immediate agglutination (Fig. 8–3) and/or hemolysis. Some activity, however, is IgG, and antibodies of this class attach to the cell surface without immediately affecting the viability. Anti-A or anti-B of the IgG class readily crosses the placenta and can cause hemolytic disease of the newborn (see later). Group O persons more often have IgG anti-A and anti-B than do A or B individuals. ABO hemolytic disease of the newborn affects almost exclusively the offspring of O mothers (see later in this chapter).

Secretors and Nonsecretors

A, B, and H substances can be found in body tissues in soluble forms (e.g., saliva). The ability to secrete ABH substances resides in the secretor (Se) gene. All secretors have H substance in their saliva. Group A, B, or AB secretors have the A substance, B substance, or both A and B substances in their saliva as well. Individuals who lack the secretor gene do not have any A, B, or H substance in their saliva, irrespective of what their ABO blood group types are. Secretor status testing can be valuable in forensic laboratories. In most whites, the incidence of the secretor gene, which manifests its activity as a dominant inheritant, is 85% (see also Fig. 8–2).

Change in ABH Types with Various Diseases. Weakening of the A antigen may occur in some persons with acute leukemia or in chronic myeloproliferative diseases with leukemic evolution. Certain cancers, particularly cancer of the colon, may be associated with the acquisition of a B antigen termed the acquired B. Thus, occasionally an individual of Group O or A phenotype may acquire a B and apparently type as B or AB, respectively, in these diseases.

The Rh System

After the ABO system, the Rh system is the group of red cell antigens with the greatest clinical importance. Unlike anti-A and anti-B, which reliably occur in normal, unimmunized individuals, Rh antibodies do not develop without an immunizing stimulus such as pregnancy or blood transfusion. The major antigen of the Rh system (D) is more likely to provoke an antibody than any other red cell antigen if introduced into a person who lacks the antigen. The D antigen is present on the red cells of 85% of whites, and a higher percentage of blacks, American Indians, and

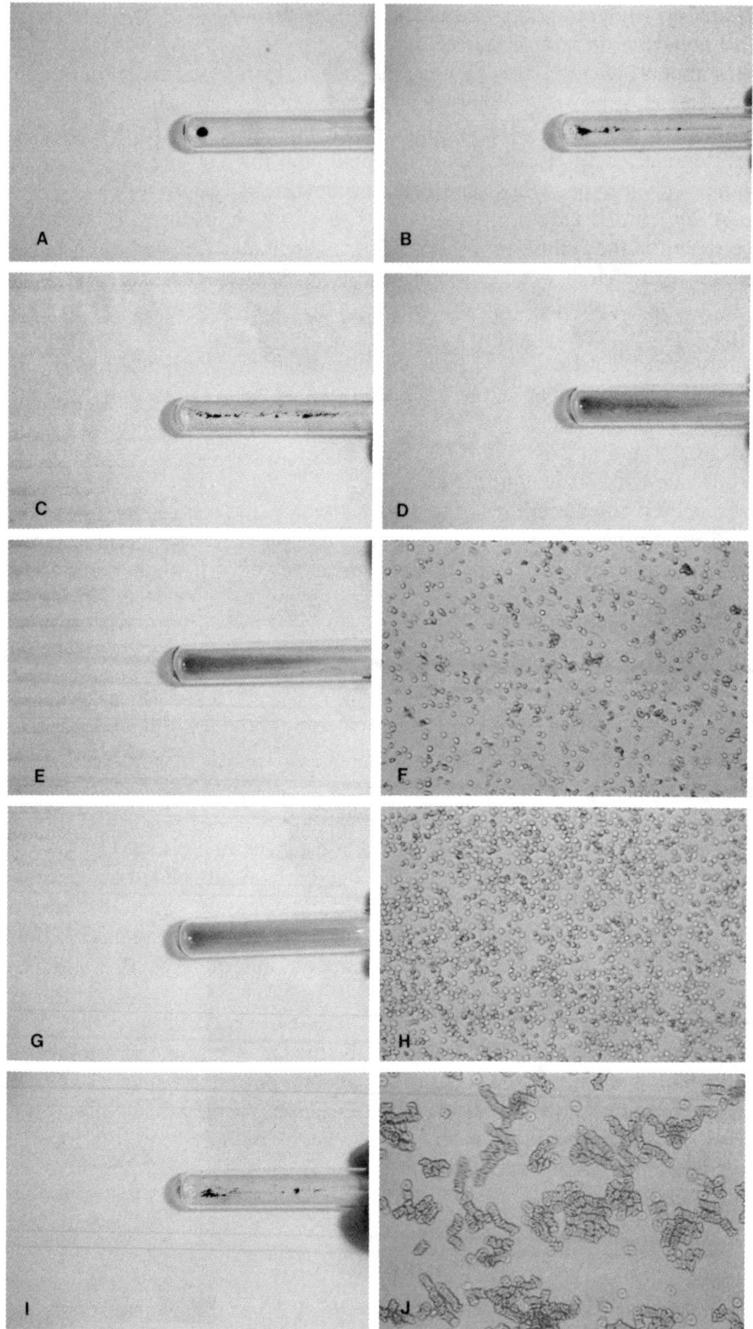

Figure 8–3. Agglutination reactions. (*A*) 4+: One solid aggregate of red cells. (*B*) 3+: Several large aggregates. (*C*) 2+: Medium-sized aggregates, clear background. (*D*) 1+: Small aggregates; turbid, reddish background. (*E*) +w (weak): Tiny aggregates; turbid, reddish background, or (*F*) +w: microscopic aggregates only (original magnification ×10; enlarged 240×). (*G*) Negative: no aggregates. (*H*) Negative: no aggregates—microscopic appearance (original magnification ×10; enlarged 240×).(*I*) Pseudoagglutination or strong rouleaux (2+). (*J*) Rouleaux: microscopic appearance (original magnification ×10; enlarged 240×). (From Harmening, D [ed]: Modern Blood Banking and Transfusion Practices, ed 2. FA Davis, Philadelphia, 1989, with permission.)

Asians. Since 15% of whites lack the antigen, they are capable of forming the antibody if exposed to D; but only 50% to 75% of Rh-negative persons exposed to large numbers of Rh-positive cells actively form an antibody. Nevertheless, no other blood group antigen has comparable immunizing potential.

Historically, Rh antigens and genes were described in two different terminologies, reflecting differences in experimental and theoretical approach. Current usage now tends toward simplification of the symbols, at written and spoken levels, with a numerical nomenclature available for highly technical communications. The American Association of Blood Banks and Bureau of Biologics of the Food and Drug Administration now use only the simpler CDE-cde (Fisher-Race nomenclature) in most publications. The Rh-Hr nomenclature remains historically and conceptually important.

Antigens of the Rh System

The Rh system includes many different antigens. Persons whose red cells possess D are called *Rh-positive,* those whose cells lack D are called *Rh-negative,* no matter what other Rh antigens are present. Besides D, there are four other Rh antigens of major clinical significance. The genes for the Rh system reside on chromosome 1. Thus, each gene controls the presence of several different Rh antigens on the red cell surface and determines a different combination of two or three major antigens, and numerous other antigens of less clinical significance.

Because it so readily provokes an identifying antibody, D was the first Rh antigen to be discovered. The other four major antigens are C, E, c, and e; antibodies to these occur less frequently but still fairly often. Many other antigens exist that are either very rare themselves, or require rare antibodies to demonstrate their presence.

Rh Genes

The Rh genes common in the United States population are given in Table 8–2. It can be seen that all these genes determine the presence of one antigen at the C-c site and one E-e site. Most also indicate the presence of D. The r gene determines a product that lacks D but possesses c and e. A single group of Rh antigens defined by their

Table 8–2. Rh GENES COMMON IN THE US POPULATION

			Frequency in US Population (%)			
Allele	**Antigens *(Rh Terminology)***	**Antigens *(CDE Terminology)***	**Whites**	**Blacks**	**American Indians**	**Orientals**
R^1	rh′, Rh_o, hr″	C, D, e	0.42	0.17	0.44	0.70
r	hr′, hr″	c, e	0.37	0.26	0.11	0.03
R^2	hr′, Rh_o, rh″	c, D, E	0.14	0.11	0.34	0.21
R^o	hr′, Rh_o, hr″	c, D, e	0.04	0.44	0.02	0.03
r′	rh′, hr″	C, e	0.02	0.02	0.02	0.02

Adapted from data in Widmann, FL (ed): Technical Manual, ed 8. American Association of Blood Banks, Arlington, VA, 1981.

alleles on one chromosome is called a *haplotype*. We do not know the specific polypeptides produced by the Rh genes, nor do we know the chemical and spatial composition that determines antigenic activity. Rh material has a high lipid content, and is a more integral part of the red cell membrane than are the ABH antigens.

Since every person has two examples of chromosome 1, everyone has two Rh alleles. These may be either identical or different. If two examples of the same allele are present on the two chromosomes, the red cell will only have one set of antigens. If two different alleles are present, there will be two haplotypes. Of the five common Rh antigens, the minimum number that a normal person could have is two—c and e, since d has not been identified and exists only by inference in the absence of D. This occurs in persons with the r gene on both chromosomes. A single cell tested with five major antibodies can have the maximum five different antigens—DCEce. This occurs with the genotype R^1R^2(CDe/cDE).

Rh-positive cells always have D as part of at least one haplotype. In routine testing, it is not feasible to distinguish cells with a single dose of D from persons who are homozygous for D (double dose). This distinction sometimes can be inferred from the presence of other antigenic factors that commonly accompany D. Rh-negative cells, which lack D, may have c or C on both, as well as e or E on both. Most Rh-negative persons have two examples of the allele r, which determines c and e, but some Rh-negative persons have less common alleles.

Rh Antibodies

As already mentioned, not every Rh-negative person exposed to Rh-positive cells develops anti-D. Transfusion immunizes more consistently than pregnancy, largely because more cells are involved. About 20% of Rh-negative mothers develop anti-D after carrying an Rh-positive infant, whereas antibody develops in between 50% to 70% of Rh-negative persons transfused with Rh-positive blood. For this reason, every reasonable effort is made to avoid giving Rh-positive blood to Rh-negative recipients. Antibodies to the other four major Rh antigens occur only sporadically. In routine transfusion practice, no effort is made to match these antigens in donor and recipient. A few people have anti-E spontaneously (i.e., without having been exposed to blood, blood products, or pregnancy). Other Rh antibodies almost never develop spontaneously.

When Rh antibodies develop, they are predominantly IgG. Some IgM appears early as part of the primary immune response, but it tends to disappear soon after the immunizing event; whereas IgG can persist for a lifetime. Rh antibodies do not, as a rule, activate complement. The usual biologic effect of Rh antibodies is to coat (opsonize) circulating cells containing the corresponding antigen and set them up for destruction by the reticuloendothelial system. When antibody attaches to cell surface antigens, systemic symptoms may occur such as hypotension and a rising temperature, vomiting, or loss of consciousness. The hematologic result is hemolysis of the antibody-coated cells in the reticuloendothelial organs, predominantly the spleen or liver. Destruction may be complete within a minute or two, or proceed slowly over hours or days. In the test tube, Rh antibodies can cause a modest degree of agglutination, but surface coating usually predominates. Agglutination is enhanced by Coombs sera (AHG), albumin, or enzyme treatment of the red cells.

Rh antibodies readily cross the placenta from mother to fetus. Historically, anti-D has been the commonest cause of severe hemolytic disease of the newborn. Passive Rh antibody prophylaxis successfully prevents antibody formation when given to an unimmunized Rh-negative woman at 28 weeks antenatally and just after the birth of an Rh-positive child. Women with anti-D existing at the time pregnancy begins are very likely to have an affected infant. Other Rh antibodies can cause hemolytic disease much less frequently, and pharmacologic means of prevention are not available (see Hemolytic Disease of the Newborn, later in this chapter).

RH IMMUNOPROPHYLAXIS

Anti-D formation in pregnant Rh-negative women can be prevented by giving a dose of preformed anti-D by injection at the time that Rh-positive cells enter the circulation or at periods of increased risk. The passive antibody interferes with the interaction between the antigen on the cell surface and the recipient's immune system. The cells are not destroyed, but they lose their ability to trigger the individual's own antibody production. Both the timing and the dosage must be correct. The usual dose is 200–300 μg at 28 weeks antenatally and at term, following delivery of an Rh-positive infant. If an Rh-incompatible blood transfusion is inadvertently given, approximately 25 μg of passive anti-D should be given for every milliliter of blood infused. The anti-D coats the circulating Rh-positive cells and apparently causes accelerated splenic destruction to the extent that the individual does not experience immunization or severe hemolytic reaction. Rh immune globulin can be given effectively at any time during the first 72 hours after Rh cells are introduced. Insufficient data exist to indicate whether this interval can be prolonged safely.

During pregnancy, if more than 50 ml of fetal cells has entered the circulation, more RhIg can be given. If an Rh-negative woman undergoes an amniocentesis, or spontaneous or induced abortion, she should similarly be protected with adequate levels of RhIg immunoprophylaxis. If a woman is administered antenatal prophylaxis, it is extremely important that this be noted in her medical history, because otherwise the presence of anti-D in a postpartum blood sample might be considered evidence for preexisting immunization. Whether or not she has received RhIg during pregnancy, the unimmunized Rh-negative woman should always receive RhIg after giving birth to an Rh-positive child (see later).

Other Blood Groups

Table 8–3 outlines some of the more common red cell antigen systems of clinical importance. A blood group system is a series of antigens controlled by allelic genes inherited independently of other genes. The ABO and Rh systems dominate the blood bank scene, but many other systems exist. Blood group antigens are clinically significant if they elicit antibodies following transfusion, if they react with antibodies in such a way that *in vivo* hemolysis occurs, or if they are implicated in hemolytic disease of the newborn. Besides ABO and Rh, the blood group systems of greatest clinical significance are Kell, Duffy, and Kidd. Other antigens and antibodies create clinical problems in relatively few cases, but often enough that their presence must be sought and acknowledged.

Red Cell Alloimmunization

Alloantibody production to red cell antigens occurs when foreign erythrocytes enter the circulation of an individual whose red cells lack the antigens. Transfusion and pregnancy are the usual ways in which red cell antigens are transferred between individuals. Immunization characteristically elicits first a relatively transient IgM antibody, and then an IgG antibody that persists for years. These IgG antibodies

Table 8–3. SOME OF THE WELL-KNOWN BLOOD GROUP SYSTEMS AND THEIR COMMON ALLELES

ABO	A, B, O, AB
Rh	C, D, E, c, e
K	K, k
Duffy	Fy^a, Fy^b
Kidd	Jk^a, Jk^b
Lutheran	Lu^a, Lu^b
MNS	M, N, S, s
Lewis	Le^a, Le^b
P	P_1, P_2
I	I, i

react best at body temperature; once an antibody is present it will hemolyze or coat cells that possess the relevant antigen. Antibody screening and crossmatching attempt to prevent such hemolytic episodes by detecting and identifying the antibodies so that antigen-positive cells will not be transfused.

Antibodies differ in their incidence, in the frequency with which they cause clinical problems, and in the methods in which they are detected in the laboratory. Patients may have several different antibodies simultaneously; this makes it difficult to identify the weaker ones and sometimes causes more specificities to be overlooked.

Sometimes antibodies weaken as time passes so that it is difficult or impossible to demonstrate that a person has been immunized. If antigen-positive cells are transfused to such a patient, the antibody very rapidly reappears. This rapid return of antibody, called an *anamnestic response,* may destroy the transfused antigen-positive cells (*delayed hemolytic transfusion reaction,* see Adverse Effects of Transfusions, later in chapter.) The Rh antibodies anti-E and anti-c are especially likely to cause delayed hemolysis, as are antibodies of the Kidd system (anti-Jk^a and anti-Jk^b). Kidd antibodies are often weak to begin with and tend to exist as one of several different antibodies in the same sensitized person.

Hemolytic reactions are rare, but antibodies are fairly frequent, occurring in 6% or more of persons with previous transfusions or pregnancies. Finding blood that lacks the one or several antigens reactive with a patient's antibodies can seriously delay transfusion, but failure to find and give compatible blood can cause even worse problems. These IgG antibodies provoked by transfusion or pregnancy can also cause hemolytic disease of the newborn (see Hemolytic Disease of the Newborn, later in chapter).

Antibody Formation without Known Stimulation

Although anti-A and anti-B are the only antibodies regularly found in the serum of unimmunized individuals, antibodies active against other red cell antigens occasionally occur in persons who have never been exposed to human red blood cells. Such antibodies are sometimes called *naturally occurring,* but a better term is *non–red cell stimulated*. The immunizing stimulus is presumably exposure to environmental material antigenically similar to red cell antigens, but no one ever knows why some people form antibodies and most do not.

Antibodies that develop without red cell stimulus are usually IgM and usually react best at temperatures of 30°C or below. Because of their low thermal optimum, they seldom cause problems in a transfusion setting. Some retain activity at 37°C and must be considered to have potential clinical significance. These antibodies, being IgM, do not cross the placenta and do not cause hemolytic disease of the newborn. The most notable and most clinically important IgM antibodies of this type, of course, are anti-A and anti-B, which can cause serious hemolytic transfusion reactions when ABO-incompatible blood is given.

Other non–red-cell-stimulated (natural) antibodies (not including ABO), usually have specificity against antigens in the systems designated Lewis, Ii, P, or MNS. In cold reactive autoimmune hemolytic anemia associated with Mycoplasma pneumoniae infections (see Chapter 3, Autoimmune hemolytic anemia, pp 116–120), anti-I is often implicated. Anti-I and anti-IH often cause laboratory problems in crossmatching because high titer examples tend to have persistent agglutinating activity even at 37°C. Lewis antibodies occur fairly commonly in the unimmunized population. *In vivo* hemolysis from anti-Le^a occurs only rarely. Most Lewis antibodies are clinically insignificant, but there is enough unpredictability that many blood bankers are reluctant to ignore them if they are active at 37°C.

ANTIHUMAN GLOBULIN SERUM TEST

Immunoglobulins, the antibody molecules themselves, are antigenic if introduced into a nonhuman host. In 1945, Coombs, Mourant, and Race injected whole human serum into rabbits; the resulting antihuman serum antibody proved remarkably useful as a laboratory reagent. The term *Coombs' serum* is still applied to antibodies that react with human globulins. Almost any protein or polypeptide fragment can be used in this manner to prepare immunoreactive reagents. Consequently, a panspecific antihuman globulin (polyspecific) or a monospecific antihuman globulin directed to a specific component of the antibody or complement can be prepared. Using these test reagents, the specific reactant antibody can be identified either coating the red cells or floating free in the serum. Antibodies against the immunoglobulin molecule or various chains or fragments are widely used in immunology. Currently, newer methodology using monoclonal antibodies is defining specific globulins with more precise specificities (see Chapter 7). In blood banking, the significant test reagent specificities are against IgG and, to a lesser degree, complement, especially C3d.

Antiglobulin serum (antihuman globulin or AHG) detects the presence of antibody or complement molecules on the red cell surface in the *direct antiglobulin test (DAT)*. Red cells can become globulin coated, either *in vivo* or *in vitro*. Most blood banks use a single antiglobulin reagent capable of detecting IgG globulin and complement (polyspecific), and then have specific reagents that react only with IgG or certain complement components (monospecific). *In vivo* coating is detected by the DAT (Table 8–4). *In vitro* manipulations are used in antibody screening, in crossmatching, and in special applications of blood typing.

The principle of the test is to amplify the presence of immunoglobulin and/or complement on erythrocytes using AHG to agglutinate (stick red cells together) the

Table 8–4. USES OF THE DIRECT ANTIGLOBULIN TEST

To Detect IgG Antibody and/or Complement:

1) On fetal RBC in hemolytic disease of the newborn.
2) On recipient RBC in hemolytic transfusion reactions.
3) On patient's RBC in autoimmune hemolytic anemia; e.g., collagen disease (SLE), lymphoproliferative disorders (CLL, lymphoma).
4) On patient RBC related to drug therapy (penicillin, quinidine, methyldopa, cephalosporin).

coated red cells, either directly *(directly antiglobun test)* or following incubation with serum-containing antibodies *(indirect antiglobulin test)*.

The Direct Antiglobulin Test

In Autoimmune Hemolytic Anemia

It is never normal for circulating red cells to be coated with immunoglobulins (IgG or IgM). In the DAT, cells are tested directly as they come from the circulation and are treated only by thorough washing to remove unbound proteins. If the polyspecific antiglobulin reagent agglutinates the cells, it is desirable to use individual reagents that can demonstrate if the coating is IgG or complement or both.

Table 8–4 lists the uses of the DAT. The usual cause of a positive DAT result is autoimmune hemolytic anemia (AIHA; see Chapter 3, pp 116–120, immune-mediated hemolytic anemia). In this condition, patients have antibodies that react with their own cells. These autoantibodies may be IgG or IgM, and nearly always react with red cells from all other persons as well as those of the patient. Red cells coated with IgG, IgM, or complement experience mechanical difficulty passing through tiny capillaries, especially in the spleen. More importantly, the globulin coating renders them liable to adhesion and phagocytosis by macrophages of the reticuloendothelial system. Coated red cells undergo accelerated destruction (hemolysis), and if the bone marrow is unable to compensate for the lost red cells, the patient becomes anemic. The causes of these conditions are discussed in Chapter 3, (immune-mediated hemolytic anemia).

Autoimmune hemolytic antibody syndromes are usually classified as cold reactive or warm reactive, depending on the thermal optimum of the autoantibody. IgM autoantibodies usually react at temperatures well below 37°C; often they attach only briefly to the red cell so that few or no IgM molecules remain to coat the cell. In their brief interaction, however, they often initiate the complement sequence activation, and various components of complement remain firmly attached to the circulating cells. These can be identified with monospecific anticomplement Coombs antisera (AHG). In cold-reactive AIHA, the antiglobulin activity is often due solely to complement. This form of AIHA occurs as a primary event in older people of both sexes, or after such infections as mycoplasma pneumonia, and infectious mononucleosis. It constitutes 20% to 25% of autoimmune hemolytic anemias.

Warm-reactive autoimmune hemolytic anemia is due to *IgG autoantibodies,* which remain on the red cell surface for as long as the red cell remains in the circulation. The condition is often a primary, idiopathic event that can affect any age group. Warm-reactive AIHA may also occur in conjunction with leukemias, lymphomas, disseminated carcinoma, or collagen vascular diseases, especially lupus erythematosus. Up to 70% of AIHA is the warm-reactive IgG type. Drug reactions are also a common cause of warm autoimmune hemolytic anemia (see Chapter 3).

Direct Antiglobulin Test without Autoimmunity

Not every positive DAT result is due to autoantibodies. In many instances, antibody coating of the red cells may occur for some unknown reason and are not associated with any apparent anemia. It has been estimated that approximately 7% of the elderly hospital population may have a positive DAT result. In some instances, these may be related to drug reactions. Drug antibodies can cause a positive DAT result because the red cell may be coated with the drug, or because an immune complex of drug and antibody attaches to the red cell surface and initiates complement activation. The antihypertensive drug alpha-methyldopa (Aldomet) produces a positive DAT result in up to 15% of patients taking it, although hemolysis rarely accompanies the phenomenon. In these cases, the antibody seems truly to be directed against the red cell membrane, but the manner in which the drug leads to the formation of antibody remains unclear.

Alloantibodies cause a positive DAT result in several other special circumstances. In hemolytic disease of the newborn, maternal IgG crosses the placenta and attaches to the fetal cells, which become coated with IgG. At birth, the cord cells are seen to have a positive DAT result, with monospecific AHG to IgG. If Rh immune globulin is inadvertently given to an Rh-positive individual, the DAT result will be positive but hemolysis, if it occurs, is mild. Similarly, transfusion of antibody-containing plasma may, on rare occasions, cause the recipient's red cells with the corresponding antigen to be coated with antibody, but significant hemolysis is extremely rare.

Delayed hemolytic transfusion reactions cause a clinically significant positive DAT result. If an antigen on transfused red cells provokes anamnestic antibody production, the resulting IgG attaches to the circulating transfused cells and causes their accelerated destruction. The DAT in these cases affects only the transfused cells, not the patient's own cells, which are negative for the antigen. This type of partial activity in any agglutination reaction is called *mixed field agglutination* (see Delayed Consequences of Transfusions and Fig. 8–3).

Antibody Screening Test (Indirect Antiglobulin Test)

It is important to know if patients or donors have any antibodies in their serum other than anti-A and anti-B. It is impossible to predict which persons will develop antibodies after immunizing exposure, or which nontransfused persons will have non–red-cell-stimulated antibodies. Standard practice calls for screening every blood sample from every patient for the presence of unsuspected antibodies prior to each transfusion. Routine screening for antibodies is also performed empirically during pregnancy to detect those antibodies likely to be associated with hemolytic disease of the newborn. Most donor bloods are also screened, although antibodies in donor plasma are much less significant. Table 8–5 is a list of the uses of the antibody screening test. The antibody screening test is sometimes called the indirect antiglobulin test or indirect Coombs' test. This is an imprecise or misleading term

Table 8–5. USES OF THE ANTIBODY SCREENING TEST

To Detect IgG Antibody:

1) In maternal serum during pregnancy and in association with hemolytic disease of the newborn.
2) In recipient's serum prior to transfusion—major crossmatch.
3) In donor serum prior to transfusion—minor crossmatch.
4) In recipient's serum after hemolytic transfusion reaction.

because antiglobulin serum (Coombs serum) is used in a variety of laboratory procedures. Therefore, the antibody screening test identifies antibody in the serum. It is a modified system that uses indicator red cells containing a variety of red cell antigens to define the presence of serum antibody by agglutination. In this system, the indicator red cells become coated with antibody *in vitro* (in the test tube during blood banking procedures [Table 8–6]).

Type and Screen

In certain surgical procedures, blood is transfused in less than 25% of cases, and in some procedures less than 10% of the time. Blood should not be crossmatched for a patient unless the chances are high that the unit will be transfused. In situations where blood is infrequently used, yet the likelihood is possible for it to be required, a type and screen system can be set up. In this manner, the blood bank determines the ABO and Rh type and performs an antibody screen on the serum. The specimen is usually held for crossmatching of donor units if needed. If the antibody screen is positive, crossmatching will be performed despite the low likelihood of the blood's being needed. If no antibodies are detected, units are generally not crossmatched; however, there is always an adequate inventory of type-specific blood available in the event that the patient actually needs to be transfused. In this situation, if blood is needed it can be issued as "partially crossmatched" blood within 15 minutes. Issuing blood in this manner is 99.9% as safe as performing the crossmatch and vastly improves the efficiency of blood banking. Even in situations where there is an incompatible crossmatch with a negative antibody screen, it is highly unlikely that the antibodies are going to be clinically significant. Tables for Transfusion Service blood order guidelines in elective surgical procedures should be established in each individual hospital, and in most instances should be established with collaboration between the blood bank physician, surgeon, and anesthesiologist (Table 8–7). If a positive antibody screen is identified and is deemed to be clinically significant, blood lacking the corresponding antigens should be available and complete crossmatching should be performed using the antihuman globulin test.

Crossmatching

Before blood is administered, the donor cells and the recipient's serum are tested for the presence of serologic incompatibility by *crossmatching.* The crossmatch is the final check that the patient does not have a circulating antibody reactive against the transfused red cells.

Table 8–6. ROUTINE INTERPRETATION OF ANTIBODY SCREENING AND CROSSMATCHING (INDIRECT ANTIGLOBULIN TEST)

Result	Interpretation
Negative antibody screen	No antibody against antigens on reagent RBCs.
Crossmatch compatible	No antibody in recipient serum against donor erythrocytes.
Positive antibody screen Alloantibody Autoantibody Drug antibody	Irregular antibody against reagent erythrocyte antigens. Identify antibody by testing with cell panels of known antigenic specificity.
Crossmatch incompatible	Recipient antibody against donor erythrocyte antigens. Identify antibody by testing with cell panels of known antigenic specificity. Select donor who lacks corresponding antigen. If crossmatch is still incompatible, multiple alloantibodies, unusual antibodies, or autoantibody artifacts are responsible.

Antiglobulin serum (AHG) markedly enhances the sensitivity of *in vitro* testing. Strong IgM antibodies usually cause grossly visible agglutination of cells possessing the relevant antigen, but weaker antibodies are difficult to detect and many IgG antibodies do not agglutinate cells no matter how strong the antibody is. All tests for antibodies, including the crossmatch, use centrifugation of serum and cells as the first phase of testing. Agglutination indicates a positive result (see Fig. 8–3). The serum and cells are then allowed to incubate, usually for 15–30 minutes, to allow any antibody that is present in the serum every opportunity to attach to the donor red cells. After unbound proteins are washed away, antiglobulin serum is added. If the serum contains an antibody that reacts with and attaches to an antigen on the cell surface, adding AHG causes the antibody-coated cells to agglutinate. If there is no agglutination after the addition of AHG, it means that no antigen–antibody reaction has occurred. The serum may well contain an antibody, but if the cells do not have the relevant antigen, the reaction will be negative and the transfused cells will be crossmatch-compatible.

Antibody screening is important, not only in a transfusion setting, but also in evaluating pregnant women for the possible occurrence of hemolytic disease of the newborn.

The crossmatch is the best available test to predict satisfactory transfusion outcome. A negative crossmatch does not, however, guarantee that the red cells will survive normally or that the patient will experience no ill effects from the transfusion.

PRETRANSFUSION TESTING

Table 8–6 outlines the interpretation of antibody screening and compatibility tests.

Pretransfusion Testing on Donor Blood

Blood drawn from the donor's vein must be processed for safe transfusion. Regardless of subsequent fractionation, the blood must be found to be free of hepatitis B surface antigen (HbsAg) and human immune deficiency virus (HIV), human T leukemia virus (HTLV) type 1, and surrogate tests must be performed to reduce the likelihood of non-A, non-B hepatitis virus transmission (see Infectious Disease Transmission by Blood Components). Testing for antibody to hepatitis C virus (HCV) will also become routinely implemented. In addition, blood is also tested for exposure to syphilis. Blood that is positive for any of these tests is never transfused. Blood found to have unexpected red cell antibody is separated into plasma and red cells. The red cells can be used for transfusion, but the plasma is either pooled for large-scale fractionation procedures or saved for reagent purposes.

Recipient's Blood

Before a patient receives blood, his or her ABO group and Rh type must be known and the patient must be tested for unexpected red cell antibodies as described above. Every blood sample received from each patient undergoes these tests, and the results are compared against previously recorded results stored in the blood bank. A person's ABO and Rh types do not change, but there is always the danger of incorrectly identified blood samples; comparing present with previous results on the "same" patient has detected many instances of mistaken identity and prevented many transfusion-associated disasters. Antibody screening tests often do change, going from negative to positive in the days, weeks, or months that follow transfusions. It is important to document if immunization has occurred.

It is not essential to test the patient's blood samples for HBsAg, for HIV, serologic tests for syphilis, or the presence of antibodies on the red cell surface (DAT). Some transfusion services perform some or all of these tests routinely, but many do not.

Compatibility Testing for Red Cells

Before blood is transfused into a patient, samples from donor and recipient should be tested for serologic compatibility. The likelihood of incompatibility is much reduced if both patient and donor have negative antibody screening test results, but no screening procedure can ensure against specific rare antibody antigen reactions. For patients with known antibodies, pretransfusion compatibility testing is crucial.

The crossmatch is the final search for incompatibility between a patient's blood and a donor's red cells. Before antibody screening tests were done routinely on donor blood, a "minor" crossmatch was also performed. The minor crossmatch tests the donor's serum against the patient's red cells. It is called minor because the rapid dilution that plasma undergoes on entering the patient's bloodstream ensures

Table 8–7. TRANSFUSION SERVICE GUIDELINES FOR ELECTIVE SURGICAL PROCEDURES*

Procedure	Requirement	Procedure	Requirement
General surgery		*Ear, nose and throat surgery*	
Cholecystectomy	T&S	Caldwell-Luc	T&S
Exploratory laparotomy celiotomy)	T&S	Laryngectomy	T&S
Ileal bypass	T&S	*Plastic surgery*	
Hiatal hernia repair	T&S	Mammoplasty	T&S
Colectomy and hemicolectomy	2 Units	Thoracoabdominal flap	T&S
Splenectomy	2 Units	*Oral surgery*	
Breast biopsy	T&S	Osteotomy	T&S
Radical mastectomy	1 Unit	Genioplasty	T&S
Modified radical mastectomy	1 Unit	Bilateral subcondylar osteotomy	T&S
Simple mastectomy	1 Unit	Vestibuloplasty	T&S
Gastrectomy	2 Units	LaFort I osteotomy	T&S
Antrectomy and vagotomy	2 Units	Anterior maxillary osteotomy	T&S
Inguinal herniorrhaphy	T&S	*Neurosurgery*	
Liver biopsy	T&S	Craniotomy	2 Units
Vein stripping	T&S	Herniated disk	T&S
Cardiovascular surgery		Ventriculoperitoneal shunt	T&S
Saphenous vein bypass	6 Units	Transsphenoidal hypophysectomy	2 Units
Open heart surgery (congenital defect)	6 Units	*Orthopedics*	
Valve replacement	6 Units	Open reduction	2 Units
Pleurodesis	T&S	Scoliosis fusion	3—4 Units
Aortobifemoral bypass	8 Units		
Thoracotomy	3 Units	Herniated disk	T&S
Closed mediastinal exploration	T&S	Arthroplasty	T&S
Resection abdominal aortic aneurysm	8 Units	Shoulder reconstruction	T&S
Carotid endarterectomy	2 Units	Total hip replacement	2—3 Units
Obstetric-gynecologic surgery		Total knee replacement	T&S
Total abdominal hysterectomy	T&S	*Genitourinary surgery*	
Exploratory laparotomy	T&S	Transurethral resection of prostate	T&S
Total vaginal hysterectomy	T&S	Radical nephrectomy	1 Unit
Vaginal resuspension	T&S	Renal transplantation	1 Unit
Laparoscopy	T&S	Penile prosthesis insertion	T&S
Repeat C-section	T&S	Patch graft	T&S
Labor and delivery requests (oxytocin drips & C-sections)	T&S	Prostatectomy	2 Units

*Modified from Boral and Henry[1].

From Widmann (ed): Technical Manual, ed 9. American Association of Blood Banks, Arlington, VA, 1985, p 408, with permission.

T&S = type and antibody screen.

that problems caused by *transfused antibody* will be minor at worst. Now that all donor blood is screened for unexpected antibodies, the minor crossmatch has become an obsolete procedure.

In the "major" crossmatch, a donor's red cells and a patient's serum are combined under conditions designed to elicit both IgG and IgM antibody activity. The cells and serum must be incubated long enough to allow minimally avid antibodies time to react. It is also necessary to add antiglobulin serum after incubation to detect antibodies that coat red cells without agglutinating them, as described above. These tests are time consuming but important. Under emergency conditions, when delaying transfusion jeopardizes the patient's life, incompletely crossmatched blood may be administered, but the crossmatch should be carried to completion. In patients who have previously been typed and screened, a partially crossmatched blood can also be released, as described above.

Many centers are now using an extended type and screen procedure to replace the major crossmatch in patients who do not demonstrate unexpected antibodies against a comprehensive polyvalent three cell reagent panel (three cell screen). An abbreviated crossmatch is performed to verify ABO compatibility. This technique has now established a proven safety record and is less labor intensive.

Selection of Blood Products

Transfused red cells must lack antigens to which the recipient has antibodies. If anti-A is present, A or AB cells cannot be given; the same applies to B or AB cells in a patient with anti-B. Although antibodies in donor plasma are far less important, occasional units of Group O blood contain potent anti-A or anti-B that can damage A, B, or AB recipient cells on transfusion. The concept of Group O as a "universal donor" applies to red cells, not to whole blood. It is good practice to give group-specific blood at all times. When this is impractical, Group A or Group B recipients can receive O red cells, and AB recipients can receive red cells of any ABO type. An O recipient can only receive Group O blood.

Since Rh antibodies are not naturally occurring, no immediate harm results from giving Rh-positive blood to an Rh-negative patient. Subsequently, however, 60% to 70% of Rh-negative recipients will develop anti-D, and the practice is considered generally undesirable. It is important to *avoid* giving *Rh-positive blood* to *Rh-negative* girls or women capable of childbearing because hemolytic disease of the newborn is almost certain to occur in any Rh-positive child they would subsequently bear. More flexibility is possible in selecting plasma products and platelet concentrates than in red cell selection. Ideally, all such products should be group-specific. In practice, transfused anti-A and anti-B rarely cause problems except in very small children and rare cases of intensively treated hemophilia. Group O plasma is more likely to be dangerous than other groups and should be the last choice for transfusing recipients of blood groups other than O.

The situation with platelet concentrates is awkward. Concentrates stored at room temperature contain at least 50 ml of plasma, which possesses antibodies that might have the potential for injuring the recipient's cells. In addition, platelets have ABH antigenic activity that can react with the recipient's antibody. Group-specific platelets are definitely the product of choice, but non–group-specific platelets are preferable to none at all.

BLOOD COMPONENT THERAPY

Cellular Components

A unit of blood consists of cellular and noncellular elements that serve diverse functions. Transfusion therapy is directed toward replacing a component or components that are deficient in a symptomatic patient. There is always some risk associated with any product, and the risk/benefit ratio should always be ascertained. Table 8–8 summarizes the use of blood and components in transfusion therapy, and also outlines some of the risks associated with each specific component.

RED CELL PRODUCTS

Red cells contain hemoglobin, which transports the oxygen that is necessary to maintain life. In the past, the only indication for transfusion was to replace or restore oxygen-carrying capacity. The bulk of transfusions are still given for this purpose.

Whole Blood. Circulating blood consists of plasma, red blood cells, white cells, and platelets. When blood is drawn from the donor, anticoagulant preservative solution is added to prevent clotting during storage. The resulting component consists of about 450 ml of blood, diluted with 63 ml of anticoagulant preservative. Since neither white cells nor platelets survive very long at refrigerated temperatures (2–6°C), stored whole blood consists, functionally, of red cells and plasma. Albumin and most globulins survive throughout storage, but the labile coagulation factors deteriorate unpredictably.

At present, refrigerated whole blood collected in CPD-A1 anticoagulant has a shelf life of 35 days. Administering whole blood augments the recipient's total blood volume and oxygen-carrying capacity and is most useful for treating large-scale blood loss. Patients with adequate blood volume but deficient hemoglobin derive little benefit from the plasma of transfused whole blood, and patients whose cardiac function is precarious may suffer congestive heart failure if given whole blood.

Metabolic changes occur both within the red cells and in the plasma on storage. These are listed in Table 8–9. The metabolic changes occurring with storage are termed the *storage lesion* and have some importance when large volumes of whole blood are replaced, as in massive blood transfusion (see Acute Transfusion Reactions). Ordinarily, metabolic changes in the red cells during surgery are not clinically important for adults. However, because of leakage of potassium from erythrocytes into the plasma during storage, as well as a drop in the erythrocyte 2,3 DPG (a major organo-phosphate protein responsible for oxygen delivery) especially after one week of storage, blood less than one week old is preferable for neonatal transfusions. Whole blood replacement is of particular value in individuals who have lost more than 25% of their total blood volume, since it provides oxygen-carrying capacity, volume expansion, and coagulation support. Perhaps the only true indication for the use of whole blood would be in massive blood replacement; however, this can generally be satisfactorily accomplished with red cells, fresh frozen plasma, and colloid or crystalloid solutions. Fresh, whole blood if available, however, would seem to be the component of choice for exchange transfusions in the newborn. If this cannot be accomplished, red cells less than seven days of age should be reconstituted with fresh frozen plasma, ideally from the same donor.

Concentrated Red Blood Cells. Red cells can be separated from the rest of the blood by centrifugation. The resulting red blood cell preparation has all the oxygen-

Table 8–8. INDICATIONS AND COMPLICATIONS OF BLOOD COMPONENT THERAPY

Cellular and Plasma Components	Content	Indications	Amount of Active Substance per Unit	Volume (ml)	Shelf Life	Dosage Effect	Precautions and Complications
RBC concentrates, PRBCs	70–80% RBCs, some plasma, WBCs, and platelets or their degradation products	Improves oxygen-carrying capacity, increases red blood cell mass for symptomatic anemia and hemorrhagic shock, preferred over whole blood to reduce complications	175–280 ml PRBC mass	250–350	ACD—21 days, CPD—21 days, CPDA-1—35 days, ADSOL—42 days	Increases Hct 3% per unit	Must be ABO compatible FR ++ UR ++ AR + H ++++ PTP ++ INF ++
Washed RBCs	>80% erythrocytes suspended in saline	Reduces febrile reactions due to leukocyte debris in patients with preformed leukocyte antibodies	200 ml PRBC mass	200–250	Open system: 24 hours	Increases Hct 3%	ABO compatible FR 0 → +/ – UR 0 AR 0 H ++++ PTP 0
Leukocyte concentrates	WBCs, platelets, some erythrocytes	Granulocytopenia with sepsis (neutrophils < 500/mm^3)	$>1.0 \times 10^{10}$ granulocytes	200–600	24 hours	Cannot be determined	FR +++ UR +++ AR ++ H 0

		unresponsive to appropriate antibiotics after 48 hours or positive blood culture; sepsis in premature infant with depleted WBC reserve					PTP +++ INF ++ (CMV↑)
Platelet concentrates (single unit random donor; single donor—apheresis, HLA matched also available)	Platelets, some WBCs and plasma	Bleeding due to thrombocytopenia or thrombocytopathy, platelet disorders, DIC, massive transfusions (6–8 units per 10 units PRBCs transfused)	At least 5.5 × 10^{10} platelets	30–60 per unit	72–120 hours at RT (20–24 °C) depending on container, 48 hours at 1–6 °C	Increases platelet count 5000–8000 per concentrate	Do not use microaggregate filter FR +++ UR +++ AR ++ PTP ++++ INF ++
FFP	Plasma, all coagulation factors, no platelets	Treatment of multiple coagulation disorders or in massive transfusions (2 units per 10 units PRBCs transfused)	0.7–1.0 units of factors II, V, VII, VIII, IX, X, XI, XII, XIII; 500 mg fibrinogen	200–250	Frozen—1 year, thawed—6 hours	Increase of 20–30% in coagulation factor activity per dose of 10–15 ml of plasma per kg body weight	UR ++++ AR +++ INF ++ Fluid overload +

Table 8–8. INDICATIONS AND COMPLICATIONS OF BLOOD COMPONENT THERAPY *(Continued)*

Cellular and Plasma Components	Content	Indications	Amount of Active Substance per Unit	Volume (ml)	Shelf Life	Dosage Effect	Precautions and Complications
Cryoprecipitated plasma AHF (CRYO); purified AHF (factor VIII) and factor IX complex also available	Fibrinogen, factor VIII:C, factor XIII, von Willebrand factor, fibronectin	Factor VIII deficiency (hemophilia A), von Willebrand disease, factor XIII deficiency, fibrinogen deficiency, consumption of fibrinogen—DIC	80 units of factor VIII:C, 200 mg fibrinogen (usually given every 15–20 hours), 40–70% of von Willebrand factor present in initial unit	10–25	Frozen—1 year (−18°C or below); thawed—6 hours; if entered or pooled—4 hours	Increase of 50–100 units of factor VIII per unit of cryoprecipitate (about 10 ml volume)	UR ++++ AR ++++ INF ++
Albumin (5%, 25%)	96% albumin, 4% globulins (α-β)	Plasma volume expansion	12.5 g albumin	50 or 250	3 years at RT, 5 years at 2–8 °C		Fluid overload ++ UR + AR 0 Very expensive

ACD = acid citrate dextrose; AHF = antihemophilic factor; AR = anaphylaxis; C = coagulant; CMV = cytomegalovirus; CPD = citrate phosphate dextrose; CPDA = citrate phosphate dextrose adenine; DIC = disseminated intravascular coagulation; FFP = fresh frozen plasma; FR = febrile reaction; H = hemolysis; Hct = hematocrit; INF = infection; PRBCs = packed red blood cells; PTP = post-transfusion purpura; RBCs = red blood cells; RT = room temperature; UR = urticarial reaction; WBCs = white blood cells.

Modified from American Association of Blood Banks. Blood Component Therapy: A Physician's Handbook. American Association of Blood Banks, Arlington, VA, 1981).

Table 8–9. SOME OF THE CHANGES OCCURRING IN BLOOD STORED IN CPD AND CPD-ADENINE SOLUTION AT 4°C

Days Stored	0	7	14	21	35
Percentage of red cells destroyed within 24 hr of transfusion	0	5	10	20	—
CPD					
Plasma pH	7.20	7.00	6.89	6.84	—
Plasma K (mmol/liter)	3.9	11.9	17.2	21.0	
Plasma Na (mmol/liter)	168	166	163	156	—
Plasma Hb (g/liter)	1.7	7.8	12.5	19.1	—
CPD-A					
Plasma pH	7.22	—	—	6.77	6.57
Plasma K (mmol/liter)	—	—	—	—	26.7
Plasma Na (mmol/liter)	—	—	—	—	15.3
Plasma Hb (g/liter)	—	—	—	—	50.6

blood by centrifugation. The resulting red blood cell preparation has all the oxygen-carrying capacity of the original unit without much plasma to dilute its therapeutic effect. This is especially important for patients with chronic anemia, congestive heart failure, or other individuals who have difficulty regulating blood volume. Red cells are more effective than whole blood in supplying oxygen-carrying capacity and raising the recipient's hematocrit. Like whole blood, refrigerated red blood cells stored in CPD-A1 have an improved shelf life of 35 days. With the use of newer additive anticoagulant solutions (Adsol and Nutricel), the shelf life can be extended to 42 days. The amount of plasma and white cells that remain in refrigerator-stored red cells is not enough to perform any physiologically useful function, but is sufficient to induce immunization or cause immune reactions in sensitized recipients. Concentrated erythrocytes are the treatment of choice in individuals who have symptomatic loss of oxygen-carrying capacity due to either acute or chronic anemia. Concentrated erythrocytes should be used only when an individual is symptomatic from the anemia, and should not arbitrarily be used to raise a hematocrit value to some set level in absence of symptoms, although it can sometimes be justified prior to surgery.

Leukocyte-Poor Red Blood Cell Concentrates. Leukocytes may be removed from red cell concentrates by means of centrifugation, mechanical separation using filters, or washing procedures using saline or glycerol. Glycerol is used as a cryopreservative agent in frozen red cells, but is subsequently washed and removed on thawing from storage. The efficiency of leukocyte removal varies with the different preparation, and it appears that frozen deglycerolized red cells contain the least number of contaminating white cells. Leukocyte removal is indicated in individuals who have experienced febrile, nonhemolytic transfusion reactions to contaminating white cells (see Acute Transfusion Reactions, later in this chapter). Centrifugation is the simplest means of removing leukocytes prior to transfusion; however, it is probably the most inefficient method. Microaggregate filtration is a very practical method of leukocyte removal, but is also relatively inefficient although newer filters are more efficacious. It should be used empirically if a patient has had a febrile nonhemolytic transfusion reaction. Individuals who have experienced more than two febrile reactions should be given washed, concentrated red blood cells. The red blood cells may be washed by centrifugation and resuspension in saline, or may be washed by the automated mechanical cell washers. Cell washing triples the cost of the red cell component. Washed red cell components are also indicated in patients with IgA deficiency who have experienced anaphylactoid reactions to plasma. Frozen, deglycerolized red cells are the components with the least number of leukocytes. In addition, this component is almost devoid of platelets and plasma.

Red cells cannot simply be placed in a freezer for storage; there must be some cryoprotective agent to prevent damage to the cell membrane. Glycerol is the agent most often used. As red cells are exposed to the glycerol solution, all traces of plasma and nearly all the platelets and white cells are removed. Red cells can be kept in a frozen state for years; on reconstitution, at least 70% of the original cells survive normally if properly transfused. The recommended shelf life of frozen cells is *three years,* but they can be stored up to *seven years.* Once the cells are deglycerolized, they have a shelf expiratory time of *twenty-four hours.* Frozen, deglycerolized red cells are indicated in individuals who have had severe reactions to leukocytes and plasma components in packed red cells, and in particular those patients who have experienced febrile reactions or anaphylactoid reactions to washed red cells. Frozen blood can also be stored for individuals who have rare blood types and for whom it is difficult to find compatible blood. Furthermore, frozen cells may also be used for autologous transfusion, although this greatly increases the costs. There is some evidence that the use of frozen, deglycerolized blood components can reduce the incidence of cytomegalovirus transmission to neonates.

Patients severely immunized to plasma proteins or white blood cells usually tolerate transfusion with deglycerolized, thawed red cells without ill effect. Frozen storage is also useful for inventory management, because red cells have a long shelf life stored in this manner. It also facilitates stockpiling bloods of rare types needed for patients with difficult antibody problems. Many centers encourage patients with complex antibody mixtures or antibodies against high-incidence antigens to store their own blood for possible future use.

Platelet Concentrates

Random and Single Donor. Two kinds of platelet preparations are currently available: a single-unit concentrate, which contains approximately 75% of the original platelets suspended in a small amount of plasma, and thrombocytapheresis concentrates from *one single donor* that contain the equivalent of 6–8 units of platelets derived from 6–8 random single donors. Hemapheresis procedures make it possible to process large volumes of blood from a single donor, since the red cells and other elements are immediately returned to the donor. Large quantities of plasma, platelets, or white cells can be harvested by means of this technique. Except for small children, adequate platelet therapy always requires infusion of multiple units. With thrombocytapheresis, all the platelets can come from a single donor, thereby reducing the number of donor exposures and consequently the risk of transfusion-transmitted infection or immunization.

One unit of random platelet concentrate consists of the platelets collected from a single whole blood unit (450 ml of blood). The platelets are separated from the whole blood after collection into a multipack and are resuspended in 50–75 ml of plasma. Platelets can be stored for up to five days at 22°C on a platelet agitator to prevent platelet clumping. Platelets have a shorter lifespan than red cells, surviving only 8–10 days *in vivo* compared with 120 days for red cells. Survival *in vitro* is also much shorter. Platelets have a maximum shelf life of up to five days, but their postinfusion survival and effectiveness decline severely during storage.

Therapeutic Effects. An average single-unit platelet concentrate contains 5.5×10^{10} platelets. Although specific figures vary widely, this is a realistic mean figure when careful techniques of donor selection, phlebotomy, preparation, storage, and transportation have been employed. In a hematologically stable patient, transfusion of one unit of platelets elevates the platelet count approximately 8–10,000/μl/square meter of body surface area. The primary indication for platelet therapy is in an individual with *symptomatic thrombocytopenia.* Clearly, thrombocytopenia has many mechanisms, and platelet transfusions are most effective where there is defective platelet production such as occurs with marrow aplasia (e.g., post-chemotherapy, or with marrow failure). Thrombocytopenia associated with secondary destruction or peripheral sequestration generally does not have the same response following platelet transfusion (e.g., ITP). When platelets are given to a bleeding patient, the therapeutic effect is measured by improved hemostasis and not necessarily by improved laboratory values. If platelet consumption (see Chapter 5) has caused the bleeding and a low platelet count, transfused platelets suffer the same entrapment and destruction as the patient's own platelets. Platelet transfusions cause only slight clinical improvement, if any, in such cases. Patients with large spleens or with autoimmune platelet destruction derive little benefit from transfused platelets. Infection or high fever from any cause also reduces the survival of the transfused platelets. Nevertheless, the evaluation of platelet increments following transfusions, particularly at one hour and twenty-four hours, is very valuable in determining the *in vivo* platelet survival. This is clinically important from the point of view of assessing whether or not the person receiving the platelet transfusion is alloimmunized to platelets and also in determining and defining the most effective platelet therapy (Table 8–10).

Platelet Antibodies. Transfused platelets can be destroyed rapidly by alloantibodies in the recipient's plasma. Platelets lack red cell antigens other than A, B, and H, but they share HLA antigens with white cells and other body tissues and have unique platelet antigens as well. Anti-A and anti-B cause much less damage to incompatible platelets than to incompatible red cells. It is desirable, but not essential, that the platelets and the patient's plasma be ABO-compatible. Antibodies to

Table 8–10. CAUSES OF POOR PLATELET RESPONSES FOLLOWING TRANSFUSION

Immune causes	
Alloimmunization:	anti-HLA antibodies
	antiplatelet specific antibodies
Autoantibodies:	Immune thrombocytopenic purpura
Drug antibodies:	Quinidine
Immune complexes	
Nonimmune causes	
Fever/septicemia	
Disseminated intravascular coagulation	
Splenomegaly	
Veno-occlusive diseases of the liver	

HLA antigens, elicited by past transfusions and multiple pregnancies, damage platelets far more than do ABO antibodies. Alloimmune antibodies to HLA antigens (or, much more rarely, to specific platelet antigens) rapidly destroy transfused, incompatible platelets. For the immunized patient who requires platelet transfusions, HLA-typed platelets are often desirable. Difficulties in antibody identification, the expense of HLA typing, and the tremendous range of HLA phenotypes among donors and recipients make it unlikely that routine type and crossmatch will precede uncomplicated platelet transfusions in the near future. Nevertheless, newer technologies associated with identifying platelet-associated antibodies are being developed. Rapid platelet crossmatching techniques using microtiter plates are under investigation. There are, of course, many other reasons why platelet transfusions may not produce the expected posttransfusional increment (see Table 8–10). The dosage of platelets given should not be an empiric dose, but should be evaluated on the basis of the underlying cause of the thrombocytopenia, the location of the bleed (in CNS bleeds the platelet count should be greater than 80–100,000/μl, whereas lower levels might be appropriate for nosebleeds in the thrombocytopenic patient). In general, platelet counts above 50,000/μl are sufficient for adequate hemostasis except with bleeding into the central nervous system. Values greater than 20,000/μl are usually satisfactory for prevention of spontaneous bleeding. Empiric use of platelet therapy for management of the thrombocytopenia associated with cardiopulmonary bypass or open heart surgery is not warranted.

White Cell Concentrates

With the availability of hemapheresis procedures, it has become possible to collect enough granulocytes to make white cell transfusions more practical. Unfortunately, the data supporting the use of white cell transfusions in septic, granulocytopenic persons are less than satisfactory. Normal blood contains so few white cells that it would take 30 or more single donor units to provide a practical transfusion dose in adults; however, fresh buffy coat granulocytes collected from one or two units of fresh, whole blood may be useful in the management of sepsis in the newborn. Leukopheresis of a single donor provides approximately 10^{10} granulocytes in 300–500 ml of plasma; about 25 ml of red cells inevitably contaminate the granulocyte product, and substantial numbers of platelets are also present.

Granulocytes concentrates are indicated only for treating documented bacterial sepsis in patients with severe granulocytopenia (less than 500 granulocytes/μl) who have not responded to appropriate antibiotic therapy for at least 48 hours and/or have a positive blood culture. Repeated infusions are always necessary, imposing a high risk of transfusion-related reactions and a very high cost. Granulocyte transfusions are rarely used in treatment regimens for leukemia, but optimal use remains controversial and they should only be used in a protocol setting. There is, however, good data supporting the use of granulocyte transfusions in the treatment of neonatal sepsis with depletion of the bone marrow reserve. The optimal granulocyte product, however, has not yet been defined.

Plasma Components

Plasma contains coagulation proteins, albumin, immunoglobulins, and innumerable other constituents. Commercial plasma fractionation makes it possible to separately recover albumin, gammaglobulins, and coagulation factors from large pools of donor plasma. Solutions of albumin or of less purified plasma proteins are used

Table 8–11. CLINICAL INDICATIONS FOR FRESH FROZEN PLASMA

1. Deficiencies of clotting factors for which specific factor concentrates are unavailable.
2. Multiple coagulation factor deficiencies in a bleeding patient.
3. Reversal of Coumadin effect or Coumadin overdose.
4. Massive blood transfusion (> 1 blood volume within several hours).
5. Antithrombin III deficiency.
6. Treatment of thrombotic thrombocytopenic purpura.

for volume expansion; when properly prepared they carry virtually no risk of hepatitis, because they are pasteurized. Similarly, albumin does not transmit HIV infection. *Coagulation factor concentrates* carry a substantial hepatitis risk because pooling plasma from large numbers of donors multiplies the risk contributed by just a few infective units. Factor VIII concentrates have a moderately high risk; concentrates of the "liver factors" (factor IX concentrates, prothrombin concentrates) have a very high risk. This may be reduced once hepatitis C testing is implemented. Newer monoclonal antibody factor VIII concentrates seem to have a very low risk of hepatitis transmission.

Fresh frozen plasma (FFP) is the liquid portion of the whole blood unit collected and frozen within 6 hours and stored at −20°C. The indications for using fresh frozen plasma are listed in Table 8–11. Because fresh frozen plasma is processed so rapidly, it contains the labile coagulation factors (VIII,V), all the other coagulation factors, and plasma proteins as well. The major indication for the use of *fresh frozen plasma* is in coagulation factor deficiency with hemostatic defects where the factor deficiency is *not well established* or is a *multiple deficiency.* Fresh frozen plasma should only rarely be used, if ever, for volume expansion. It can, however, be satisfactorily used to reconstitute red cells for exchange transfusion in the newborn. It is also used as a replacement solution. Because it has the same hepatitis risk as whole blood, because it potentially contains antibodies to the recipient's white cells or plasma proteins, and because it takes 20–30 minutes to thaw before infusion, it is *not* a more desirable colloid source for volume expansion than albumin.

Single donor plasma and *cryoprecipitate-poor plasma* are byproducts of component preparation and are often less costly than FFP. The levels of labile coagulation factors are more variable than in FFP, but these products have the same content of stable coagulation factors, albumin, bactericidal material, opsonins, and other constituents. Many donor centers do not keep these products in inventory because they pool all their available plasma for use in industrial processing.

CRYOPRECIPITATE AND FACTOR VIII CONCENTRATES

Donor centers can prepare transfusion products from the plasma of *individual donors;* these have a low risk of disease transmission. *Cryoprecipitate* is a gelatinous residue obtained by freezing and slowly thawing freshly drawn plasma. It contains 80–100 IU of factor VIII, and about 250 mg of *fibrinogen* in a volume of 10–15 ml/unit. Cryoprecipitate is useful in treating minor or moderate bleeds in patients with factor VIII deficiency. If very high factor VIII concentrations are needed, as for life-threatening hemorrhage, for surgical procedures, or to overcome an inhibitor to factor VIII, the commercial concentrates are more convenient and more effective. Fresh frozen plasma and cryoprecipitate are the only transfusion products that contain *fibrinogen*. Cryoprecipitate is also the best available source of *von Willebrand factor,* which is not present in commercial concentrates of factor VIII. Commercial concentrates of factor VIII also carry a greater risk of hepatitis transmission, although with the more recently introduced heat treatment procedures, this risk may be somewhat decreased and even further reduced with the monoclonal antibody-prepared VIII concentrates. Heat treatment, in conjunction with HIV screening, appears to reduce, if not eliminate, the likelihood of transfusion-transmitted AIDS with this component. Cryoprecipitate is indicated in patients with mild hemophilia who do not respond to 1-deamino-(8-D-arginine)-vasopressin (DDAVP) infusion (see Chapter 6—Hemophilia). It is also useful in the management of hypofibrinogenemic states and in disseminated intravascular coagulation with consumption of fibrinogen. Factor VIII concentrates, of course, can be stored in the home setting and be reconstituted and infused directly at the first sign of bleeding. These concentrates, therefore, have revolutionized the home management of the hemophiliac. With concerns related to AIDS, however, the use of the factor VIII concentrates had declined substantially. Since the introduction of the heat-treated factor VIII concentrates and monoclonal antibody-purified factor VIII, home management using this component has again increased.

Factor IX Concentrate

This component contains concentrates of the vitamin K–dependent factors II, VII, IX, and X that are derived from pools of thousands of donors. This component, therefore, has similar risks to factor VIII concentrate; however, it is prepared from plasma fractionation rather than cryoprecipitation. These products are the treatment of choice for bleeding or prophylaxis in *Christmas disease patients (factor IX deficiency).* This component is also heat treated, as is factor VIII. Some factor IX concentrates also contain small amounts of activated coagulation factors and therefore can be useful in the management of hemophilic patients with inhibitors to factor VIII.

Serum Globulin Preparations

Commercial plasma fractionation can also concentrate gammaglobulin for administration to patients with severe humoral antibody deficiency. Plasma pools containing high titers of specific gammaglobulins may be used as hyperimmune gammaglobulin serum preparations for the management of individuals who have been exposed to varicella-zoster (VZIG) or hepatitis B (hepatitis B immune serum globulin). Table 8–8 is a summary of blood component therapy, its indications, and complications.

Autologous Transfusion

The safest transfusion uses the patient's own blood. Before an elective operation, many individuals can donate several units of blood for their own later use. With appropriate iron supplementation and clinical surveillance, it is possible to draw two or more units of blood, even as much as one unit/week, in the 35 or 42 days before the operation. Samples collected in this manner are stored in a liquid state; however, if frozen storage is available, the time between phlebotomy and autologous transfusion can be extended indefinitely. Autologous transfusion should always be indicated for any individual going for *elective surgery* for whom blood is likely to be used. Half-units can even be collected from smaller persons, or even adolescents going for surgery, despite the fact that they may fail to qualify as regular blood donors.

A procedure that is useful in harvesting patients' own blood is that which occurs during surgery termed *intraoperative salvage.* In this manner, blood lost at surgery is filtered and washed and can be reinfused back into the patient. Another technique of autologous transfusion is using preoperative hemodilution to the extent that blood lost at surgery contains less red cells. Autologous donations have the major advantage that they eliminate the risk of transfusion-transmitted disease and alloimmunization. This type of blood product should always be offered to all qualified patients.

Irradiated Blood Products

Graft vs. host disease (GVHD) is a rare complication of transfusion therapy that occurs exclusively in immunocompromised patients (see Graft vs. Host Disease, later in chapter). In this condition, the viable transfused T-lymphocytes attack the host's cells. Exfoliative dermatitis, diarrhea, liver inflammation, and marrow aplasia are the main clinical features. Posttransfusion GVHD is almost always fatal.

Graft vs. host disease can be prevented by irradiating the blood components given to persons at risk. Radiation is usually performed by placing the blood unit in a gamma radiation field with an exposure of 1500–3000 rad. This dose kills lymphocytes but does no harm to erythrocytes, platelets, or granulocytes. The blood itself is not radioactive and can be given to any recipient. Table 8–12 is a list of those patients who require irradiated blood products.

THERAPEUTIC HEMAPHERESIS

Therapeutic *hemapheresis* involves the exchange of ''diseased'' blood or components with ''healthy'' blood or components. *Plasmapheresis* refers to the removal of

Table 8–12. PATIENTS WHO REQUIRE IRRADIATED BLOOD

Absolute Indications	Relative Indications	No Definite Indications
Allogeneic and autologous bone marrow transfusions	Intrauterine transfusions	Nonpremature neonates
Congenital immunodeficiency syndrome	Neonatal exchange transfusions	Solid tumors
	Hodgkins and non-Hodgkins lymphoma	AIDS
	Acute leukemia	Aplastic anemia Agammaglobulinemia CGD

AIDS - acquired immunodeficiency syndrome; CGD = chronic granulomatous disease.

plasma and replacement with plasma or plasma substitutes, and has been reportedly successful in the diseases listed in Table 8–13. *Cytapheresis* is the term used to describe the removal of cellular components (thrombocytapheresis—platelets, leukocytapheresis—white cells, and erythrocytapheresis—red cells). The mechanisms of injury in certain diseases involve the presence of harmful circulating plasma or cellular factors, which may be removed by mechanical means. A notable example is the hyperviscosity syndrome, where an excess amount of abnormal viscous plasma may induce clinical symptoms. Removal of the abnormal plasma and replacement by crystalloid or colloid substitutes can effectively reduce these symptoms. The efficiency of plasmapheresis is substantially better when the abnormal compound or substance is distributed in the intravascular fluid. In this situation, a single plasma exchange may remove up to 90% of the factor (e.g., hyperviscosity syndrome due to macroglobulinemia). However, in many conditions where plasmapheresis has been used, pathogenesis is uncertain and the effectiveness or utility has been undefined.

Hemapheresis may be accomplished by means of continuous flow or intermittant flow cell separators. The blood volume of the patient must be estimated, and a CBC, coagulation screen, and electrolyte evaluation need to be obtained. In this manner, replacement solutions can be titrated accordingly, and electrolytes replaced to keep the patient as physiologic as possible. Specific laboratory tests may be performed in specific diseases (e.g., serum viscosity levels prepheresis and postpheresis may be monitored in patients with hyperviscosity syndrome). Similarly, in individuals with myasthenia gravis, one might monitor the titer of acetyl choline receptor antibodies. Table 8–14 lists the laboratory determinations commonly monitored during plasmapheresis.

ADVERSE EFFECTS OF TRANSFUSIONS

Adverse reactions to blood component transfusions are classified as acute or delayed (see Table 8–13). These transfusion reactions are defined as any unexpected or unfavorable symptom or clinical sign occurring in a patient during or immediately following the administration of a blood component. Delayed reactions may occur days to many years after the transfusion. The clinical interpretation of whether a transfusion reaction has occurred must be made with the understanding of 1) the patient's condition, 2) any underlying primary disease, 3) the type of component that has been administered, 4) the volume administered, and 5) whether the patient previously had a positive antibody screen. Whenever a decision is made to transfuse a patient, the potential side effects must be weighed against the likely benefits. Reactions in common with other intravenous solutions may further complicate a blood transfusion and include: 1) pyrogens, 2) bacterial contamination, 3) circulatory overload, 4) air embolism, and 5) thrombophlebitis.

General Complications

Pyrogenic substances are toxins capable of evoking a fever. Following an intravenous infusion of pyrogens, fever will occur. Pyrogens were formerly a problem with intravenous solutions or intravenous administration sets. Pyrogens are now strictly prevented by quality control in industry and are no longer a significant problem.

Bacterial contamination may complicate a blood transfusion or may occur in other intravenous solutions that serve as culture mediums (e.g., high sugar solu-

Table 8–13. INDICATIONS FOR THERAPEUTIC HEMAPHERESIS

Benefit	Disease	Component Removed
Plasmapheresis definite	Hyperviscosity syndromes	Abnormal protein
	Myasthenia gravis	Anticholinesterase antibody
	Goodpasture's syndrome	Antiglomerular basement membrane antibody
Plasmapheresis probable	Hyperlipidemia	Excess lipids and abnormal lipoproteins
	Thrombotic thrombocytopenic purpura	Platelet aggregating toxic factors
	Acute and chronic inflammatory demyelinating polyneuropathy (Guillain-Barre syndrome)	Antibody/Immune complexes
	Essential cryoglobulinemia	Cryoglobulins
Plasmapheresis possible	Renal transplant rejection	Antibody/cytotoxic lymphocytes
	Systemic lupus erythematosus	Immune complexes
	Rh isoimmunization	Anti-Rh antibodies
	Immune thrombocytopenic purpura	Antiplatelet antibody
	Autoimmune hemolytic anemia	Anti-RBC antibody
	Protein-bound toxins	Toxin bound to plasma proteins (e.g., mushroom poisoning)
	Rapidly progressive nephritis	Immune complexes (without anti-GAM)
Cytapheresis definite	Hyperleukocytosis with leukostasis	Excessive myeloid precursors (AML and CML)
	Hemorrhagic thrombocythemia	Excess abnormal platelets
Cytapheresis probable	Sickle cell complications	Sickled erythrocytes
Cytapheresis possible	Renal transplant rejection	Cytotoxic lymphocytes
	Chronic lymphocytic leukemia	Abnormal lymphocytes

Adapted from Sacher, RA and Ruma, TA: Therapeutic hemapheresis. In Henry, JB (ed): Clinical Diagnosis and Management by Laboratory Methods. WB Saunders, Philadelphia, 1984, p 1043.

tions). Organisms may grow in the solution, and when infused into a patient they may evoke a serious reaction mimicking a hemolytic transfusion reaction.

Circulatory overload occurs particularly in patients with chronic anemia and in the elderly or those with heart disease. The clinical features are mostly cardiopulmonary symptoms, and management is to stop or slow the infusion and administer diuretics. Circulatory overload is one of the commonest complications of blood component administration.

Table 8–14. LABORATORY DETERMINATIONS COMMONLY MONITORED DURING PLASMAPHERESIS

CBC with differential white count
Platelet count
Serum calcium
Prothrombin time
Partial thromboplastin time
Serum viscosity
Serum electrolytes
Serum protein electrophoresis, quantitative immunoglobulins
Hepatitis B surface antigen (Hb_sAg)
Human immunodeficiency virus antibody

Adapted from Sacher, RA and Ruma, TA: Therapeutic hemapheresis. In Henry, JB (ed): Clinical Diagnosis and Management by Laboratory Method. WB Saunders, Philadelphia, 1984.

Thrombophlebitis, or inflammation of the walls of the veins, may occur if an intravenous site has been used for extended periods or if large needles are placed in small veins. Clinical features include pain, redness, and tenderness at the infusion site. Intravenous lines should be replaced regularly, and the infusion site must be inspected frequently.

Acute Transfusion Reactions

Acute complications of blood components may be categorized into those that are not associated with preformed immune antibodies (immunoglobulins), and those where preformed antibodies are responsible for damaging transfused blood components. These are referred to as nonimmunologic and immunologic (antibody-mediated) transfusion complications, respectively (Table 8–15).

NONIMMUNE REACTIONS

Hemolytic. Destruction of donor red cells by the patient and the release of hemoglobin from inside of the erythrocytes (hemolysis) usually results from patients' preformed antibodies (see below). Occasionally bacteria may contaminate blood transfusions if strictly aseptic techniques are not followed during collection of the donated blood. Release of bacterial enzymes can cause hemolysis of red blood cells. Blood is a very favorable culture medium for these organisms, and therefore must be refrigerated and kept between 2 and 6°C. Organisms such as coliforms, pseudomonas, and others may grow even under these temperature conditions. Prior to release from the blood bank, blood is always inspected for visible hemolysis to screen against this complication. However, if infused into a patient, this may evoke the clinical features of an immediate hemolytic transfusion reaction with shock, fever, and the release of the bacterial endotoxins. In any fever associated with transfusions, this rare complication must be considered and the transfusion stopped. Once the specimen is submitted to the blood bank, routine Gram stains and cultures are performed on the posttransfusion specimen and bags returned to the blood bank.

Aggregates. Under conditions of storage, white cell and platelet debris and minimal amounts of fibrin may develop. If transfused into a patient, these may

Table 8–15. SPECIFIC COMPLICATIONS OF BLOOD COMPONENTS

Acute Transfusion Reactions	Delayed Transfusion Reactions
Nonimmune	Delayed nonimmune
Hemolytic (bacterial contamination)	Infection
Aggregates and pulmonary infiltrates	Iron overload
Metabolic	Delayed immune
	alloimmunization
Immune (antibody-mediated)	Delayed hemolytic
Non-hemolytic	Graft vs. host disease
Febrile	Posttransfusion purpura
Urticarial	
Anaphylactoid	
Leukocyte agglutinin reactions	
Acute hemolytic	
Incompatible transfusion	

occlude the microcirculation in the lungs and cause pulmonary distress. They are believed to be one of the causes of adult respiratory distress syndrome following massive blood replacement. A routine blood filter usually removes these aggregates so they are not transfused into the patient. Cellular components in particular must always be infused using a standard blood filter (150 μm). In situations of massive blood replacement, these filters may have to be changed after 3–4 units have been infused, to prevent cellular debris from entering the lungs and impeding pulmonary circulation.

Metabolic. Electrolyte and metabolic changes occur while blood is stored (see Table 8–9). Potassium leaks out of the erythrocytes, red cells continue to undergo anerobic metabolism, and the anticoagulant solutions may cause metabolic imbalances. This is called the "storage lesion" and refers to the changes occurring in blood during storage. Metabolic effects of transfusion include hyperkalemia, hypocalcemia, citrate toxicity, acidosis, hypernatremia, and hypothermia. The larger the amount of blood transfused, the more clinically significant these electrolyte problems may become (see Whole Blood).

ANTIBODY-MEDIATED ACUTE TRANSFUSION REACTIONS

Immune antibodies may be directed against the erythrocyte (hemolytic) or nonerythrocyte, cellular, and noncellular (nonhemolytic) components.

Acute Hemolytic Transfusion Reactions. These are the most serious, but fortunately one of the least common, transfusion reactions. They arise mostly because of major ABO incompatibilities due to clerical or administrative errors. When anti-A and anti-B destroy incompatible red cells, hemolysis occurs immediately, usually in the circulation itself. This is because the isohemagglutinins, anti-A and anti-B, are IgM antibodies that efficiently bind to A and/or B antigens on the erythrocytes and rapidly activate complement. Most other antibodies attach to the surface of transfused compatible cells, coating them for removal by the extravascular reticuloendothelial cells. Pretransfusion crossmatching reduces the danger of hemolysis; however, it is apparent that, no matter how accurate the pretransfusion testing is, if the wrong sample is tested or the wrong blood is administered to the patient, these severe hemolytic reactions may occur. No serologic subtleties are involved when group A blood is given to a group O patient. It is sheer carelessness. Occasionally, crossmatching fails to demonstrate very weak or atypical antibodies that later cause hemolysis, but hemolytic reactions on this basis are very uncommon.

Clinical Spectrum. Hemolytic transfusion reactions often begin with a rising temperature, shaking chills, and falling blood pressure. Other symptoms include palpitations, anxiety, substernal pain, flank pain, and warmth and tenderness at the site of infusion. These events are the result of widespread interaction between antibody and antigen. The major and severe clinical sequelae result from hypotension, disseminated intravascular coagulation, and renal failure. Damage is especially likely to occur if flow rates are low and the tubular urine is highly concentrated.

Most fatalities occur in the anesthetized patient, since the patient cannot complain about the immediate and distressing symptoms. This situation may be recognized only by a drop in blood pressure and the presence of diffuse bleeding from the surgical wounds.

Disseminated intravascular coagulation occurs as a result of the complement activation, with subsequent activation of the coagulation cascade and intravascular thrombin generation (see Chapter 6). Fibrinogen is converted to fibrin in the vascular system. Additionally, the fibrinolytic system is also activated and fibrin and fibrinogen breakdown occurs, also within the vascular system. Coagulation factors are consumed and a coagulopathy develops. Bleeding occurs because of consumption of normal coagulation factors, poor clot formation, and enhanced lysis of the weak clots. In addition, platelets may also be consumed and microangiopathic hemolytic anemia may develop as the red cells become scythed and chopped by the fibrin strands (see Chapter 3—MAHA [see Color Plate 14]).

Renal failure occurs as a result of occlusion of the renal tubules by antibody-coated red cell membranes and acute tubular necrosis (ATN). In addition, an early manifestation may be evidence of the release of hemoglobin from the damaged red cells *(intravascular hemolysis).* As the red cells are destroyed, hemoglobin is released into the plasma. Although a large protein, hemoglobin readily crosses the glomerular filter and hemoglobinuria commonly follows hemolysis. Free hemoglobin itself does not produce renal damage. Renal failure is a result of the combined effects of hypotension, massive antigen–antibody reaction, and intravascular coagulation. Antibody-coated erythrocyte membrane fragments produce occlusion of the renal tubules with oliguria, diminished glomerular filtration from the shock, and marked tubular dysfunction. Treatment is aimed at reestablishing renal blood flow and blood pressure control, forced diuresis to flush out the occluded renal tubules, and correction of the coagulation abnormalities. In view of critical blood volume problems, strict attention to fluid control is mandatory. To prevent post-hemolytic renal failure, blood pressure should be maintained and brisk diuresis established for the next several hours. This may involve the use of the osmostic diuretic mannitol or the loop diuretic furosemide (Lasix).

Some IgG antibodies can also produce acute hemolytic transfusion reactions (anti-Jk^a, Jk^b, anti-Duffy, Kell, etc.). *IgG-coated cells* are usually destroyed in the reticuloendothelial cell *(extravascular hemolysis)* and not in the circulation, with the exception of anti-Jk^a and Jk^b. Plasma hemoglobin levels rise only if cell destruction is so massive that it overloads the capacity of the reticuloendothelial system for hemoglobin disposal (see section on Hemolytic Anemia, Chapter 2). If extravascular destruction occurs gradually, the only sign that there has been a transfusion reaction may be a drop in hematocrit or failure to achieve the expected rise in hematocrit following the transfusion (see Delayed Hemolytic Reactions).

Laboratory Examination. At the first suspicion of a hemolytic transfusion reaction, the transfusion must be discontinued, but the intravenous line or catheter should be kept patent. Verification of the patient's name and blood type must be performed. *Mislabeling* and *misidentification* cause most transfusion disasters. Diagnosing this cause is easy enough; however, it may be more difficult to ascertain how and why the mistake occurred.

Laboratory investigation requires examination of the patient's posttransfusion blood. A sample of clotted blood must be sent to the laboratory, where the crossmatch and pretransfusion sample is verified. It is examined for the presence of free hemoglobin in the serum. The pretransfusion and posttransfusion samples are compared. The presence of antibody-coated cells is tested by the performance of the direct antiglobulin test (see The Direct Antiglobulin Test). If this result is positive, the blood bank will then verify the nature of the antibody coating the red cells. Absence of ABO incompatibility and negative test results make it unlikely that a hemolytic reaction has occurred. If the results are positive, further studies must be performed, including an administrative evaluation as to how the problem occurred.

ACUTE NONHEMOLYTIC REACTIONS

Febrile Reactions. A febrile reaction is defined as 1 °C or more rise in temperature during or immediately after the transfusion.

Certain patients, in particular persons who have received multiple transfusions and women who have had multiple pregnancies, may become immunized to blood proteins or other cells, including platelets and white cells. If these people are given blood transfusions, they may mount an immune attack against these transfused components that elicits fever and shaking chills and is termed a *febrile (nonhemolytic) reaction.* The clinical features are usually headaches, general malaise, and a rapid rise in temperature of less than 24 hours' duration. The shaking chills are often the most distressing symptom. More often these reactions are relatively mild. Since bacterial contamination and hemolytic reactions may mimic this milder cause of fever, the transfusion must be stopped and evaluated for these possibilities.

Most often, however, these reactions are caused by white cell antibodies and are unrelated to hemolysis. These antibodies can be specific for granulocyte antigens, or may react with HLA antigens common to nearly all tissues. It is not practical to attempt matching of the recipient against the donor's white cells. Simply, this type of reaction may be prevented by using microaggregate filters or newer leukocyte filters particularly for red blood cell components or the use of washed or deglycerolized red cells (see Concentrated Red Blood Cells, pp 283–284). Leukocyte removal from platelets is more complicated and requires centrifugation sufficient to concentrate the leukocytes yet maintain good numbers of platelets in the plasma. Microaggregate filtering cannot be used for this purpose since the filters will trap platelets as well, however, new third-generation leukocyte filters are now available for platelet concentrate. These filters allow passage of platelets yet restrict most of the leukocytes. Patients may require premedication with an antipyretic and/or hydrocortisone.

Urticaria. Itching, hives, and urticaria are also commonly seen in patients who have received multiple blood products (up to 3% of all transfusions). They occur as a result of allergies in the recipient to proteins in the donor blood. The mechanism is an immediate hypersensitivity to transfused blood proteins affected by IgE (histamine-releasing) antibodies. Therefore, this can often be premedicated or treated by means of antihistamines. In most instances, if the patient's vital signs are stable, the transfusion may simply be slowed and antihistamines administered. If the patient has a more severe reaction, including bronchospasm, the transfusion may have to be stopped. Stopping of a transfusion is a clinical decision. If patients have severe cutaneous reactions to blood components with hypotension, a more severe immunologic reaction must be suspected, such as an anaphylactoid reaction.

Anaphylactoid Reactions. Approximately 1 in 4,000 people have low or deficient IgA levels. These people may develop naturally occurring IgA antibodies. Deficiency of IgA is often associated clinically with recurrent infections of the body tracts, since this antibody is the prime humoral antibody lining body cavities. Recipients of blood products should always be questioned regarding recurrent respiratory or gastrointestinal infections or a history of hypogammaglobulinemia. These patients may also develop immune anti-IgA antibodies that avidly bind to IgA in transfused blood. Under these circumstances, an immune complex activation of complement cascade occurs and the patient manifests a severe anaphylaxis (see Immunology section). These patients must either receive blood that is deficient in IgA from rare donor registries or must receive blood that has been treated to remove plasma by extensive washing or following freezing and deglycerolization.

Delayed Consequences of Transfusions

These may be defined as any side effect of blood component administration occurring 24 hours or more following infusion. Again, this group may be classified according to whether they are antibody mediated or not. By far the commonest delayed effect of transfusion is infectious disease transmission. Immune antibodies may produce delayed effects, including delayed hemolytic reactions, graft vs. host disease, and posttransfusion purpura (see Table 8–15).

Delayed Hemolytic Reactions

These occur when an immune antibody previously undetectable in pretransfusion testing is reinduced by exposure to the same antigens in the transfused blood. The recipient has immune memory that, following exposure to the transfused cells containing the antigen, evokes an amplified immune response (anamnestic response). A delayed hemolytic reaction is diagnosed by failure to achieve a sustained increment in hemoglobin or hematocrit following the transfusion. Other effects of the hemolysis (which is usually extravascular) may occur, including the demonstration of the antibody by screening, coating of transfused red cells several days after the transfusion by the antibody (positive DAT), and elevated bilirubin, LDH, and even reversible renal failure. The antibodies mostly involved in this type of reaction include anti-Rh antibodies (c and E) and anti-Duffy and anti-Kidd. A recipient who has had such a reaction should be given the information. This should always be written down and carried with the person, and future transfusions must be negative for these specific antigens.

Graft vs. Host Disease

Graft vs. host disease is a rare complication that may occur in immunocompromised patients or following intrauterine transfusions. Transfused lymphocytes may attack the host (recipient) and cannot be rejected due to the immunoincompetence of the patient. The clinical manifestations of diarrhea and exfoliative dermatitis may occur. This is avoided by the use of irradiated blood (see Irradiated Blood Products).

Posttransfusion Purpura

Posttransfusion purpura is a rare delayed consequence of transfusion associated with a thrombocytopenia developing one week following transfusion. It is seen in persons who lack the platelet antigen PLA-1 and have anti–PLA-1 preformed antibodies. Exposure to PLA-1–positive platelets causes immune adherence of antibody/antigen complexes to their own platelets and subsequent sequestration and thrombocytopenia. These recipients must always receive PLA-1–negative blood components.

Transfusion Hemosiderosis

A unit of concentrated red blood cells contains 250 mg iron. Since the body stores of iron are only 500–1500 mg, six transfusions may saturate these stores. Once this occurs, iron is deposited in other parenchymal cells in various organs (e.g., liver, pancreas, skin, and heart). Iron overload syndromes occur particularly in persons who have received over 100 units of red cell transfusions. Individuals receiving so many transfusions include patients who are critically dependent on transfusion support for life (e.g., thalassemia, sickle cell anemia, myelofibrosis [see Iron Overload Syndromes, Chapter 2]). These patients usually die from cardiac failure due to iron deposition in the cardiac tissues. Iron overload from transfusions may be retarded by the use of iron chelation therapy.

Infectious Disease Transmission by Blood Components

Table 8–16 is a list of diseases transmitted by blood transfusion. Although in recent times AIDS has preoccupied concerns about transfusion-transmitted diseases, hepatitis transmission continues to be the most frequent serious infectious complication of transfusion therapy. Several viral diseases, however, can be transmitted by blood transfusion. Transfusion-transmitted viral infections have increased because of the use of pooled plasma components and also greater reliance on transfusion support for transplantation and treatment of cancer patients. Transfusion-

Table 8–16. INFECTIOUS DISEASES TRANSMITTED BY BLOOD TRANSFUSION

Viruses	
Cell-free (plasma) viruses	Hepatitis B virus
	Hepatitis A virus
	Non-A, non-B hepatitis (Hepatitis C virus)
Cell-associated viruses	HIV (human immunodeficiency virus)
	CMV (Cytomegalovirus)
	EBV (Epstein-Barr virus)
	Other retroviruses (HTLV-1, HTLV-2, etc.)
Spirochetes	*Treponema pallidum* (syphilis)
Protozoans	Malaria
	Babesia
	Chagas' disease (Trypanosomiasis)
Bacteria	

transmitted viruses usually have long incubation periods. Prevention of transfusion-transmitted infections is one of the main thrusts of modern blood banking and pretransfusion testing.

Human Immunodeficiency Virus (HIV, HTLV-III, LAV)

The transmission of the HIV virus by blood products to produce the acquired immunodeficiency syndrome (AIDS) is a worldwide concern. Recipients of blood products collected in the United States from 1978 to early 1985 are particularly at risk.

Since April 1985, blood components collected in the United States have been screened for the presence of antibody to the HIV. Donors are screened using a serologic test that detects the presence of anti-HIV using an enzyme-linked immunosorbent assay (ELISA) system. This test is very sensitive. The diagnosis of posttransfusion HIV is made by obtaining a positive test of the antibody to HIV in the recipient. Seroconversion is thought to occur 6–8 weeks following infection.

There are several tests for HIV antibody that measure IgG or total antibody. The ELISA is the most common test. The source of the antigen is inactivated virus that has been grown in a human lymphoid cell line but also contains other antigens in the cell line (HLA antigens). The ELISA antibody test is the initially performed test, and donors who are positive with this test are excluded from future donations. The test is usually performed in duplicate, and if one of the results is positive, an additional test is performed. If again positive, the donor is termed *repeatedly reactive* and the sample is sent to be confirmed by another test called the *Western blot* test. If the Western blot sample is negative, or if two of the three initial ELISA tests are negative, the test is considered to be a negative test. The confirmatory Western blot test utilizes the principle of immunoblotting and separation of the viral antigens so that specific antiviral antibodies can be identified. It is used to confirm all positive ELISA tests since the ELISA has a high false-positive rate. Approximately one in every thousand donors is positive (repeatedly reactive) initially, of which two in ten thousand is Western blot positive (confirmed positive) (see also p 545).

The method uses the electrophoretic separation of viral proteins and glycoproteins, followed by nitrocellulose blotting and fixation of the antibody. Patient sera are applied and incubated either with peroxidase-conjugated goat antihuman IgG followed by staining, or with radioimmunoprecipitation. Seropositivity is considered in the presence of a specific envelope protein for the virus termed gp-41 band, or gp-120 in its absence and in the presence of antibody to the viral core proteins p24 and p55. More sensitive and specific assays for both IgG and IgM antibody are now being developed using recombinant DNA protein methods.

Transfusion-transmitted HIV infection has effectively been eliminated from the blood supply by means of these testing methods. Donor education and specific predonation questions regarding high-risk groups are still used as additional safeguards. There is a theoretical possibility that a viremic, seronegative donor (window of seronegativity) who does not consider himself to be part of a high-risk group may donate a unit of blood that is eventually transfused. This occurrence is estimated as less than one in 100,000 transfusions. Pooled plasma products used in the treatment of hemophilia are now additionally heat treated, pasteurized, or refined by monoclonal antibody to prevent transfusion-transmitted HIV. These processes effectively remove the potential for viral transmission.

Hepatitis C Virus (HCV, Non-A, Non-B Hepatitis). This is currently the most common type of hepatitis today, with an incidence approaching 2% to 4% following a single-unit transfusion. The organism responsible for the transmission of non-A, non-B hepatitis has now been identified and is called Hepatitis C. Since there were no specific tests for this condition, certain surrogate tests had been used as a means of reducing the likelihood of transfusion-transmitted non-A, non-B hepatitis. The two main surrogate tests are the antibody to the hepatitis B core antigen (anti-HBc) and the liver enzyme alanine aminotransferase (ALT; serum glutamic-pyruvic transaminase [SGPT]), both of which reduced the likelihood of non-A, non-B hepatitis by 40%. The critical cutoff exclusion values for ALT at which donors should be excluded were not well established; therefore, donors may have been excluded who were otherwise perfectly healthy. The ALT levels may also be increased nonspecifically in obesity, following exercise, and with certain medications. The major clinical features of HCV hepatitis are subclinical, and jaundice is infrequent. Raised serum enzymes are typically fluctuant and may be missed. The major significance is the tendency to develop progressive liver disease. One of the major complications of HCV hepatitis is the development of chronic active hepatitis and, subsequently, postnecrotic cirrhosis. Formerly, a diagnosis of non-A, non-B hepatitis could only be made after serologic studies had excluded hepatitis A, B, CMV, EBV, and HIV. The introduction of the HCV antibody test has been a major breakthrough in infectious disease screening prior to blood transfusion and may reduce transfusion-transmitted hepatitis to less than 1%. Fifteen to twenty percent of the patients with non-A, non-B hepatitis may develop cirrhosis.

Hepatitis B Virus. Jaundice with raised enzymes occurring 6–12 weeks after transfusion is more commonly produced by hepatitis B transmission by blood products. Screening of blood donors for the presence of hepatitis B virus has effectively reduced this likelihood to less than 1:1000 transfusions. It may produce a spectrum of liver disease ranging from a fulminant hepatitis to a mild, subclinical infection. The incidence has greatly decreased since the abolition of paid donors and the institution of screening procedures for hepatitis B virus (see Hepatitis; Virology section, p 544).

Cytomegalovirus and Epstein-Barr Virus. These viruses reside within granulocytes and mononuclear cells and cause a viral illness with hepatitis. Individuals at risk for transfusion-transmitted CMV infections are persons who lack antibody to the cytomegalovirus (CMV seronegative) and who are immunocompromised, such as neonates and bone marrow transplant recipients. The use of CMV seronegative blood products is the most effective means of preventing this complication. Other methods have been the use of blood products that are depleted of white cells, including frozen deglycerolized blood. The prevalence and the likelihood of transfusion-transmitted CMV infection varies across geographic regions. It is still uncertain whether transfusion-transmitted CMV infections occurs because of reactivation of dormant virus in the transfused cells or the transfusion of active virus from the donor.

Hepatitis A Virus. Posttransfusion hepatitis A is a rare event. The incubation period is 28 days, which is shorter than both hepatitis C and hepatitis B.

HEMOLYTIC DISEASE OF THE NEWBORN

Definition and Pathophysiology

Hemolytic disease of the newborn (HDN), also termed erythroblastosis fetalis, is a syndrome of hemolytic anemia and jaundice occurring as a result of the destruction of antibody-coated (sensitized) erythrocytes in the infant. In this syndrome, the mother develops immune (IgG) antibodies from a transplacental hemorrhage (TPH) of incompatible fetal cells. These antibodies are harmless to the maternal cells, but cross the placenta into the fetal circulation and attack antigens present on the fetal erythrocytes. Depending on the severity of red cell destruction in the fetus or newborn, a spectrum of disease ranging from hydrops fetalis (fetal congestive cardiac failure) to a milder jaundice in the newborn period may develop.

When any fetal blood group factor inherited from the father is not possessed by the mother, there is the possibility of a maternal alloimmune reaction. Depending on the degree of antigenicity involved, this transplacental passage may lead to HDN. Blood group incompatibility for the Rhesus D antigen was formerly the major cause of HDN. The overall incidence of HDN due to anti-Rh_0 (D) has dramatically changed, and deaths from Rh-HDN are now uncommon. There has been, concommitant with this decrease, a relative rise in the frequency of mothers with other antibodies to Rhesus antigens and to antigens of the non-Rhesus systems. The immunologic conditions for ABO HDN occur most commonly, and group A or B infants born to group O mothers often have maternal IgG antibody on their cells. However, ABO HDN is rarely serious, although infants may have mild disease.

PATHOPHYSIOLOGY OF HDN

Immunization. All pregnancies are associated with the passage of some fetal blood cells into the mother. This is particularly evident at 28 weeks, and occurs more especially at birth. This passage is termed *transplacental hemorrhage* (TPH) and may especially be seen to occur with antenatal procedures such as amniocentesis (sampling the amniotic fluid of the fetus), or manually changing the position of the baby from a breech position. Transplacental hemorrhage may also occur with spontaneous or induced abortions. Fetal cells comprise surface antigens from both parents. If the mother lacks erythrocyte antigens possessed by the father and transferred to the fetus, and if TPH occurs, the mother is likely to become immunized to these cells. The mother then develops, initially, IgM antibodies, and subsequently IgG antibodies to these foreign antigens. Since IgG antibodies are capable of being transported across the placenta, if the antibodies are directed to erythrocyte antigens on the fetal cells, they may undergo immune adherence to the erythrocytes of the fetus. These cells are now coated with antibody (opsonized), and are then capable of being removed by the reticuloendothelial system of the fetus, where they are destroyed. Extravascular hemolysis then occurs. There are two main effects:

1. As the increased numbers of red cells are destroyed, hemoglobin is liberated and undergoes conversion to bilirubin and other bile pigments that diffuse across the placenta back into the mother's circulation. The mother's liver readily conjugates and excretes the fetal bilirubin. Some bile pigments leak back into the amniotic fluid and are not directly excreted. Sampling of the amniotic fluid may therefore give an index of the severity of hemolysis.

2. If the fetal bone marrow cannot compensate for the shortened red cell survival, progressive anemia develops. As the hemoglobin drops, tissue oxygenation declines and a severely anemic fetus may go into congestive heart failure and develop systemic edema. The fetus with severe HDN may die of congestive cardiac failure around the time of delivery. This disorder is called *hydrops fetalis,* which emphasizes the edematous appearance of these stillborn infants. The fetal bone marrow responds to the hemolytic process by increasing red cell production in an attempt to maintain adequate erythrocyte levels and avoid anemia. The marked increased in erythropoiesis causes many immature nucleated red cells to circulate prematurely. Erythroblasts may then be seen in the fetus' circulation and sometimes the term *erythroblastosis fetalis* is used to describe this situation.

Rh Hemolytic Disease of the Newborn

In Rh-HDN, the development of anti-D antibodies by the mother occurs following exposure to the Rh-positive (D cells) of the fetus. Pregnancy and childbirth are the immunizing events, since Rh-positive blood almost never is given to an Rh-negative woman of childbearing age. In regard to other antibody specificities, either transfusion or prior pregnancies may be the immunizing stimuli. Rh hemolytic disease of the newborn (Rh-HDN) was formerly the most common cause of HDN, and at one time was responsible for close to 50% of all perinatal deaths. In Rh-HDN, laboratory testing for the detection of such antibodies is used to determine the clinical strategy: intrauterine transfusion, premature delivery, or term delivery. Exchange transfusions may be needed after birth, as determined by the bilirubin and/or degree of anemia.

Anti-D, in practical terms, is the only antibody for which HDN is severe and creates serious risk to the fetus. When anti-D is present, it is important to perform all available procedures to evaluate the fetus' condition. Titering the antibody may be useful in indicating the timing for amniocentesis, to assess fetal risk, and to determine a strategy for management during pregnancy.

Prevention of Rh Hemolytic Disease of the Newborn

One of the major accomplishments of the last 25 years has been the almost total conquest of Rh-HDN. This success has occurred because of recognition of the Rhesus-D antigen in the pathogenesis of the disease, and widespread use of passive antenatal and postnatal anti-Rh IgG immunotherapy.

All Rh_o(D)-negative mothers who are nonimmunized (negative irregular antibody screen), who are pregnant, or who have any procedure associated with an increased likelihood of transplacental bleeding should receive RhIg prophylaxis. If the blood group of the father is known to be Rh_o(D)-negative, RhIg immunoprophylaxis can be avoided. The appreciation that antenatal TPH can occur has prompted the administration of RhIg at 28 weeks of pregnancy in women who are unimmunized. This has allowed a reduction in the incidence of Rh sensitization in pregnancy from 1.8% (the level associated with only postpartum RhIg therapy) to less than 0.07% of all Rh-negative women. Administration of antenatal RhIg is not associated with any significant adverse clinical effects on the infants. Infants may, however, have weakly positive direct antiglobulin tests. More transplacental bleeding occurs during delivery, and is sufficiently covered by routine administration of postpartum RhIg. The usual dose of 300 μg is sufficient to cover a 15 ml TPH of fetal erythrocytes. Usually less than 1 ml of fetal erythrocytes cross the placenta during delivery, and even less during pregnancy. However, occasionally a large TPH may occur. This can be detected by the *rosette screening test,* and then quantitated by the *acid-resistant hemoglobin test (Kleihauer-Betke test).*

Diagnosis of Transplacental Hemorrhage

Rosette Test. This test uses the principle that if fetal D-positive cells cross the placenta into the maternal circulation, a sample of blood taken from a D-negative mother will have a minor population of D-positive cells. If reagent anti-D is added to the blood specimen, coating of the D-positive cells occurs and microscopic agglutination may be seen. To amplify the test, further reagent D-positive cells are then added and appear as a rosette of agglutinated cells when examined microscopically. The finding of rosettes is evidence that a transplacental hemorrhage of D-positive cells has occurred. This test is a qualitative test, and does not quantitate the amount of TPH.

Acid-Resistant Hemoglobin Test for Fetal Hemoglobin (Kleihauer-Betke Test). This test uses the principle that fetal hemoglobin is more resistant to acid pH than adult hemoglobin. If a sample of blood is taken from a mother who has had a transplacental hemorrhage, a small population of fetal cells will be present in her circulation. If this blood is placed in an acidic solution and a stained blood smear is made, fetal cells will show preservation of hemoglobin staining, whereas adult cells will appear as ghosts. The relative percentage of *stained to unstained cells* is determined. This ratio is multiplied by the correction factor for maternal blood volume, then the amount of fetomaternal hemorrhage (FMH) in milliliters is quantitated. This test is used to evaluate a large TPH, and to accurately calculate the dosage of RhIg needed.

It is imperative that every immunized Rh_0(D) woman is identified and given Rh immune prophylaxis. At the initial visit to the obstetrician, an ABO and Rh type and the presence or absence of irregular antibodies must be determined. Rh immune prophylaxis is then given at 28 weeks and again at delivery. At the time of delivery, if the infant is Rh positive, a rosette test for the detection of TPH should be performed. If the test is negative, routine administration of RhIg should be given. If the test is positive, the degree of FMH is quantitated by means of the acid-resistant fetal hemoglobin test. Other tests such as the enzyme-linked antiglobulin test also are being used in some centers.

Laboratory Management of the Immunized Rh-Negative Pregnancy

Irregular Antibody Screen. Immunization, as detected by a *positive irregular antibody screen,* with the identification of the anti-D antibody, represents a challenge of management of a high-risk pregnancy. For all practical purposes, other antibodies are not generally associated with intrauterine death, and consequently do not need the degree of laboratory management or monitoring that is needed in women who have Rh sensitization. Once an anti-D is identified, the *antibody titer* needs to be evaluated. The titration is performed by consecutively diluting the antibody and letting it react with the known antigen-positive cells. The titer represents the lowest dilution with which reactivity occurs. Titer is important in this situation, since it determines the need for fetal amniotic fluid sampling.

Amniotic Fluid Analysis. Amniotic fluid is usually straw colored and is the fluid in which the fetus is suspended *in utero.* Analysis of the amniotic fluid for bilirubin concentration can give an indication of the degree of HDN. A specific test called the delta OD 450 is usually performed in this situation. This represents the optical density difference at the wavelength of light at which bilirubin exhibits maximal light absorption. This difference quantitates to the degree of bilirubin concentration. When this value is plotted on a graph and related to gestational age, a strategy of management can be appreciated. Three zones are identified (Fig. 8–4), called the low, moderate, and severe risk zones. A value in the severe risk zone means that fetal death is imminent. These values can be used to determine whether intrauterine transfusions or premature delivery or term delivery is appropriate. In addition, analysis of the amniotic fluid can provide information on the fetal lung maturity. Measurement of the phospholipids *lecithin and sphingomyelin (L:S) ratio* gives an accurate reflection of fetal lung maturation that can determine a strategy for premature delivery or intrauterine transfusion (see Chapter 17).

Intrauterine Transfusions. Intrauterine transfusions are the mainstay of therapy for infants who are too premature to deliver and who have severe erythroblastosis fetalis. Blood used for this procedure is usually packed Group O Rh_o(D)-negative blood that is irradiated. The blood is irradiated to prevent the rare complication of graft vs. host disease, since these ill premature infants have an immature immune system (see Irradiated Blood Products). Intrauterine transfusions can be given either through the intraperitoneal route or by percutaneous intraumbilical exchange transfusion (PUBS). All these procedures are performed under direct ultrasound guidance.

The major questions that the laboratory can answer in the management of Rh sensitization are:

1. Does the pregnant woman have an antibody capable of producing HDN?
2. What is the likelihood that an intrauterine transfusion is needed?
3. What is the likelihood that premature delivery may be indicated?
4. What is the likelihood that exchange transfusions might be needed after birth?

LABORATORY MANAGEMENT OF THE NEONATE WITH HDN

General Laboratory Testing. At delivery, the infant severs connections with

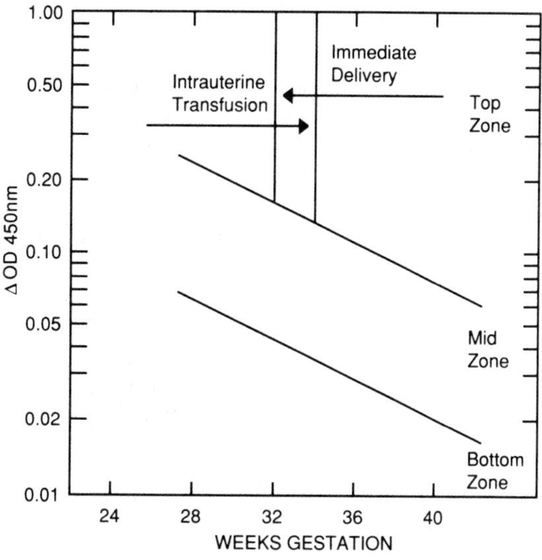

Figure 8–4. Liley graph for collecting data from amniotic fluid studies. Intrauterine transfusion should be done if the OD value is in the top zone prior to 32 weeks' gestation. After 34 weeks, top zone values indicate immediate delivery. Either intrauterine transfusion or immediate delivery may be indicated for top zone OD between 32 and 34 weeks, depending on studies of fetal maturity. (From AABB Technical Manual,[18] p 485, with permission.)

the mother's circulation and becomes an independent individual. This removes the source of incoming antibody but deprives the infant of an important route for bilirubin disposal. Anemia may also be a significant clinical problem in these infants. Since the infant's antibody-coated cells continue to be destroyed, excessive amounts of bilirubin continue to be produced. Before it can be excreted by the liver, bilirubin must be *conjugated* within the liver cells by the addition of glucuronic acid (see Chapter 12). *Unconjugated bilirubin* is soluble only in fat solvents and not in aqueous solution. Conjugation requires an enzyme, glucuronyl transferase, which develops slowly as the liver matures. Premature infants have a less efficient liver capacity and have very little enzyme; full-term infants, only a limited amount of enzyme. When excessive quantities of bilirubin are produced, the infant's liver cannot conjugate it rapidly enough to excrete it. The result is that unconjugated bilirubin accumulates in the infant's bloodstream.

Unconjugated bilirubin is highly lipid soluble and tends to be deposited in cells of the developing nervous system. The mature nervous system is not damaged by unconjugated bilirubin, but the infant's neurons can undergo severe, permanent damage. *Kernicterus* is the name given to localized bilirubin deposits in the brain. In severe untreated HDN, accumulation of bilirubin may deposit widely throughout the brain tissue, leading to permanent damage and even death. The immediate goal for treating an increasing bilirubin from HDN is to remove the source of bilirubin (i.e., antibody-coated red cells) and subsequently to remove excessive accumulation of unconjugated bilirubin.

Exchange Transfusion. Exchange transfusion refers to the replacement of most or all of the neonate's erythrocytes and plasma with compatible erythrocytes and plasma (or plasma components) from donor sources. Listed in Table 8–17 are the *indications for exchange transfusions.* The procedure of exchange transfusion is accomplished usually through the umbilical vein, and replaces the infant's blood volume with 85–100 ml/kg of whole blood. Aliquots of 15 ml of blood are removed and infused successively until the total volume is exchanged. It is critically important that the clinical and laboratory parameters are monitored during this procedure. These include fluid volume infused and removed, serum, electrolytes, hemoglobin, and bilirubin levels. Usually Group O Rh_0(D)-negative blood is used and is irradiated if the infant has received an intrauterine exchange transfusion. The blood must be compatible with both the infant and the maternal serum. Blood should be as fresh as possible, and preferably less than five days old (maximum, seven days). Potassium values should be determined in the blood used for exchange, and if higher than normal, the red cells should be washed and reconstituted with fresh frozen plasma. When performed by experienced personnel, complications are infrequent, usually less than 1%.

Table 8–17. EXCHANGE TRANSFUSION INDICATIONS

Hemolytic disease of the newborn
Rh hemolytic disease
ABO hemolytic disease
Other antibodies
Hyperbilirubinemia
Respiratory distress syndrome
Neonatal sepsis
Disseminated intravascular coagulation
Miscellaneous

Hemolytic Disease of the Newborn Due to Other Maternal Antibodies

The commonest cause of mild HDN is anti-A or anti-B. The reasons for this are that most anti-A and anti-B antibodies are IgM class and therefore incapable of crossing the placenta; however, Group O individuals often may have anti-A or anti-B antibodies of the IgG class as well. Why these IgG antibodies occur in some Group O people and not in others is unknown. Neither pregnancy nor blood transfusion is needed as an immunizing event. It is also unclear why Group A people do not have IgG anti-B and vice versa. A fetus whose erythrocytes are Group A, B, or AB, and whose mother is Group O with IgG anti-A or B antibodies, may suffer red cell hemolysis. However, in view of the relatively low likelihood of severe HDN in these patients, neither immune prophylaxis nor antibody titering and screening is warranted unless determined by a previously severe obstetrical history.

Many other immune antibodies have been implicated in HDN, some causing severe disease in the infant; more recently, because of the declining incidence of Rh HDN, these antibodies are relatively more important. Anti-c, anti-E, and anti-K are next most frequent. Evaluation for ABO HDN is appropriately made after delivery when an infant manifests symptoms of clinical jaundice. Laboratory testing entails establishing neonatal–maternal incompatibility. The presence of anti-A, anti-B, or other antibodies in the serum or in red cell eluates from cord blood samples is considered diagnostic. It is extremely unlikely that intrauterine transfusions or premature delivery will be needed for antibodies other than anti-D.

Routine Antenatal Laboratory Testing

Antibody screening tests in the early or middle part of pregnancy detect antibodies likely to cause HDN, but does not identify IgG, anti-A, or anti-B in Group O women. Any woman whose earlier pregnancies were affected by HDN must be carefully observed in subsequent pregnancies. For each specific antibody capable of inducing hemolytic disease of the newborn, a critical titer can be developed at each hospital. This represents the value of the diluted serum above which no cases of hemolytic disease of the newborn have occurred. For example, a titer of 1:32 of anti-D will react with D-positive cells when diluted 32 times. Maternal titers have some correlation with severity of disease in the infant; however, this is not consistent.

HLA ANTIGENS AND ANTIBODIES

The HLA antigens, which historically are derived from human leukocyte antigens, are a complex system of polymorphic antigens comprising at least five groups and three classes. This antigenic system is important because it relates to histocompatibility (tissue compatibility for transplantation) and immune responsiveness (see also Chapter 7). Specific genetic material located on the short arm of chromosome 6 is inherited from each parent and is expressed as an HLA haplotype. The five different antigens belonging to the HLA system are closely linked in this region, which also contains genes for several enzymes and serum proteins, including components of complement. Because of its complexity, the term "locus" is inappropriate for this chromosomal segment; it is usually described as the HLA region or major histocompatibility complex (MHC). The five different series of antigens constituting the HLA system are designated A, B, C, D, and DR (Fig. 8–5). There are 23 distinct antigens in the A group, at least 49 in the B, 8 in C, and 19 in D, as well as 16 in DR (1984 workshop). Each chromosome includes genes that define a single antigen in each of the five groups; the assortment of HLA genes present on a single chromosome and transmitted as a single unit is called *haplotype.* Since every cell except the erythrocyte possesses two examples of chromosome 6, each person has two haplotypes, one from each parent. Within a single sibship (family of siblings), there can be only two maternal haplotypes and two paternal haplotypes, making a maximum of four different *genotypes* that the offspring can possess. The variety of haplotypes in the general population, however, is extremely variable and very diverse.

The HLA antigens consist of two main classes and a lesser third class. *Class I-HLA* antigens consist of the A, B, and C antigens, which are present on the surface membranes of virtually all cells except mature red blood cells. The D and DR antigens seem to reside only on B-lymphocytes and macrophages. They are called *class II antigens.* The class I antigens consist of two chains—an alpha chain, which is glycosylated and subdivided into three regions termed alpha-1, alpha-2, and alpha-3, and a beta chain, which consists of the beta-2 microglobulin (a plasma globulin). The alpha chain is a transmembrane chain, whereas the $beta_2$ microglobulin is situated on the cell surface. The alpha-3 portion of the alpha chain seems to have a close homology with the F_c portion of the immunoglobulin G. There is obviously, therefore, a very close and as yet ill-defined relationship between these class I antigens and the immune response or synthesis of specific antibodies.

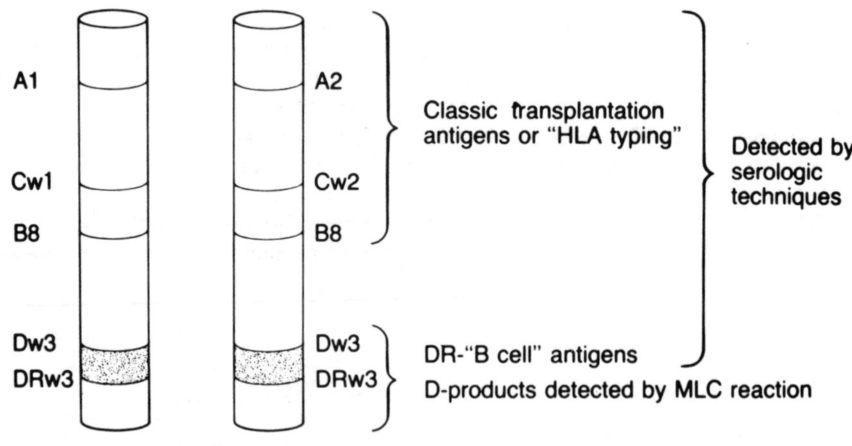

Figure 8–5. Schematic representation of the HLA Loci on the short arm of chromosome 6. (From Miller and Rodey,[11] with permission.)

The *class II antigens* consist of an alpha chain and a beta chain, both of which are transmembrane and are divided up into two sections termed alpha-1 and alpha-2 and beta-1 and beta-2. These antigens are on the surface of all B-lymphocytes, and their role is as yet uncertain. The class II antigens have a close homology with some of the serum complement components. There is, therefore, a complex interrelationship between the immunoglobulins, the surface antigens on these reactive cells, and complement. It is therefore not surprising that these antigens are involved in tissue rejection or recognition of foreign tissue, and are therefore important in transplantation biology. Haplo-identical grafts, in particular bone marrow transplants, have a much lower likelihood of graft rejection or graft vs. host disease (a syndrome in which cells from the grafted tissue attack the recipient host's tissue). The D antigens and DR antigens appear to be very important in this regard.

HLA Testing

Human leukocyte antigen typing is much more complicated than testing for red cell antigens. Most reagent antibodies come from persons immunized through transfusions or pregnancies; however, monoclonal antibody methodology is supplying specific commercial monoclonal antibodies to define specific HLA types. The number of antigens that must be studied on each lymphocyte is greater than that for red cells, and different examples of single antigens exhibit different levels of reactivity. Each cell sample must be examined against a battery of antisera so all relevant antigens are excluded. The overall reactivity determines antigenic interpretation, not just the results of one or a few individual reactions.

Human leukocyte antigen testing usually uses agglutination or cytotoxicity as endpoints. Agglutination procedures are easier, but less sensitive, less specific, and more susceptible to false-positive results. The class I antigens are identified by their reactivity with specific antibodies, and cytotoxicity is the usual endpoint for these serologic tests. Cytotoxicity testing uses complement-binding antibodies that are allowed to attach to the cells during incubation in a complement-free system. Adding active complement to the surface-bound antibody initiates complement fixation that causes lethal damage to the cell. Cell death is most easily demonstrated by adding a macromolecular dye to the medium. Viable cells are able to exclude the large dye molecules. Because a dead cell loses this barrier function, the dye enters and stains the entire dead cell. As the reaction between antibody and cell-surface antigen increases in strength and specificity, the number of stained cells in the suspension increases. This permits a degree of qualitative comparison between serum samples that contain different combinations of antibodies. An example of such a technique is the "trypan blue dye exclusion technique."

The HLA-radiolabeled D antigens are identified by DNA synthesis as determined by the incorporation of the pyrimidine base thymidine, following reactivity of lymphocytes from the recipient and the donor. Radioactive thymidine incorporation is determined by measuring the counts of radioactivity per minute, with the higher values being indicative of mismatches. The corollary is when unknown lymphocytes are reacted with known lymphocytes and low reactivity is determined, the HLA-D type can be inferred. The HLA-D locus antigens are very complex and include other serotypes, including HLA-DR, DP, and DQ. The functions of these antigen systems are as yet unknown. They do, however, allow closer tissue typing and presumably better transplantation-graft matches. Type I antigens, in particular, HLA-A and HLA-B, as well as type II (DR), are generally easily measured and available in many laboratories. Mixed lymphocyte testing for HLA-D antigens is not readily available in most laboratories, neither are antibodies for detection of the C antigens. Any one individual can have no more than two A antigens and two B antigens, coded for on chromosome 6. If it is possible to determine or to infer which pairs are transmitted together, the results are given as two haplotypes; for example, A2B8-A1B5. If there is not enough information to permit these conclusions, the results are expressed in general terms, as, for example, A1A2, B5B8.

INTERPRETATION

Human leukocyte antigen phenotype is the notation of the surface markers detected in histocompatibility testing of a single individual. The HLA genotype represents a precise determination of the antigens represented by the MHC genetic DNA on chromosome 6, determined by family studies. The term haplotype refers to an antigenic makeup of a single chromosome, 6 MCH complex (Fig. 8–6).

Linkage Disequilibrium and Antigen Distribution

Certain combinations of HLA antigens are more common than others. Some antigens are far more common or far rarer in one population or race than in others, and some combinations of antigens have strikingly high prevalence in specific populations.

The most common HLA-B antigens in American whites, for example, are B7, B8, and B12, with frequencies of 0.23, 0.20, and 0.24, respectively. In American blacks, the most common of the B series are Bw17 (0.26), Bw35 (0.32), and a specificity characterized as 1AG (0.34). This contrasts with African blacks, whose most common B antigens are B7 (0.18), Bw17 (0.33), and 1AG (0.31).

In American whites, association often exists between HLA-A1 and B8, A3, and B7, and Aw25 and B18. American blacks also have frequent associations of A1 and B8; but in African blacks, Aw30 and Bw42 are also frequent. This genetic characteristic of the MHC, where two alleles of different loci are co-associated with a higher frequency than the predicted frequencies, is called *linkage disequilibrium.* Linkage disequilibrium can extend to more than two loci; for example, HLA-A1-B8-DR3. The occurrence of these genetic frequencies, therefore, is greater than that which might be expected with random frequency expression.

Adding further to the complexity is the observation that locus recombination can occur with a possible frequency of 1%. When crossing over occurs, the C, B, and D loci remain together but separate themselves from the A locus. The portion of the region responsible for extent and intensity of immune responsiveness lies between B and D, most closely linked to D (see Fig. 8–6).

Clinical Applications of HLA Testing

There are four main areas of clinical medicine where HLA testing is important: 1) organ transplantation, 2) transfusion medicine, 3) disease associations, and 4) paternity testing and parentage assignment.

ORGAN TRANSPLANTATION

Human leukocyte antigen typing is only one aspect of donor selection for organ transplantation. Donor's ABO group should be compatible with that of the recipi-

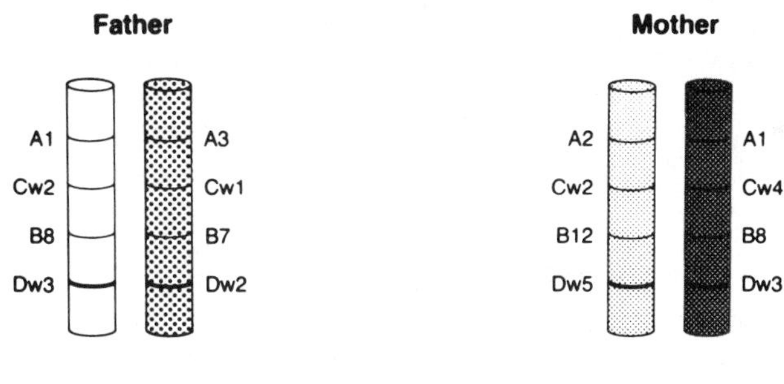

Figure 8–6. Human leukocyte antigen alleles on the same chromosome are called a haplotype. Haplotypes segregate together during meiosis; only 4 haplotypes may result from a mating. (From Miller and Rodey,[11] with permission.)

ent, and the recipient should be free from serum antibodies that react *in vitro* with the prospective donor's red or white cells. If there is sufficient time, and viable cells are available from prospective donor and recipient, mixed lymphocyte cultures (MLC) are useful in ruling out cell-mediated sensitization between donor and recipient. Transplantation workers are uncertain whether simple matching of HLA-A and HLA-B antigens is important when donor and recipient are unrelated.

When donor and recipient are blood relatives, HLA matching improves the chances of graft survival. Monozygotic (identical) twins, of course, share not only HLA antigens but all their genetic material. Nontwin siblings have only a limited genetic pool from which to receive phenotypic profiles. The more alike the tissues are with regard to HLA matching, the better the graft is likely to survive. In siblings, 2-haplotype matches give better results than 1-haplotype matches, all other things being equal. One-haplotype matches are better than complete HLA disparity. If no siblings are available with 2-haplotype or 1-haplotype, the patient's parents or children should be considered as potential donors. With parents and offspring, 1-haplotype matches necessarily must be identical; the other, of course, will generally be completely different.

When donor and recipient are unrelated, HLA matching provides much less predictive information. Graft survival is not much improved by using tissue from donors who share one or several A and B antigens with the recipient. However, in patients with preformed HLA antibodies, it is important to use tissue negative for the relevant antigen in selecting the donor.

The enormous polymorphism of the HLA system has many important implications in marrow transplantation. For about one in ten transplants, a parent is homozygous for a specific haplotype, and the phenotypic identity should always be confirmed by family segregation studies. In unrelated donor–recipient transplants, it must be appreciated that mutants or variants can exist that cannot be detected by serology, but detected only by cellular techniques. In this regard, 10% of individuals who are HLA-A2 (not red cell group A2) seropositive carry one out of four different HLA-A2 variants that can only be recognized by cellular techniques. A lack of appreciation of these potential mismatches can lead to severe graft vs. host reactions. There is also the existence of splits or subgroups of different HLA alleles. Each HLA molecule may carry an unknown number of different epitopes.

The evaluation of recipient serum for antibodies to donor leukocytes is important prior to transplantation and transfusion, since evidence indicates that presensitization to HLA antigens may cause rapid rejection of transplanted tissues. In a family, there is a one in four chance that two haplotypes segregate in the same way, and therefore a one in four probability that two siblings will have identical HLA haplotypes. Similarly, there is also a one in four probability that no haplotype will be shared between two siblings. It is apparent that a parent and a child can share only one haplotype, since the child must have received the other haplotype from the other parent. Therefore, it is a remote possibility that an identical match will occur between a child and a parent. Similarly, other parental relatives are unlikely to have identical haplotypes with any given child.

Bone marrow transplantation is used to treat patients with severe aplastic anemia, various types of leukemia, and immunodeficiency syndromes, and is being more widely used in salvage management of various types of lymphomas and other cancers. Two major problems that occur that are referable to HLA incompatibility are *graft rejection* and *graft vs. host disease.* In the former, foreign identity of the HLA types is recognized by the host, who rejects the graft. This is more of a problem in solid organ transplantation than in bone marrow transplantation. The reason is that bone marrow recipients are conditioned by intensive radiation therapy and chemotherapy to ablate their immune systems. This creates another problem in situations where histocompatibility is not optimal, namely *graft vs. host disease.* In this situation, the viable transplanted cells attack the host's cells by virtue of incompatibility between antigens. Graft vs. host disease produces a severe immune attack against particularly rapidly dividing cell populations, namely the gastrointestinal tract, skin, and bone marrow. There is a much lower incidence of both graft rejection and graft vs. host disease in HLA-identical transplants. Rejection of marrow is unlikely if the patient is identical for HLA-A, B, C, D, and DR determinants, as well as low reactivity with the mixed lymphocyte reaction (MLR). ABO compatibility is also important, since ABO-incompatible marrow transplants may require more blood component support and have delayed engraftment.

In renal transplantation, it appears that those donors who are well matched for HLA-B and DR alleles are associated with better graft survival. The HLA-B alleles are highly associated in linkage disequilibrium with DR alleles. Careful matching for HLA-B and DR alleles can provide a much greater likelihood of renal transplant survival.

TRANSFUSIONS

Blood transfusions are a common cause of alloimmunization to HLA antigens, since even concentrated red cell transfusions contain many contaminating platelets, granulocytes, and lymphocytes. Leukocyte-depleted blood (buffy coat poor, washed, and frozen deglycerolized red cells) contain far fewer leukocytes, and are therefore less likely to produce alloimmunization. Platelet concentrates, however, are highly immunogenic. Immunocompetent recipients of multiple platelet transfusions frequently develop antibodies to either HLA antigens, or specific platelet antigens, or both. Once antibodies develop, platelets that contain the relevant antigens are rapidly destroyed. Granulocyte transfusions that are used occasionally in the treatment of neonatal sepsis are also highly immunogenic.

Intensive chemotherapy for malignant disease and in preparation for bone marrow transplantation has caused a massive increase in the usage of platelet transfusions. The majority of these patients require multiple platelet transfusions to prevent and treat thrombocytopenic bleeding. These patients may be exposed to many different donors with many HLA phenotypes; therefore, alloimmunization is frequent. The clinical effect, of course, is that there is a marginal or no response to platelet transfusions, and methods are suggested to reduce the degree of alloimmunization. One such method is platelet crossmatching (see Blood Component Therapy). This is a technically difficult procedure, and is not routinely used in most laboratories. Matching for HLA antigens between the platelet donor and the recipient is used in individuals who are alloimmunized and who fail to get appropriate responses to platelet transfusions. Clearly, this limits the number of donors available, and although HLA-matched platelets are the most desirable product, they are logistically extremely difficult to obtain. Much current practice is aimed at reducing the number of donors to whom the patient is exposed, in an attempt to reduce alloimmunization. Similarly, depleting blood of contaminating leukocytes may also facilitate a reduction of alloimmunization. A complicating factor is that non-HLA platelet-derived antigens are not well understood. They may also be contributing to the degree of sensitization and lack of platelet response. It does appear, however, that platelets are less immunogenic if one or several HLA antigens are common to donor and recipient. When blood relatives are available as donors, complete HLA matching may be possible. In this case, reduction of donor exposure may allow decreased immunogenicity and sensitization. Even the use of unrelated donors with matching antigens is often better than completely random transfusion. Practical considerations do, however, complicate this provision. Technology and reagents exist for typing platelet donors, but the process is expensive and demanding on reagents needed and time consumed.

Antibody development becomes obvious when a patient no longer shows hemostatic improvement, or there is a reduced increment in the platelet count after platelet transfusion. At that point, the antibody must be identified and compatible donors found if further transfusions are to be effective. Screening for HLA antibodies and definition of HLA phenotypes is the most appropriate next step.

The kinds of white cell antibodies that cause febrile transfusion reactions are not necessarily the same as those that destroy platelets. If a patient who repeatedly has febrile reactions is given platelet transfusions, the posttransfusion platelet response should be observed carefully. If platelet survival and therapeutic benefit are poor, the antibody must be identified and compatible platelets given.

HLA and Disease Association

Determining associations between diseases and HLA antigens is difficult because there is such a variety of phenotypes and varied disease presentations. Two major approaches are possible: 1) to compare the frequency of a specific antigen in a group of unrelated patients exhibiting the disease with the antigen frequency of a control population (of the more than 80 HLA specificities, only approximately 20 are associated with diseases), and 2) to study families with known haplotypes to see if a particular disease reliably occurs in individuals with a particular haplotype. In this way genetic factors coded within or near HLA complex antigens may be evaluated to confer susceptibility to the development of the disease. This susceptibility may be related to altered immunologic responsiveness.

The best association between disease and HLA involves rheumatologic disorders and the antigen HLA-B27. *Ankylosing spondylitis,* a clearly defined subcategory of arthritis, is very closely tied to HLA-B27. This antigen occurs only in populations native to the northern hemisphere. Worldwide, more than 90% of patients with ankylosing spondylitis are positive for B-27, compared with 2.8% of control populations. Ankylosing spondylitis is virtually nonexistent in populations that lack B27. In populations possessing the antigen, the relative risk that a person having the antigen will also have the disease ranges from 49 in American blacks to more than 300 in Japan. Other arthritic syndromes, notably Reiter's syndrome (urethritis, arthritis, and conjunctivitis), juvenile rheumatoid arthritis, and arthritic complications of psoriasis, show positivity with HLA-B27, in descending order.

Associations have emerged between diseases of possible autoimmune etiology and antigens at the B and D loci. Myasthenia gravis, Addison's disease, and chronic active hepatitis are modestly associated Dw3, and Sjogren's syndrome has a fairly strong association with this allele. Insulin-dependent diabetes mellitus has been linked with B8 and Bw15, and with Dw3 and Dw4. The nature of these associations suggests that one or two diabetogenic genes resides somewhere around or between the B and D loci, but their effect does not become apparent unless external influences also coincide.

Research is continuing in the associations of HLA typing and disease, and in particular in the understanding of the pathogenesis and immune relationships.

PATERNITY TESTING/PARENTAGE ASSIGNMENT

Human leukocyte antigen typing is well suited for parentage studies because the antigens are fully developed at birth, they are transmitted in simple codominant mendelian fashion, and great phenotypic diversity exists among unrelated individuals. Used in conjunction with red cell phenotyping, and even independently, HLA testing provides a precise means of parentage exclusion as well as probability inclusion. If the HLA phenotypes of a child and the parent are known, it becomes possible to assess fairly accurately whether or not a given individual is the other parent. Up to 75% of falsely accused men have been excluded from paternity with HLA testing alone, in jurisdictions that allow HLA testing results as evidence. Strong (but by no means absolute) statistical support also can be presented that a given man *is* the father if the haplotype matches that of the putative father. This is especially true if the haplotype is uncommon in the population under study.

REFERENCES

1. Boral, LI and Henry, JB: The type and screen: A safe alternative and supplement in selected surgical procedures. Transfusion 17:163, 1977.
2. Braunstein, AH and Oberman, HA: Transfusion of plasma components. Transfusion 24:281, 1984.
3. Dodd, RY and Barker, LF (eds): Infection, Immunity and Blood Transfusion. In Clinical and Biological Research, Vol 182. Alan R. Liss, New York, 1985.
4. Giblett, ER: Blood group alloantibodies: An assessment of some laboratory practices. Transfusion 17:299, 1977.
5. Grindon, AJ: The decision to transfuse: Role of the immunohematology laboratory. Lab Med 13:270, 1982.

6. Holland, EA and Sacher, RA: Use of Blood Products. Monograph 82, American Academy of Family Physicians, 1982.
7. Issitt, PD and Crookston, MC: Blood group terminology: Current conventions. Transfusion 24:2, 1984.
8. Lewis, M: Recent advances in blood groups. Clin Lab Med 2:137, 1982.
9. Luban, NLC and Keating, LJ (eds): Hemotherapy of the Infant and Premature. American Association of Blood Banks, Arlington, VA, 1983.
10. Menitove, JE and Aster, RH: Transfusion of platelets and plasma products. Clin Haematol 12:239, 1983.
11. Miller, WV and Rodey, G: HLA without tears. American Society of Clinical Pathologists, Chicago, 1981.
12. Mollison, PL: Blood transfusion. In Clinical Medicine, ed 7, Blackwell Scientific Publications, Oxford, 1983.
13. Race, RR and Sanger, R: Blood Groups in Man, ed 6. Blackwell Scientific Publications, Oxford, 1975.
14. Sandler, SG: In Sandler, SG and Silvergleid, A (eds): Autologous Transfusion. American Association of Blood Banks, Arlington, VA, 1983, p 8.
15. Schmidt, PJ (ed): Standards for Blood Banks and Transfusion Services, ed 11. American Association of Blood Banks, Arlington, VA, 1984.
16. Tomasulo, PA and Lenes, BA: Platelet transfusion therapy. In Menitove, JE and McCarthy, LJ (eds): Hemostatic Disorders and the Blood Bank. American Association of Blood Banks, Arlington, VA, 1984.
17. Warrier, AI and Lusher, DM: DDAVP: A useful alternative to blood components in moderate hemophilia-A and von Willebrand's disease. J Pediatr 102:228, 1983.
18. Widmann, F (ed): Technical Manual of the American Association of Blood Banks, ed 9. Arlington, VA, 1985.
19. Office of Medical Applications of Research, National Institutes of Health: Consensus Conference: Fresh frozen plasma: Indications and risks. JAMA 253:551, 1985.
20. Capon, SM and Sacher, RA: Hemolytic transfusion reactions: A review of mechanisms, sequelae and management. J Intensive Care Med 4:100–111, 1989.

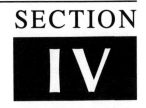

CLINICAL CHEMISTRY

OUTLINE

CHAPTER 9

TESTS

CHAPTER 9

GENERAL CHEMISTRY

SERUM CHEMISTRY ANALYSIS

The blood transports a large number of chemical substances throughout the body between organs and into the tissues. These substances reflect metabolic processes and disease states. Alterations in their concentrations are frequently useful in diagnosis and the planning and monitoring of therapy.

Those substances typically measured in serum fall generally into the following categories:

1. *Normally present* with a *function* in the circulation: glucose, sodium, potassium, chloride, bicarbonate, total proteins, albumin, calcium, magnesium, phosphorus, triglycerides, cholesterol, hormones (thyroxine, cortisol), vitamins (folate, B_{12}), individual proteins (haptoglobin, transferrin, immunoglobulins)
2. *Metabolites* (nonfunctioning waste products in the process of being cleared): urea, creatinine, uric acid, ammonia, bilirubin
3. Substances *released* from cells as a result of *cell damage* and *abnormal permeability* or abnormal *cellular proliferation* (usually enzymes/proteins): lactate dehydrogenase, alanine aminotransferase, aspartate aminotransferase, creatine kinase, amylase, gamma glutamyl transferase, alkaline phosphatase, acid phosphatase, ferritin
4. Drugs and toxic substances: antibiotics (aminoglycosides), cardiac (antiarrhythmics, digoxin), antiasthmatic (theophylline), anticonvulsants, salicylates, alcohol, and other substances of abuse

This chapter deals with several of the analytes most commonly measured in serum. Other special chemical tests performed on serum are described in separate chapters: Chapter 5, coagulation proteins; Chapter 10, acid-base balance and electrolytes; Chapter 11, enzymes; Chapter 12, liver functions; Chapters 16 and 17, hormones and other endocrine markers; Chapter 18, drugs and toxic substances.

A special word should be said about *sample type*. The portion of the blood that is in equilibrium with tissues and that contains substances emanating from tissues is the *plasma*. Therefore, almost all blood chemistry measurements are performed on plasma or more typically on serum that is obtained after a blood sample has been clotted and the clot separated by centrifugation. Serum is equivalent to plasma with the fibrinogen removed (see Chapter 5). The use of serum instead of plasma also precludes contamination of the specimen with an anticoagulant that may interfere with one or more tests. Some substances do localize in erythrocytes and therefore are usually measured in whole blood. These include such determinations as blood gases (oxygen), the metal lead, and the drug cyclosporin. However, the vast majority of chemical substances in the plasma either are excluded from erythrocytes and the other blood cells or are at much different concentrations intracellularly than extracellularly. Thus, precautions should always be taken to prevent or minimize hemolysis in the collection of serum. Hemolysis can falsely elevate serum levels of *potassium* and *lactate dehydrogenase* in particular and may also cause methodologic interference in other tests due to release of the pigment hemoglobin.

Serum has become the almost universally employed sample for chemistry testing. To facilitate its collection and preparation, most commercial blood drawing tubes have a vacuum sealed with a red rubber stopper (i.e., red-topped tube). These tubes may contain a fine powder or other nondissolving material that enhances clot formation at the contact phase of coagulation. Some of these tubes also have at the bottom a gel that settles out between the clot and the serum (serum separator tubes) on centrifugation, thereby protecting the integrity of the serum sample separate from cells in the clot. (These tubes cannot be used for blood bank serology; see Chapter 8.)

Ever greater demands for faster turnaround times in critical care situations and for simplified sample preparation in satellite sites and physician office laboratories have led to new strategies for using whole blood directly from a fingerstick drop or venipuncture samples anticoagulated with heparin. Future developments in blood chemistry testing will most likely emerge in the fields of sample collection and analysis, whereas the actual tests and their interpretation should remain very much as detailed in this text. Emphasis is given to those substances most commonly measured.

CARBOHYDRATE METABOLISM

Oxidative metabolism of *glucose* provides most of the energy used in the body. Glucose is a simple six-carbon sugar. Glucose in the diet is largely present as *disaccharides* (i.e., chemically bonded to another sugar molecule: *sucrose* is glucose plus fructose; *lactose* is glucose plus galactose; *maltose* is two glucose molecules) and as the complex polysaccharide starch. The disaccharides are broken down into their constituent monosaccharides by enzymes in the mucosa of the small intestine called *disaccharidases.* These enzymes *(lactase, sucrase,* and *maltase)* are entirely specific for a single disaccharide. The starch is broken down by *amylase* secreted from the pancreas and also by the salivary glands. Sugars are absorbed by the intestine in the form of monosaccharides.

Glucose metabolism generates pyruvic acid, lactic acid, and acetylcoenzyme A (acetyl-CoA) as intermediary compounds. The complete oxidation of glucose yields carbon dioxide, water, and energy that is stored as the high-energy phosphates compound adenosine triphosphate (ATP).

If not immediately metabolized to produce energy, glucose can be stored in liver or muscle as *glycogen,* a polymer consisting of numerous glucose residues in a form available for subsequent release and metabolism of glucose. The liver can also convert glucose through other metabolic pathways into *fatty acids*, which are stored as *triglycerides*, or into *amino acids* for use in protein synthesis. Because of its large volume and its content of enzymes for multiple metabolic conversions, the liver plays a pivotal role in distributing glucose for immediate energy need or for storage and structural purposes as well. If glycogen becomes depleted and available glucose is insufficient for energy needs, the liver can synthesize glucose from fatty acids, and also from amino acids (gluconeogenesis).

The energy for most cellular and tissue functions derives from glucose. Alternative energy generation can derive from metabolism of fatty acids, but this pathway is less efficient than burning glucose and creates acid metabolites that can be harmful if allowed to accumulate. Therefore, glucose in the blood is controlled by several homeostatic mechanisms that in health maintain levels in the range 70–110 mg/dl in the fasting state. Following ingestion of a meal with a heavy glucose load, blood glucose normally does not exceed about 170 mg/dl. Many hormones participate in maintaining adequate blood glucose levels in steady-state conditions or in response to stress (Table 9–1). Measurement of blood glucose is frequently performed to monitor the overall success of these regulatory mechanisms. Pronounced deviation from normal, either too high or too low, indicates faulty homeostasis and should initiate a search for the etiology.

Glucose Measurement

Sample Type

Historically, blood glucose values were given in terms of whole blood, but most laboratories now measure the serum glucose level. Because erythrocytes have a higher concentration of protein (i.e., hemoglobin) than serum, serum has a higher water content and consequently more dissolved glucose than does whole blood. To convert from whole-blood glucose, multiply the value by 1.15 to give the serum or plasma level.

Collection of blood in clot (red-top) tubes for serum chemistry analysis permits the metabolism of glucose in the sample by blood cells until separated by centrifugation. Very high white cell counts can lead to excessive glycolysis in the sample with substantial reduction in glucose level. Ambient temperature at which the blood sample is kept prior to separation also affects the rate of glycolysis. At refrigerator temperatures, glucose remains relatively stable for several hours in blood. At room temperature, a loss of 1–2% of glucose/hour should be expected. This loss is not significant for hospital laboratories that process blood samples soon after they are drawn. However, if blood samples are sent a long distance to reference laboratories, there may be opportunity for substantial loss of glucose to glycolysis by the blood cells. This problem can be circumvented by using *fluoride*-containing (gray-top) tubes that inhibit glycolysis, thereby preserving the glucose level even at room temperature. Gray-top tubes are generally employed when glucose levels are to be used for diagnostic purposes (e.g., in the initial diagnosis of diabetes). Red-top serum separator tubes also preserve glucose in samples once they have been centrifuged to isolate the serum from the cells. Serum separator tubes are generally used for the majority of glucose determinations (e.g., both outpatient screening and inpatient monitoring of intravenous [IV] fluid therapy), since other analytes can be measured on the same serum samples. Particular care should be given to drawing blood samples from the arm opposite the one in which an intravenous line is inserted, to prevent contamination of the sample with intravenous fluids. As little as

Table 9–1. HORMONES THAT INFLUENCE BLOOD GLUCOSE LEVEL

Hormone	Tissue of Origin	Metabolic Effect	Effect on Blood Glucose
Insulin	Pancreatic β cells	1. Enhances entry of glucose into cells 2. Enhances storage of glucose as glycogen, or conversion to fatty acids 3. Enhances synthesis of proteins and fatty acids 4. Suppresses breakdown of protein into amino acids, of adipose tissue into free fatty acids	Lowers
Somatostatin	Pancreatic D cells	1. Suppresses glucagon release from α cells (acts locally) 2. Suppresses release of insulin, pituitary tropic hormones, gastrin, and secretin	Raises
Glucagon	Pancreatic α cells	1. Enhances release of glucose from glycogen 2. Enhances synthesis of glucose from amino acids or fatty acids	Raises
Epinephrine	Adrenal medulla	1. Enhances release of glucose from glycogen 2. Enhances release of fatty acids from adipose tissue	Raises
Cortisol	Adrenal cortex	1. Enhances synthesis of glucose from amino acids or fatty acids 2. Antagonizes insulin	Raises
ACTH	Anterior pituitary	1. Enhances release of cortisol 2. Enhances release of fatty acids from adipose tissue	Raises
Growth hormone	Anterior pituitary	1. Antagonizes insulin	Raises
Thyroxine	Thyroid	1. Enhances release of glucose from glycogen 2. Enhances absorption of sugars from intestine	Raises

Adapted from Howanitz and Howanitz[5] and Guyton.[3]

10% contamination with 5% dextrose (D5W) will elevate glucose in a sample by 500 mg/dl or more. Arterial, capillary, and venous blood have comparable glucose levels in a fasting individual, whereas after meals venous levels are lower than those in arterial or capillary blood.

Methodology

There are two different major methodologies that have been used to measure glucose. The older one is a chemical method that exploits the nonspecific *reducing property of glucose* in a reaction with an indicator substance that acquires or changes color on its reduction. Since other compounds also present in blood are reducing substances (e.g., urea, which can build up to appreciable levels in uremia), glucose measurement can be 5–15 mg/dl erroneously higher by reducing methods than by more accurate *enzymatic methods* that are highly specific for glucose. These enzymatic methods generally employ the enzymes *glucose oxidase* or *hexokinase,* which act on glucose but not on other sugars and not on other reducing substances. The enzymatic conversion of glucose to product is now quantitated on automated chemistry analyzers by a color change reaction as the last of a series of coupled chemical reactions or by the consumption of oxygen on an oxygen-sensing device. By making several measurements over a period of minutes, modern chemistry analyzers can calculate the rate of the reaction, which is proportional to concentration of glucose. This kinetic analysis is technically preferable to endpoint analysis, by which only the final amount of product is measured. In general, kinetic analysis is superior to endpoint for many common chemical measurements due to the shorter time period required for each assay and also because interferences in endpoint assays can frequently be nullified in measuring reaction rates.

Outside of the clinical laboratory, there are presently available several brands of personal glucose monitors that diabetic patients can use for measuring their own glucose levels in a drop of blood from a fingerstick. These glucose meters are extremely useful for providing fast and frequent feedback to the patient for changing medication and therapy. The present generation of these personal glucose meters has the disadvantage that low hematocrit falsely elevates the glucose result and conversely, high hematocrit falsely lowers the result. This hematocrit effect (and a similar one for high or low protein in serum) is probable cause for many discrepancies noted between glucose values measured in blood samples sent to a hospital laboratory and simultaneously performed by a patient on a personal glucose meter. It is therefore recommended that each patient using a glucose meter for personal monitoring should at periodic intervals have that measurement checked against a laboratory with a full quality control program to insure that the meter results are within acceptable limits (within ±15% of the laboratory result).

Whereas the measurement of blood glucose concentration provides information about immediate glucose homeostasis, evaluation of long-term glucose control (e.g., over the previous few weeks) is available from measurement of *glycosylated hemoglobin* in erythrocytes. Hemoglobin is glycosylated spontaneously in the circulation with larger amounts formed when blood glucose levels are high. Glycosylated hemoglobin is measured by electrophoretic or chromatographic methods on a lysate of washed erythrocytes (see Chapter 16, Endocrinology).

Clinical Correlation

The *fasting blood glucose* level gives the best indication of overall glucose homeostasis, and most routine determinations should be done on fasting samples.

Table 9–2. CAUSES OF ABNORMAL GLUCOSE LEVELS

Reference Range, Fasting Serum Glucose: 70–110 mg/dl
Persistent hyperglycemia:
Diabetes mellitus
Adrenal cortical hyperactivity (Cushing's syndrome)
Hyperthyroidism
Acromegaly
Obesity
Transient hyperglycemia:
Pheochromocytoma
Severe liver disease
Acute stress reaction (physical or emotional)
Shock
Convulsions
Persistent hypoglycemia:
Insulinoma
Adrenal cortical insufficiency (Addison's disease)
Hypopituitarism
Galactosemia
Ectopic insulin production from tumors
Transient hypoglycemia:
Acute alcohol ingestion
Drugs: salicylates, antituberculosis agents
Severe liver disease
Several glycogen storage diseases
"Functional" hypoglycemia
Hereditary fructose intolerance

Conditions that affect glucose levels are shown in Table 9–2. They reflect abnormalities in the multiple control mechanisms of glucose regulation.

The metabolic response to a carbohydrate challenge is conveniently assessed by the postprandial glucose level drawn two hours after a meal or a glucose load. In addition, the glucose tolerance test, consisting of serial timed measurements after a standardized amount of oral glucose intake, is used to aid in the diagnosis of diabetes. These applications are given more detailed consideration in the section on the pancreas (see Chapter 16).

Other Sugars

High blood and urine *fructose* levels occur in patients with any of several relatively uncommon enzyme deficiencies *(essential fructosuria)*. When reducing methods were used for glucose determinations, *fructosemia* was readily detected as an unexpectedly high blood sugar level. Now that most tests use glucose-specific enzyme techniques, fructosemia will be diagnosed only if specifically sought. Patients with hereditary fructose intolerance (deficiency of fructose-1-phosphate aldolase) experience severe hypoglycemia and hypophosphatemia after exposure to fructose or to table sugar (sucrose), which consists of one glucose and one fructose moiety. Lack of a different fructose-related enzyme impairs the ability to synthesize glucose from other sugars; hypoglycemia develops if there is no glycogen available as a reserve source of glucose.

Galactosemia results from deficiency of any of several galactose-metabolizing enzymes. Because severe mental and physical changes accompany prolonged galactosemia in infancy, it is important to test newborn infants for the presence of excess galactose. Screening tests are done on urine, but galactose will be detected only if the test is done after the infant begins to ingest milk. More definitive blood tests are indicated if screening results are abnormal.

The deposition and retrieval of glucose into and out of glycogen involve myriad enzymes; congenital deficiency states have been identified for a great many of these. Collectively designated *glycogen storage diseases* have an overall incidence of 1 in 40,000, with diverse clinical signs and population distribution. Definitive diagnosis requires enzyme analysis, but screening procedures include measuring fasting blood glucose and observing responses to glucose load, to glucagon infusion, to muscular exertion, and to other stimuli.

For additional discussion of carbohydrate abnormalities, see Chapter 16.

NONPROTEIN NITROGENOUS COMPOUNDS

This group of chemical substances refers to low molecular weight compounds that contain nitrogen and are distinguished from proteins. Nonprotein nitrogen (NPN) includes urea, creatinine, uric acid, ammonia, and amino acids. These compounds are by-products of protein or nucleic acid metabolism. They are present in concentrations of milligrams/deciliter or less because of ready clearance into the urine. In the past, before specific analyses were available, NPN measurement was used as an index of renal function. However, modern assays for the individual compounds has made NPN determination obsolete.

Urea

METABOLISM

Amino groups are exchanged between amino acids as catalyzed by *aminotransferases* in many tissues of the body. In addition, amino groups are removed from amino acids in the transformation and recycling of the amino acid pool. The liberated amino groups are converted to ammonia that travels to the liver where it is incorporated into *urea* in a metabolic pathway referred to as the urea cycle. Urea is a small molecule with the following chemical structure:

$$H_2N-\overset{\overset{\displaystyle O}{\|}}{C}-NH_2$$

Urea
molecular weight = 60 daltons

Urea diffuses freely into both intracellular and extracellular fluid. It is concentrated in the urine for excretion. In stable nitrogen balance, about 25 g urea is excreted daily. Levels in the blood reflect the balance between production and excretion of urea.

Measurement

Chemical methods for determining urea have been largely replaced by enzymatic methods utilizing *urease* and therefore are highly specific for urea. By convention in the United States, urea assays are calibrated and values expressed as the nitrogen content of the molecule, also referred to as *blood urea nitrogen* or BUN. Normal serum concentration of BUN is roughly 5–20 mg/dl. In other countries, values are expressed as total weight of urea instead of nitrogen content. Nitrogen contributes $^{28}/_{60}$ to the total weight of urea; the concentration of urea can be calculated by multiplying BUN concentration by $^{60}/_{28}$, or 2.14.

Clinical Considerations

Blood urea nitrogen derives from breakdown of protein, primarily dietary in origin. Men have slightly higher mean values than do women. Blood urea nitrogen is usually on the high side of the normal range in otherwise healthy individuals whose diet is heavy in protein on a long-term basis. Low levels of BUN are not generally considered abnormal. They may be due to low protein in the diet or to expansion of plasma volume. More serious is liver damage so severe that the organ is not able to synthesize urea from ammonia in the circulation.

The condition of high urea levels is called *uremia.* Its most common cause is renal failure resulting in impaired excretion. *Azotemia* refers to elevation of all the low molecular weight nitrogenous compounds in renal failure. *Prerenal uremia* means an elevation of BUN due to some mechanism acting prior to filtration of the blood by the glomeruli. These causes include markedly reduced blood flow to the kidney as in shock, dehydration, or increased catabolism of protein such as massive bleeding into the gastrointestinal tract with digestion of the hemoglobin and its absorption as protein in the diet. *Postrenal uremia* occurs when there is obstruction of the lower urinary tract in the ureters, bladder, or urethra that prevents excretion of urine. The urea in the backed-up urine can diffuse back into the blood stream. *Renal* causes of uremia include diseases or toxicities that affect either the glomeruli and renal microvasculature or the renal tubules. Causes of elevated BUN are listed in Table 9–3.

Table 9–3. COMMON CAUSES OF UREMIA

Prerenal:
- Reduced blood flow to kidney
  - Shock, blood loss, dehydration
- Increased protein catabolism
  - Crush injuries, burns, fever, hemorrhage into soft tissues or body cavities, hemolysis

Renal:
- Acute renal failure
  - Glomerulonephritis, malignant hypertension, nephrotoxic drugs or metals, renal cortical necrosis
- Chronic renal disease
  - Glomerulonephritis, pyelonephritis, diabetes mellitus, arteriosclerosis, arteriolosclerosis, amyloidosis, renal tubular disease, collagen-vascular diseases

Postrenal:
- Ureteral obstruction by stones, tumor, inflammation, surgical misadventure; obstruction of bladder neck or urethra by prostate, stones, tumor, inflammation

Creatinine

METABOLISM

Creatinine is the endproduct of creatine metabolism. Creatine is present mostly in skeletal muscle, where it is involved in energy storage as *creatine phosphate* (CP). Creatine phosphate is converted to creatine in the synthesis of ATP from ADP catalyzed by the enzyme creatine kinase (CK).

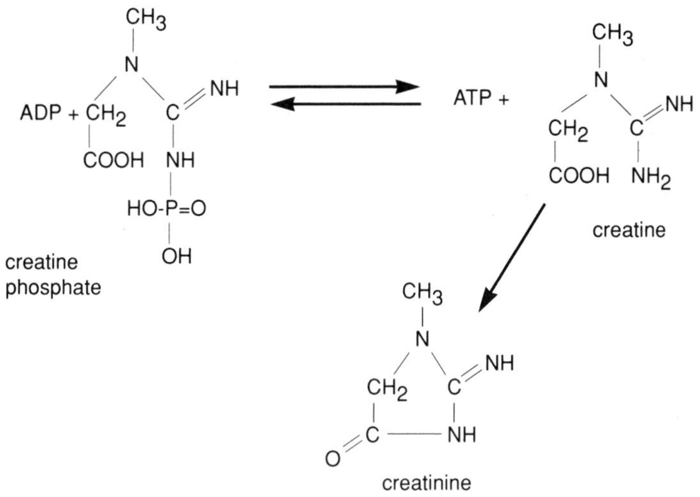

$$\text{ADP} + \underset{\text{creatine phosphate}}{CH_3\text{-}N(CH_2COOH)\text{-}C(=NH)\text{-}NH\text{-}P(=O)(OH)_2} \rightleftharpoons \text{ATP} + \underset{\text{creatine}}{CH_3\text{-}N(CH_2COOH)\text{-}C(=NH)\text{-}NH_2}$$

$$\downarrow$$

$$\underset{\text{creatinine}}{CH_3\text{-}N(CH_2\text{-}C(=O)\text{-}NH\text{-}C(=NH))}$$

This reaction continues as energy is utilized and CP is regenerated. In the process, small amounts of creatine are irreversibly converted to creatinine, which is removed from the circulation by the kidneys. The amount of creatinine generated in an individual is proportional to the mass of skeletal muscle present. Reference values for creatinine are 0.6–1.3 mg/dl for men and 0.5–1.0 mg/dl for women.

The daily generation of creatinine remains fairly constant, with the exceptions of crushing injury or degenerative disease that cause massive damage to muscle. The kidneys excrete creatinine very efficiently. Levels of blood flow and urine production affect creatinine excretion much less than they affect urea excretion because temporary alterations in blood flow and glomerular activity are compensated by increased tubular secretion of creatinine into urine. Blood concentration and daily urinary excretion of creatinine in an individual fluctuate very little. Consequently, serial measurements of creatinine excretion are useful in determining whether 24-hour urine specimens for other analyses (e.g., steroids) have been completely and accurately collected.

CLINICAL CONSIDERATIONS

Blood creatinine becomes elevated when renal function declines. If slow loss of renal function occurs simultaneously with slow loss of muscle mass, the concentration of creatinine in serum may remain stable, but 24-hour excretion (or clearance) rates would be lower than normal. This pattern may happen in aging patients. Thus, a better index of renal function is *creatinine clearance,* which takes into account both serum creatinine and the quantity excreted in a day (see Chapter 19, Urine).

Elevated levels of BUN in a patient with normal creatinine indicate a nonrenal cause for the uremia (usually prerenal). Blood urea nitrogen rises more steeply than creatinine with declining renal function. With dialysis or successful renal transplantation, the urea falls more rapidly than creatinine. With severe long-term renal impairment, urea levels continue to climb, whereas creatinine levels tend to plateau, perhaps due to excretion across the alimentary tract.

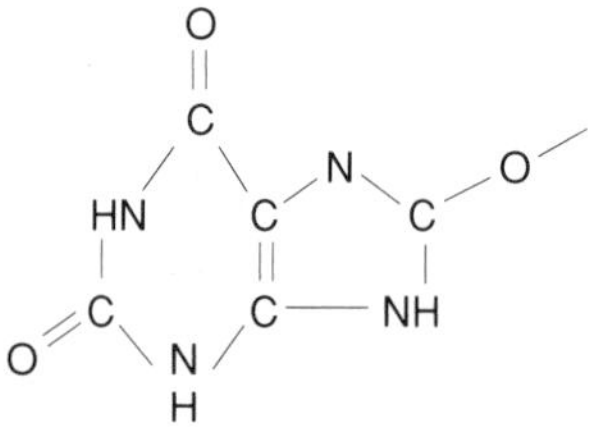

Uric Acid

Uric Acid

METABOLISM

Uric acid is produced as the endproduct of purine metabolism in humans. Purines (adenine and guanine) are constituents of nucleic acids. Purine turnover is occurring continuously in the body with RNA and DNA synthesis and degradation, so that substantial amounts of uric acid are produced even in the absence of dietary purine intake. Uric acid is synthesized primarily in the liver, a reaction catalyzed by the enzyme xanthine oxidase. Uric acid then travels through the blood to the kidneys, where it is filtered, partially reabsorbed, and partially further secreted before final excretion in the urine. On a low-purine diet, daily excretion is about 0.5 g; on a normal diet, excretion is about 1 g daily. Organ meats, legumes, and yeast are especially high in purines.

HYPERURICEMIA

Uric acid is poorly soluble in water, and urate crystals readily precipitate from urine with high concentrations of urate to produce urate kidney stones. Similarly, patients with high blood uric acid levels often deposit urate crystals in soft tissues, especially joints. This clinical syndrome is *gout.* The crystals in tissues cause an inflammatory response, with release of enzymes from leukocytes and local tissue damage that leads to an acid environment favorable to formation of more urate crystals, and so forth, in a renewed cycle. The result is painful swollen and inflamed joints. Urate stones sometimes occur in patients with gout, but normouricemic persons (i.e., normal uric acid levels in the blood) may have urate stones if urinary levels of uric acid are excessive.

Both the amount of uric acid produced and the efficiency of renal excretion affect serum urate levels. Uric acid production is increased by idiopathic mechanisms associated with gout. It is also increased in proportion to cell turnover due to the degradation of nucleic acids, as with leukemia or other malignancies with a large cell mass. Cytolytic therapy of malignancies should be expected to result in extremely high levels of uric acid for periods of days. In such instances it is necessary to take special precautions to prevent acute renal failure due to precipitation of

Table 9–4. FACTORS AFFECTING SERUM URIC ACID LEVELS

Reference Range: 4–8.5 mg/dl for Men; 2.7–7.3 mg/dl for Women
Increased production, raised serum levels:
Idiopathic mechanisms associated with primary gout
Excessive dietary purines (organ meats, legumes, anchovies, etc.)
Cytolytic treatment of malignancies, especially leukemias and lymphomas
Polycythemia
Myeloid metaplasia
Psoriasis
Sickle cell anemia
Decreased excretion, raised serum levels:
Alcohol ingestion
Thiazide diuretics
Lactic acidosis
Aspirin doses <2 g/day
Ketoacidosis, especially diabetes or starvation
Renal failure, any cause
Increased excretion, lowered serum levels:
Probenecid, sulfinpyrazone, aspirin doses above 4 g/day
Corticosteroids and ACTH
Coumarin anticoagulants
Estrogens
Decreased production, lowered serum levels:
Allopurinol

From Woo and Cannon,[15] with permission.

urates in the kidneys. Renal failure, of course, causes uric acid and also urea and creatinine to accumulate. Thiazide diuretics and low doses of aspirin diminish urate excretion. Allopurinol, probenecid, corticosteroids, and large doses of aspirin increase urate excretion.

Although symptoms of gout occur during periods when blood urates are high, many people have hyperuricemia without gouty symptoms or urinary problems, indicating that multiple factors probably modulate urate precipitation. *Primary gout* occurs due to overproduction of uric acid or impaired renal tubular excretion. *Secondary gout* results from excessive urate production following massive nucleic acid turnover or from acquired renal disorders that diminish urate excretion. These conditions affecting serum urate levels are shown in Table 9–4.

TREATMENT

Uric acid production can be reduced by administering the drug, allopurinol, which inhibits xanthine oxidase activity, thereby lowering serum urate level without imposing an increased excretory load on the kidneys. The uricosuric agents probenecid and sulfinpyrazone lower serum urates by increasing the uric acid content of urine, which could lead to stone formation. Patients taking these agents must maintain a high volume of alkaline urine to keep the urates in solution. Colchicine, a drug long used to treat gouty arthritis, affects neither production nor excretion of urate, but rather alters the phagocytic response of leukocytes to urate crystals in tissue.

Other NPN Compounds

Ammonia and *amino acids* constitute most of the remaining low molecular weight nitrogenous compounds. Ammonia is discussed under liver functions tests (see Chapter 12). It is not measured as a screening test but rather for special instances such as hepatic failure causing encephalopathy. The 20 different amino acids are likewise not usually measured except in special circumstances for the evaluation of some congenital or acquired abnormalities in the metabolism of specific amino acids or in the evaluation of some causes of liver failure.

BILIRUBIN

Metabolism

The normal metabolic processing of hemoglobin after its release from aging erythrocytes leads to production of the small molecule heme (see Chapter 2). Breakdown of muscle also results in the production of heme in a lesser amount as myoglobin is degraded. Heme in turn loses its iron atom and is oxidized to form the yellow pigment bilirubin, which is highly insoluble in water. Bilirubin does bind to albumin, enabling it to be transported throughout the body. In this form, the molecular species is termed *unconjugated bilirubin.* As it circulates through the liver, hepatocytes perform the following functions:

1. uptake of bilirubin from the circulation,
2. enzymatic conjugation as bilirubin glucuronides, and
3. transport and excretion of conjugated bilirubin into the bile for elimination from the body.

Congenital defects in each of these metabolic steps are recognized clinically:

1. defect in uptake: Gilbert syndrome,
2. defect in hepatic glucuronyl transferase: Crigler-Najjar syndrome, and
3. defect in transport extracellularly: Dubin-Johnson syndrome.

The intracellular conjugation of glucuronic acid onto two sites of the bilirubin molecule confers negative charge to it, thereby making *conjugated bilirubin* soluble in aqueous phase. If there is obstruction or other failure to excrete this conjugated bilirubin, it will re-enter the circulation, where it can accumulate. Functioning hepatocytes will attempt to take up conjugated bilirubin as they do the unconjugated form in step 1. A further chemical change can occur when conjugated bilirubin remains in the circulation at high levels for a prolonged time. In that instance, there is spontaneous formation of a covalent bond between conjugated bilirubin and albumin. This chemical species will not be taken up by the liver and has a long half-life in the circulation. The various chemical species of bilirubin have been designated as follows:

- alpha bilirubin—unconjugated
- beta bilirubin—monoconjugated
- gamma bilirubin—diconjugated
- delta bilirubin—covalently bound to albumin

Once bile enters the intestine, colonic bacteria convert bilirubin to *urobilinogen,* a collective term for several colorless compounds that subsequently undergo oxidation to the brown pigment *urobilin.* Urobilin is excreted in the feces, but urobilinogen is in part reabsorbed through the intestine, and through the portal circulation is picked up by the liver and re-excreted in bile. Since urobilinogen is freely water soluble, it can also pass out through the urine if it reaches the kidneys.

Measurement

Although bilirubin is normally only a minor constituent of bile (outweighed 20 to 1 by the bile salts), measurement of bilirubin in serum is relatively simple to perform in the laboratory, and is frequently used as a sensitive indicator of hepatic functions. For clinical purposes, bilirubin is expressed as two components. These are the unconjugated insoluble form referred to as *indirect* or *prehepatic* and the conjugated soluble form described as *direct* or *post-hepatic.* Direct bilirubin is measured by a specific chemical reaction (diazotization) without any modification since it is water soluble. Indirect bilirubin is not quantitated separately, but instead is calculated as the difference between *total bilirubin* and the direct fraction. Measurement of total bilirubin involves solubilization of the unconjugated form before chemical quantitation. For health screening examinations, total bilirubin measurement usually suffices, since a major increase in direct bilirubin would also be reflected in the total. Most clinical laboratories report only direct and total bilirubin (which are the actual measurements), leaving calculation of the indirect fraction to the physician.

Optimal serum specimens for bilirubin determination should be free from hemolysis, lipemia, or other sources of abnormal pigment or turbidity that could interfere with the optical detection of the colored product in some methods of bilirubin analysis. Exposure of a specimen to light can reduce serum bilirubin concentrations. This effect is particularly important in monitoring neonatal jaundice, where the actual level is very important but the specimens are usually small (e.g., microcollections from heel sticks) thereby allowing incident light to penetrate further and denature bilirubin throughout a stored sample. Phototherapy of infants is also used clinically to lower bilirubin levels in the patient.

Clinical Considerations

Jaundice is the visible yellow discoloration of skin and sclerae that arises when serum total bilirubin levels exceed 2.0 or 2.5 mg/dl. Table 9–5 lists clinically significant causes of hyperbilirubinemia. In the serum of adults, the expected range of direct bilirubin is up to 0.3 mg/dl, and that of total bilirubin is 0.1–1.2 mg/dl. Occasionally, healthy adults have normal direct bilirubin with a total of 2.0 mg/dl or greater. Such individuals may have a mild defect in the uptake of bilirubin by the liver, a variation of *Gilbert's syndrome.* This degree of unconjugated hyperbilirubinemia may be exacerbated in Gilbert's syndrome by the fasting state.

Neonatal "physiologic" jaundice reflects both increased loads of hemoglobin breakdown and immaturity of the liver in its ability to conjugate bilirubin. Any hemolytic abnormality can be expected to increase the flow of bilirubin through its metabolic intermediates (prehepatic jaundice). In patients with normal hepatic function, an increased load of bilirubin from hemoglobin will result in a mild increase of indirect bilirubin typically not above 5 mg/dl, but the direct bilirubin will likely remain normal if the liver's excretory capacity is intact. As a consequence of more

Table 9–5. CAUSES OF HYPERBILIRUBINEMIA

Reference Range: 0.3–1.1 mg/dl Total; 0.1–0.4 mg/dl Direct
Increased indirect (unconjugated) bilirubin:
Hemolysis; hemoglobinopathies; spherocytosis; G-6-PD deficiency; autoimmunity; Hemolytic transfusion reaction
Red cell degradation: hemorrhage into soft tissues or body cavities; inefficient erythropoiesis; pernicious anemia
Defective hepatocellular uptake or conjugation: viral hepatitis; hereditary enzyme deficiencies (Gilbert, Crigler-Najjar syndromes); hepatic immaturity, in newborns
Increased direct (conjugated) bilirubin:
Intrahepatic disruption: viral hepatitis; alcoholic hepatitis; chlorpromazine; cirrhosis
Bile duct disease: biliary cirrhosis; cholangitis (idiopathic, infectious); biliary atresia
Extrahepatic bile duct obstruction: gallstones; carcinoma of gallbladder, bile ducts, or head of pancreas; bile duct stricture, from inflammation or surgical misadventure

conjugated bilirubin in the intestines, there will be greater amounts of urobilinogen in the gut with reabsorption and excretion into the urine.

Hepatic testing is discussed further in Chapter 12. Generally, the direct and indirect fractions are used to determine whether liver disease primarily involves hepatocellular function (hepatic jaundice) (e.g., high total bilirubin, low direct) or a post-hepatic block (e.g., high total bilirubin, high direct) (post-hepatic jaundice). Frequently a patient with liver disease can go through different stages in which hepatic or post-hepatic *jaundice* predominate.

Elevation of direct bilirubin in serum for whatever reason permits this water-soluble species to pass into the urine, where it appears a bright yellow and can be detected on dipstick analysis as "bile" (see Urinalysis, Chapter 19).

Biliary obstruction with prolonged elevation of conjugated bilirubin in serum leads to the formation of delta bilirubin. This species of bilirubin molecule has only recently been recognized. Its significance comes in monitoring the timely descent of serum bilirubin after surgical correction of biliary obstruction (e.g., gallstones). Instead of leaving the circulation once biliary excretion is re-established, delta bilirubin can remain elevated (reacting as direct bilirubin) for weeks despite normal hepatic function. Thus, delta bilirubin must be recognized as a possible cause of persistent direct hyperbilirubinemia that has no pathologic repercussion.

CALCIUM, MAGNESIUM, AND PHOSPHORUS

Calcium and magnesium both occur as divalent cations (Ca^{2+} and Mg^{2+}) in aqueous solution. The reference range for serum calcium is 9–11 mg/dl or 4.5–5.5 mEq/liter. For serum magnesium, the reference range is 1.8–3.0 mg/dl or 1.3–2.1 mEq/liter. Roughly one half of the total calcium and magnesium circulates as free ions in plasma, while the remaining amount is bound by charge interaction to negatively charged proteins—predominantly albumin. The free fraction is physiologically active. The bound fraction is not active and does not play an immediate role in the

Table 9–6. CONDITIONS THAT AFFECT SERUM CALCIUM

Reference Range: 9–11 mg/dl, 4.5–5.5 mEq/liter
Causes of hypercalcemia:
Hyperparathyroidism, primary
Hyperparathyroidism, secondary to renal disease
Ectopic production of PTH-like material
Malignant tumors, mechanisms various or unknown
Sarcoidosis, mechanism unknown
Skeletal immobilization
Vitamin D intoxication
Hyperthyroidism
Excessive calcium intake (milk-alkali syndrome)
Causes of hypocalcemia:
Hypoparathyroidism, usually due to operation
Unresponsiveness to PTH (pseudohypoparathyroidism)
Vitamin D deficiency
Unresponsiveness to vitamin D (vitamin D–resistant rickets)
Malabsorption syndromes: calcium, phosphate, vitamin D, or combination
Acute pancreatitis

patients, leading to confusion and inability to communicate. Hypercalcemia is sometimes present in hyperthyroidism.

Hypocalcemia, as measured in the laboratory, can be a consequence of *reduced albumin* levels. In this situation, the fraction of bound calcium is reduced independently of the ionized fraction, which should remain normal. *True hypocalcemia* frequently develops as a serious medical emergency in *pancreatitis* due to sequestration of ionized calcium in the damaged tissue and surrounding fluid. Hypocalcemia produces neurologic irritability, commonly manifesting with tetany (muscular spasm and twitching, especially evident in the hands and facial muscles). This severe form of hypocalcemia requires immediate correction with intravenous calcium infusion. Patients suffering from chronic renal disease usually must take calcium supplements in the diet. Surgical removal of the parathyroids (as with complete thyroidectomy) also results in lifelong hypocalcemia requiring continuous replacement therapy. Various causes of calcium abnormalities are listed in Table 9–6.

Disorders of Phosphate Homeostasis

The equilibrium between serum phosphates and intracellular phosphate stores is determined largely by carbohydrate metabolism and blood pH. Phosphate is essential for the insulin-mediated entry of glucose into cells by a process involving phosphorylation of the glucose plus the co-entry of potassium. Acidotic diabetic patients who have lost phosphates and water by solute diuresis may experience a sudden drop in serum phosphate levels when treated with insulin and fluid expansion. Even normal individuals will show a slight reduction of the serum phosphate levels after a meal of carbohydrates.

endocrine control of calcium. Calcium participates in blood coagulation and skeletal and cardiac muscle contractility and in multiple membrane and c functions. Both calcium and magnesium are important in neuromuscular condu and activation.

Phosphorus is measured in body fluids as a mixture of the phosphates HPO_4^{-2} $H_2PO_4^{-1}$, which change in relative concentrations as one of the buffering system the blood (see Acid-Base Balance, Chapter 10). Results are reported as milligran deciliter (reference range, 2.4–4.7 mg/dl), but not as milliequivalents because difference in valences on the phosphate species. Phosphates, along with sugar moi ties, form the backbone of both nucleic acids RNA and DNA. Phosphates are als essential for intracellular storage and conversion of energy (ATP, creatine phosphate), for the intermediary compounds of carbohydrate metabolism, and in regulatory compounds such as 2, 3-diphosphoglycerate, which modulates the dissociation of oxygen from hemoglobin.

Metabolism

Calcium and phosphorus are generally considered together in routine clinical evaluations. These ions are in a continuous flux that is controlled by action of *parathyroid hormone (PTH), vitamin D,* and *calcitonin.* The amount present in serum at any one time is small compared with the major reservoir within bone. Serum levels do reflect overall mineral metabolism and, hence, the activity of the parathyroid glands. Parathyroid hormone secretion into the blood is stimulated by lowering the calcium concentration (actually the free or "ionized" fraction of calcium). Parathyroid hormone acts to elevate calcium levels by increasing the resorption of calcium from bone and suppressing loss of calcium into the urine. Vitamin D promotes absorption of calcium and phosphorus by the intestine and accelerates turnover of the minerals in bone.

Calcium phosphate has a solubility limit that restricts how high each can rise before the other is suppressed in a reciprocal relationship. This effect is strikingly important in renal disease that causes chronically elevated serum phosphate levels. In that situation, the serum calcium level (in particular the ionized calcium) will fall. However, the resulting hypocalcemia in turn stimulates PTH secretion that mobilizes calcium from deposits in bone. Long-term consequences include serious demineralization of the skeleton and secondary hyperparathyroidism with hyperplasia of that gland.

Magnesium levels usually parallel those of calcium when abnormalities occur. However, there is no large body reservoir from which to mobilize magnesium in order to replenish it as there is for calcium. Thus deficiency states of magnesium can arise and may require dietary supplementation to correct.

Clinical Considerations

Disorders of Calcium Homeostasis

Parathyroid disease, metabolic bone diseases, and disorders of *vitamin D metabolism* are usual causes of serum calcium abnormalities (Chapter 16). *Hypercalcemia* is a common problem in some *malignancies* with and without bone involvement, in *multiple myeloma* (lytic lesions of bone), and in the granulomatous disease *sarcoidosis.* Hypercalcemia can produce startling changes in the mental abilities of

Disorders of Magnesium Homeostasis

Magnesium levels usually fall in parallel with reduction in calcium due to their similar binding onto albumin. Malabsorption and starvation can lead to magnesium deficiency with serum levels reflecting depletion of body stores only late in the course. Chemical correction of calcium loss sometimes may not produce the expected clinical improvement of neurologic or cardiac status of a patient until a coexisting deficiency of magnesium is recognized and treated. Disorders of magnesium can also exacerbate the effect of potassium abnormalities (both hyperkalemia and hypokalemia).

Measurement

Calcium, magnesium, and phosphorus measurements must be done on serum to avoid interferences from anticoagulants used to collect plasma. Clot formation in those samples is prevented by agents that chelate calcium. Calcium can be measured by atomic absorption spectroscopy, by dye-binding with color change, or by ion-selective electrodes. Whole blood or plasma samples collected into heparin, which does not chelate calcium, can be used for ionized calcium measurements that reflect the physiologically active calcium. Such determinations are useful in evaluating parathyroid function and also for the acute monitoring of patients undergoing cardiac surgery or other high-risk procedures. We should expect to see ionized calcium measurements used with greater frequency in many clinical situations as the instrumentation to do so becomes more readily available at the bedside.

Special consideration must be given to obtaining high-quality, fresh specimens for ionized calcium measurements. Alkaline conditions cause ionized calcium to bind to proteins due to more negative charge on the protein molecules. Conversely, acidosis causes an elevation of hydrogen ions, which displace calcium from proteins, thereby increasing the ionized fraction. For accurate measurement, the sample should be drawn without prolonged venous stasis, which can cause local acidosis. Atmospheric contact will allow carbon dioxide to escape from both whole blood and serum specimens on even brief storage, resulting in rising pH of the sample (alkalosis). Thus, ionized calcium determinations should either be done quickly (e.g., on whole blood) or will require re-equilibration of a sample to physiologic pH.

Both phosphorus and magnesium are measured with dye-binding methods, although magnesium can also be measured with atomic absorption spectroscopy.

It has become more widely recognized recently that total body deficiency of magnesium can develop despite normal levels of magnesium in serum. This is because magnesium is predominantly an intracellular ion. Such a deficiency state is best diagnosed by administering a test load of magnesium and then measuring the percentage that is retained in the body versus excretion in urine. Normal individuals should have retentions below 20%, whereas whole body deficiency will lead to magnesium retentions substantially greater than 20%.

LIPIDS

Lipids are carbon- and hydrogen-containing compounds that are mostly hydrophobic: insoluble in water but soluble in organic solvents. Biologically important groups are the *neutral fats,* the *conjugated lipids,* and the *sterols.* Neutral fats consist of fatty acids (primarily oleic, linoleic, stearic, arachidonic, and palmitic) in the form of *triglycerides* (i.e., three fatty acid molecules esterified to a single glycerol molecule). Adipose tissue has stores of triglycerides that serve as a pool of readily available lipids. The conjugated lipids result from the joining of phosphate or sugar groups to lipid molecules. These phospholipids and glycolipids are integral constituents of the cell wall structure. Sterols also serve as structural building blocks in cells and membranes and as constituents of hormones and other metabolites. *Cholesterol* is the sterol of major biologic significance.

Due to their insolubility in water, lipids require special transport mechanisms for circulation in the blood. Free fatty acids occur in only small amounts in the blood and generally bind in a loose complex with albumin. The major lipid components found in plasma are triglycerides, cholesterol, and phospholipids. They exist and are transported in blood as *lipoproteins,* very large macromolecular complexes of those lipids with specialized proteins *(apolipoproteins)* that help in their packaging, solubility, and metabolism.

Metabolism

Body stores of energy are primarily in the form of *fatty acids.* As they enter and leave triglyceride molecules of adipose tissue, fatty acids provide the substance for conversion to glucose (gluconeogenesis) as well as for direct combustion to generate energy. Fatty acids can originate in the diet, but also derive from excess glucose that the liver and adipose tissue can convert into storable energy.

Cholesterol has two sources: dietary and that endogenously synthesized in the body. Cholesterol is an important constituent in the assembly of cell membranes. Much cholesterol also goes toward synthesis of bile acids and the steroid hormones (e.g., cortisol, estrogens, androgens). In the normal biologic process, cholesterol undergoes synthesis, degradation, and recycling. Consequently, the dietary component of cholesterol is probably not necessary for essential metabolic reactions.

The *phospholipids, lecithin, sphingomyelin,* and *cephalin* are major components of cell membranes and also act in solution to alter fluid surface tension (e.g., surfactant activity of the fluid in the lungs). The circulating phospholipids originate in liver and intestine with widespread synthesis in lesser amounts. The circulating phospholipids can participate in cellular metabolism and also in blood coagulation.

Lipids in the circulation are organized into large particles with apolipoproteins characteristic of each class of lipid particle. These apolipoproteins aid in the solubilization of the lipids and also in their transfer from the gastrointestinal tract to the liver, which contains specific receptors for apolipoproteins. Thus, the metabolism and clearance of lipids is directly regulated by the apolipoproteins.

Lipids in the circulation are organized into complex particles of different sizes that also contain different amounts of cholesterol, triglycerides, and protein, resulting in different densities characteristic of each lipoprotein type. The largest and least dense of lipoproteins are *chylomicrons,* followed by *very-low-density lipoproteins (VLDL), low-density lipoprotein (LDL), intermediate-density lipoproteins (IDL),* and *high-density lipoproteins (HDL).* Most of the triglycerides of nonfasting plasma reside in the chylomicrons, whereas in fasting plasma samples, the triglycerides are mostly in the VLDL. The majority of plasma cholesterol is contained in LDL. A smaller fraction (15–25%) of cholesterol is in the HDL.

The *dietary* or *exogenous pathway of lipid transport* involves absorption of triglycerides (TG) and cholesterol (Ch) through the intestine, with formation and release of chylomicrons into the lymph and subsequently into the blood by way of the thoracic duct. The chylomicrons release triglycerides to adipose tissue as they circulate. In addition, the apoliprotein B48 on the surface of chylomicrons activates *lipoprotein lipase (LPL)* found in the vascular endothelial cells. Lipoprotein lipase cleaves free fatty acids from the triglycerides, thereby reducing chylomicrons in size to remnants ultimately taken up by the liver. The free fatty acids so liberated are in turn taken up by muscle and adipose cells.

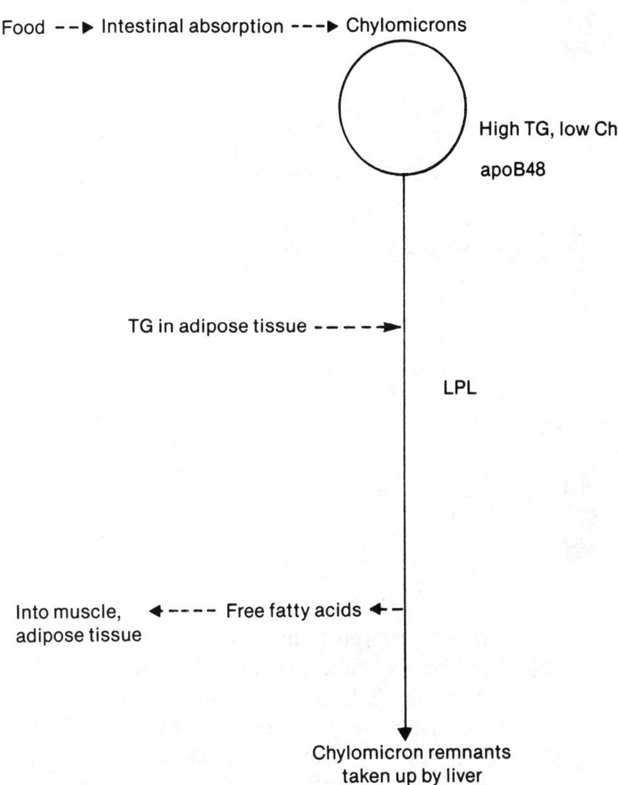

In the endogenous pathway, there is synthesis of triglycerides from fatty acids by the liver with secretion of VLDL that contain apolipoproteins B100 (which is commonly referred to as apoB in clinical measurements) and E. These VLDL particles are also modified by LPL as they circulate, leading to production of IDL that can either be removed by the liver through apoE (as remnants) or can lose the apoE in that process to become LDL. The cholesterol-rich LDL particles can be taken up by the liver (70%) or into other tissues (30%) where the cholesterol goes into membranes, steroid synthesis, or deposits (atheromas).

ENDOGENOUS LIPID PATHWAY (SYNTHESIS)

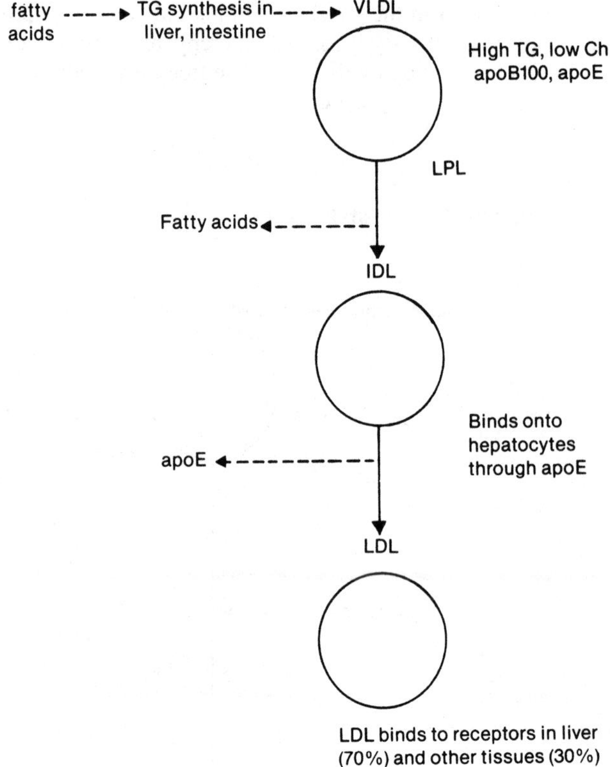

This pathway of synthesis, transport, and deposition is modulated by HDL particles that can mobilize cholesterol from tissues and reintroduce it for continued metabolism or excretion. *Nascent HDL particles* containing phospholipid, apoA1, and other apolipoproteins are synthesized and released by the liver. As these particles circulate, they pick up cholesterol from tissues, thereby becoming the HDL_3 fraction. *Lecithin cholesterol acyl transferase (LCAT)* catalyzes the esterification of this cholesterol in HDL_3, converting these particles to HDL_2. This fraction of cholesterol can be transfered to VLDL to participate in the metabolism of membrane and steroid synthesis. It can also be taken up by the liver and then excreted into bile.

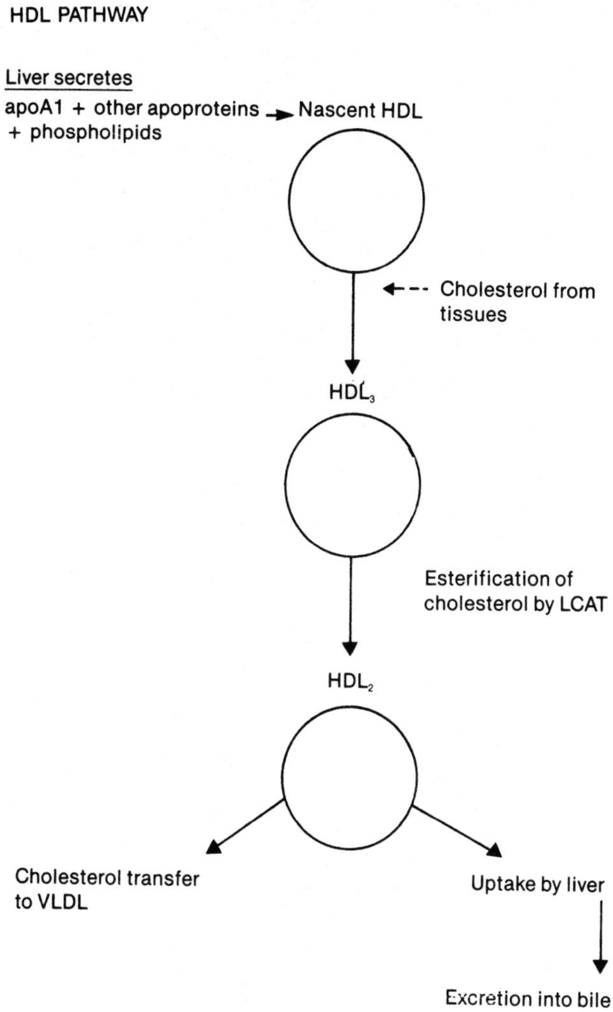

HDL PATHWAY

Liver secretes

apoA1 + other apoproteins → Nascent HDL
+ phospholipids

← Cholesterol from tissues

HDL_3

Esterification of cholesterol by LCAT

HDL_2

Cholesterol transfer to VLDL

Uptake by liver

Excretion into bile

The efficiency of these pathways for lipid transport and clearance depends on concentrations of available apolipoproteins and also on the lipid load presented to the body by diet. The importance of HDL as a means of clearing cholesterol from tissues is emphasized by the deficiency state of HDL (Tangier disease), in which cholesterol forms extensive deposits in tissues. Conversely, high levels of HDL serve to protect against development of atherosclerosis due to cholesterol deposits.

Measurement and Fractionation

The most relevant measurements of serum lipids are total cholesterol, triglycerides, and *cholesterol fractionation* into the *high-density* lipoprotein (HDL) fraction with calculation of the low-density lipoprotein (LDL) fraction of cholesterol. In addition, clinical laboratories now have the capacity to quantitate *apolipoprotein A1* (apoA1) and *apolipoprotein B* (apoB) in serum samples. Free fatty acids (FFA, also called nonesterified fatty acids, NEFA) and phospholipids are not usually quantitated in serum except in cases of specific metabolic diseases.

Measurement of total cholesterol has been done in the past by colorimetric chemical methods that demonstrate interferences from other substances. Today, most cholesterol methods use the enzyme cholesterol oxidase and are much more specific. The major technical problem in assuring standardization between different cholesterol assays is the relative insolubility of cholesterol, which limits its availability to the enzymatic reagents during the period of analysis. There is presently a major emphasis nationally to establish cholesterol standards to bring all laboratories into agreement on this assay.

Triglycerides are measured by hydrolytic removal of the fatty acids and then quantitation of the liberated glycerol. Since triglycerides can contain a variety of different fatty acids in unpredictable mixtures (probably dependent on diet), triglyceride determination must be standardized against a defined material that can differ in average composition from the samples being analyzed. Comparability is then based on the glycerol content.

Cholesterol fractionation is based on the separation of individual lipoproteins according to density by ultracentrifugation. Pure fat is less dense than water; lipids are less dense than proteins; and triglycerides are less dense than phospholipids and cholesterol. The least dense lipoproteins are those with the highest triglyceride content. Chylomicrons are lipoproteins with very high triglyceride content and a specific gravity less than that of plasma. Chylomicrons will rise to the top of a volume of plasma under conditions favorable to separation of fat from water (e.g., refrigeration overnight). The next most dense lipoprotein class is very-low-density lipoprotein (VLDL), followed by LDL and HDL. The composition of the major lipoprotein categories is given in Table 9–7.

The appearance of serum after 12 to 16 hours of refrigeration gives quick, useful information about chylomicron and VLDL content of serum with excessive triglycerides. This is summarized in the last column of Table 9–8. Freshly separated hyperlipemic serum is uniformly milky or opalescent. In chilled serum, excessive chylomicrons float to the top, appearing like a layer of cream. Uniform turbidity in the refrigerated serum indicates elevated VLDL content. Several different patterns may be seen: uniform turbidity means elevated VLDL without significant chylomicrons; "cream" atop a turbid specimen means elevation of both chylomicrons and VLDL; and "cream" atop a clear specimen means chylomicronemia without excess VLDL.

Since ultracentrifugation is not a practical method for clinical laboratory use, alternative techniques have been developed to study cholesterol fractionation. One such technique is electrophoresis that separates as follows: chylomicrons at origin, LDL at beta, VLDL as pre-beta, and HDL as alpha (Fig. 9–1). Frederickson, Goldstein, and Brown[2] have classified six distinct lipoprotein distribution phenotypic patterns by this means (see Table 9–8). These phenotypes have been correlated with genetically determined abnormalities (familial hyperlipoproteinemia) and with a variety of acquired conditions (secondary hyperlipoproteinemias) outlined in Table 9-9. Phenotype descriptions have proven useful in classifying diagnoses and in